Find videos demonstrating ultrasound anatomy and pathologies in *Atlas of Head and Neck Ultrasound* online at MediaCenter.thieme.com!

Simply visit MediaCenter.thieme.com and, when prompted during the registration process, enter the scratch-off code below to get started today.

This book cannot be returned once this panel has been scratched off.

Ultrasound is a dynamic procedure – find videos that help you understand head and neck ultrasound anatomy and identify pathologies shown in the *Atlas of Head and Neck Ultrasound* online at MediaCenter.thieme.com!

For an overview of the available content, see the List of Videos on pages XII and XIII.

System requirements:

	WINDOWS	MAC	TABLET
Recommended Browser(s) **	Microsoft Internet Explorer 8.0 or later, Firefox 3.x	Firefox 3.x, Safari 4.x	HTML5 mobile browser. iPad — Safari. Opera Mobile — Tablet PCs preferred.
	*** all browsers should have JavaScript enabled*		
Flash Player Plug-in	Flash Player 9 or Higher* ** Mac users: ATI Rage 128 GPU does not support full-screen mode with hardware scaling*		Tablet PCs with Android OS support Flash 10.1
Minimum Hardware Configurations	Intel® Pentium® II 450 MHz, AMD Athlon™ 600 MHz or faster processor (or equivalent) 512 MB of RAM	PowerPC® G3 500 MHz or faster processor Intel Core™ Duo 1.33 GHz or faster processor 512MB of RAM	Minimum CPU powered at 800MHz 256MB DDR2 of RAM
Recommended for optimal usage experience	Monitor resolutions: • Normal (4:3) 1024×768 or Higher • Widescreen (16:9) 1280×720 or Higher • Widescreen (16:10) 1440×900 or Higher DSL/Cable internet connection at a minimum speed of 384.0 Kbps or faster WiFi 802.11 b/g preferred.		7-inch and 10-inch tablets on maximum resolution. WiFi connection is required.

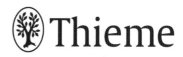

Atlas of Head and Neck Ultrasound

Heinrich Iro, MD
Professor
Medical Director
Department of Otolaryngology—Head and Neck Surgery
Friedrich-Alexander University Hospital Erlangen—Nuremberg
Germany

Alessandro Bozzato, MD
Attending Physician
Department of Otolaryngology—Head and Neck Surgery
Friedrich-Alexander University Hospital Erlangen—Nuremberg
Germany

Johannes Zenk, MD
Professor
Deputy Medical Director
Department of Otolaryngology—Head and Neck Surgery
Friedrich-Alexander University Hospital Erlangen—Nuremberg
Germany

With contributions by

Gert Hetzel, Werner Lang, Deike Strobel

523 illustrations

Thieme
Stuttgart · New York

Atlas of head and neck ultrasound / edited by Heinrich Iro, Johannes Zenk, Alessandro Bozzato ; contributors, Gert Hetzel, Deike Strobel, Werner Lang.

   p. ; cm.

 Includes bibliographical references.

 ISBN 978-3-13-160351-7 (alk. paper)

 I. Iro, H. (Heinrich) II. Zenk, Johannes. III. Bozzato, Alessandro.

 [DNLM: 1. Head–ultrasonography–Atlases. 2. Neck–ultrasonography–Atlases. 3. Ultrasonography–methods–Atlases. WE 17]

  617.5'107543--dc23

                   2012020092

For more information on Siemens ultrasound systems, visit: www.siemens.com/ultrasound

© 2013 Georg Thieme Verlag KG,
Rüdigerstrasse 14, 70469 Stuttgart, Germany
http://www.thieme.de
Thieme Medical Publishers, Inc., 333 Seventh Avenue,
New York, NY 10001, USA
http://www.thieme.com

Cover design: Thieme Publishing Group
Typesetting by Prepress Projects, Perth, UK
Printed in China by Asia Pacific Offset, Hong Kong

ISBN 978-3-13-160351-7
eISBN 978-3-13-169701-1

Preface

Since the first application of ultrasound in the examination of the head and neck in the second half of the last century, technical advances in this dynamic imaging modality have led to a greater understanding of the anatomy and pathology in this area.

Digital imaging processing and state-of-the-art transducer technology now yield an image quality with submillimeter resolution, which enables even the smallest tissue changes to be seen and which, for certain indications, is superior to that of computed tomography (CT) and magnetic resonance imaging (MRI). New procedures, such as tissue harmonic imaging, compound imaging, elastography, panoramic views, and contrast-enhanced ultrasound, together with color Doppler scanning, combined in one system, provide information not only on the appearance of an organ but also on its function and activity.

CT and MRI are claimed to give a comprehensive picture of the head and neck. However, the disadvantages of these methods, in comparison with ultrasound, are obvious: an imaging technique that is not universally and immediately available causes delay in the diagnostic and therapeutic management. Furthermore, it is essential to have all the necessary information available in order to interpret the findings; that is to say, the clinical history, laboratory findings, clinical findings on examination, and the results of the endoscopy. It is principally the treating physicians who are in possession of all this information and who are also in a position to perform the ultrasound scans themselves, thus enabling them to assess the findings in the overall context.

The more extensive and complicated the technical possibilities, the more difficult it is to adjust system parameters and interpret the data obtained. A thorough grounding in the technical basics, anatomical landmarks, and typical constellations of the findings is indispensable.

For this reason, ultrasonography is a method that depends greatly on the examiner; one of our aims in producing the atlas is to counteract this frequently voiced criticism. The fact is, however, that ultrasound is no less, but equally no more dependent on the examiner than are CT and MRI. Experience comes only with practice. We have therefore tried to provide a practical manual that is as relevant as possible for routine application.

During their more than 20 years' experience, the authors have provided continuing professional education and ultrasound courses to try to overcome the problems and stumbling blocks that continue to beset the use of this fascinating method of examination.

This atlas is intended not only to give beginners a systematic introduction to the basics of head and neck ultrasonography but also to provide more experienced users with the opportunity of gaining further in-depth knowledge. We have chosen the layout especially to give rapid access to everyday problems. The comprehensive text in Section 1 on ultrasound basics should also provide a step-by-step introduction to the individual topics. To provide an overall picture of the ultrasound appearance of the head and neck, we have also included more complicated interdisciplinary topics, such as the thyroid gland and blood vessels. As far as possible, we have used images from the latest ultrasound systems, so that the findings demonstrated are of optimal quality. In addition to static images on the pages of the book, we can also present the material as video clips so that readers can check their understanding of the material. Thus the web-based part of the atlas offers the reader further access to typical findings. These video clips allow one to identify anatomy, allow pathology to be seen even more clearly, and illustrate the particular advantages of ultrasonography as a dynamic procedure.

Thanks to its noninvasive nature and high informational value, we consider ultrasound to be an indispensable component in the diagnosis and treatment of conditions of the head and neck. And this is confirmed by more than 3500 examinations performed every year in our department at our clinic.

Heinrich Iro
Alessandro Bozzato
Johannes Zenk
November 2012

Acknowledgments

An atlas of this type cannot be produced without the cooperation and support of colleagues both within and outside of the department. We thank Markus Grunewald, MD, PhD for his preparation of the internet platform and for pictorial material we thank Dr. Nils Klintworth and Konstantinos Mantsopoulos. In addition we would like to thank the Ultrasound Division, Healthcare Sector of Siemens AG, and Mr. S. Konnry of Thieme Verlag for his outstanding assistance with the project.

Contributors

Dipl. Ing. Gert Hetzel
Siemens AG Healthcare Sector
Siemens Germany

Werner Lang, MD
Professor
Department of Vascular Surgery
Friedrich-Alexander University Hospital Erlangen–Nuremberg
Germany

Deike Strobel, MD
Professor, Attending Physician
Department of Internal Medicine
Friedrich-Alexander University Hospital Erlangen–Nuremberg
Germany

Abbreviations

AACE	American Association of Clinical Endocrinologists	**ICA**	internal carotid artery
ARFI	acoustic radiation force impulse	**IJV**	internal jugular vein
ATA	American Thyroid Association	**IMT**	intima–media thickness
BCC	basal cell carcinoma	**MALT**	mucosa-associated lymphatic tissue
bTSH	basal TSH	**MEN2**	multiple endocrine neoplasia
CCA	common carotid artery	**MI**	mechanical index
CCDS	color-coded duplex sonography	**MIP**	maximum intensity projection
CEA	carcinoembryonic antigen	**MRI**	magnetic resonance imaging
CHD	coronary heart disease	**NASCET**	North American Symptomatic Carotid Endarterectomy Trial
CI	compounding imaging	**NTM**	nontuberculous mycobacteria
CPS	contrast pulse sequence	**PEIT**	percutaneous ethanol injection therapy
CRP	C-reactive protein	**PET-CT**	positron emission tomography–computed tomography
CT	computed tomography	**PI**	phase inversion (in Chapter 14)
CW	continuous wave	**PI**	pulsatility index (in Chapter 2)
DGC	depth gain compensation	**PRF**	pulse repetition frequency
ECA	external carotid artery	**PSV**	peak systolic velocity
ECST	European Carotid Surgery Trial	**PW**	pulsed wave
ENT	ear, nose, and throat	**RI**	resistance index
ESR	erythrocyte sedimentation rate	**TB**	tuberculosis
FFT	fast Fourier transform	**TGC**	time gain compensation
FNAB	fine-needle aspiration biopsy	**THI**	tissue harmonic imaging
FNAC	fine-needle aspiration cytology	**TPO Ab**	antibodies to thyroid peroxidase
GSM	grayscale median	**VA**	vertebral artery

Table of Contents

III   Advanced Ultrasound Methods and Outlook

List of Videos

I General Considerations

1 Basic Principles of Ultrasound
Gert Hetzel

Knowledge of the physical and technological principles of ultrasound is the key to understanding sonographic images and findings and for evaluating the opportunities and limits of the method.

Physical Principles of B-mode Ultrasound Scanning

The sound wave is a purely mechanical wave. Reflections of transmitted ultrasound waves from features deep inside tissues are the basis of ultrasound diagnostics. These are processed into a sectional image corresponding to a section of the human body.

Influence of the Ultrasound Frequency

The definition of "ultrasound" is with reference to the human hearing range, which is 16 Hz to 20 kHz. Diagnostic ultrasound uses a frequency range between 2 MHz and 30 MHz (**Fig. 1.1**).

For most of today's applications in the field of ear, nose, and throat (ENT), center frequencies between 5 and 18 MHz are used, typically 7.5 MHz. This range offers the required penetration and high spatial resolution.

The propagation velocity of ultrasound waves depends on the material in which they propagate. A mean sound wave velocity of $c = 1540$ m/s (a value averaged from different soft tissues and standardized internationally; close to the sound wave velocity in water) is assumed for the different types of tissue in the human body. If the run time of a sound signal is measured, a reflection can be clearly allocated to the place of its origin with a given sound wave velocity.

Frequency (f) and velocity (c) determine the wavelength (λ) of the propagating sound wave:

$$\lambda = c/f$$

For example:

$$f = 7.5\,\text{MHz} \quad \text{implies} \quad \lambda = 0.2\,\text{mm}$$

The wavelength λ is the theoretical limit of resolution, which can never be fully reached. Since the wavelength is shorter for higher sound frequencies, the maximum reachable resolution will be higher with higher sound frequencies.

The frequency is an important factor influencing image quality.

Ultrasound is attenuated when passing through tissues, for example, by absorption. **Absorption** (attenuation) is the loss of sound energy—for example through its conversion into heat—and increases with increasing travel distance through the medium. Absorption depends on a tissue-specific absorption constant and the ultrasound frequency (**Fig. 1.2**).

Owing to this frequency-dependent attenuation of sound energy, the depth of penetration in a tissue depends not only on the tissue but importantly on the frequency.

Absorption losses can be compensated, within certain limits, by depth-dependent echo amplification control (**DGC**, depth gain compensation; or **TGC**, time gain compensation) within the ultrasound system.

The depth of **penetration** is the maximum distance between the ultrasound transducer and the deepest structures inside the tissue that can still be imaged without interference by noise. As noted, the frequency substantially influences the penetration: the depth of penetration is *inversely proportional* to the frequency. For this reason, certain working frequency ranges have proven advantageous, depending on the specific application. High frequencies are suitable for imaging near-surface structures, whereas lower frequencies are suitable for greater field depths.

Generation of Ultrasound

Piezoelectric Effect

When an electrical voltage is applied to a piezoelectric element, the element will mechanically deform. Conversely, an electrical voltage will be generated by the mechanical deformation of a piezoelectric element. Piezoelectric elements are used for ultrasound generation (**Fig. 1.3**). Alternating electrical pulses induce these elements to oscillate. The frequency of oscillation depends on the structure (e.g., thickness) and the technological features of the element. Conversely, when

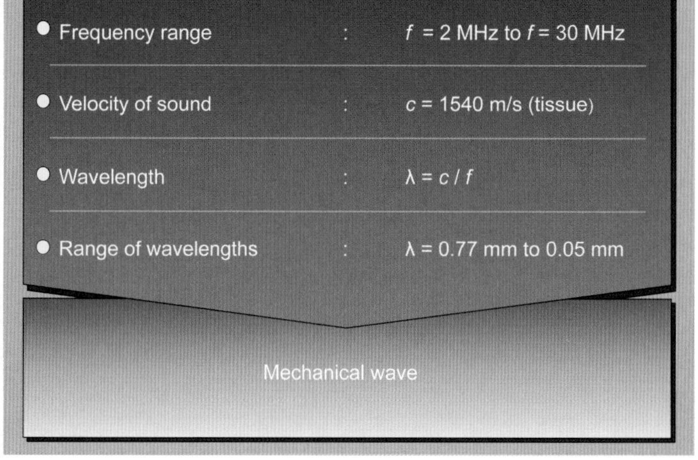

Frequency range	:	$f = 2$ MHz to $f = 30$ MHz
Velocity of sound	:	$c = 1540$ m/s (tissue)
Wavelength	:	$\lambda = c / f$
Range of wavelengths	:	$\lambda = 0.77$ mm to 0.05 mm

Mechanical wave

Fig. 1.1 Frequency and wavelength relationships. (Courtesy of Siemens AG.)

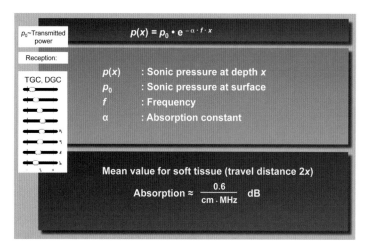

Fig. 1.2 Frequency-dependent attenuation of ultrasound according to the law of absorption. DGC, depth gain compensation; TGC, time gain compensation. (Courtesy of Siemens AG.)

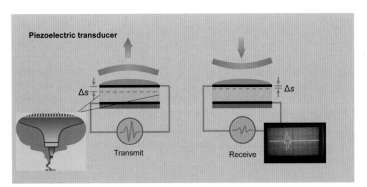

Fig. 1.3 Generation of ultrasound waves; the piezoelectric effect. Δs indicates the difference in thickness with application of a voltage to a piezoelectric material. (Courtesy of Siemens AG.)

the acoustic pressure of the ultrasound echo strikes the piezoelectric element, it generates an electrical signal of amplitude proportional to the acoustic pressure.

Very thin ceramic plates coated with a thin layer of electrical contact material on both sides are used for ultrasound transducers. Damping material is added on the back, with the effect that the transmitted and received pulses are kept to very short duration to achieve good spatial resolution. The accommodation of the probe to the body surface is obtained with one or several layers of coupling media so that the acoustic energy of the transmitted and echo pulses experiences minimum loss (to provide greater sensitivity).

Pulse-Echo Technique

An ultrasound transducer (probe) is a combined ultrasound transmitter and receiver. An electrical pulse excites the transducer element (pulse length 0.5–2 cycles; e.g.: <1 μs). The resulting acoustic pressure wave is propagated into the tissue and is reflected by a target object. The returning sound wave, again, generates an electrical signal in the ultrasound transducer element. The time (t) between the transmission of the pulse and receiving the echo is a measure of the distance x from the sound element to the reflecting object (pulse-echo method; **Fig. 1.4**). All ultrasound systems assume a mean sound wave velocity inside the tissue of $c = 1540$ m/s for image construction and display. Because of its higher sound wave velocity, in the image bone appears thinner than would the same depth of soft tissue.

Physical Laws of Sound Propagation

Reflections are generated when waves propagate through tissues of different acoustic impedances (**Fig. 1.5**). The acoustic impedance of a medium is defined as the product of the density of the medium (tissue) and the sound wave velocity of the tissue (which is tissue dependent). A reflection is generated at each discontinuity of impedance between tissues or features. The magnitude of the reflected part of the ultrasound wave (the echo) increases with the difference between the impedances.

The **impedance** value of soft tissue is similar to that of water; impedance values of air or bone are very different from this value.

With large differences in impedance at tissue–air or tissue–bone interfaces, the sound energy is reflected almost totally: objects lying behind the interface cannot be detected by ultrasound. With smaller differences in the impedances of the tissues, the penetrating sound beam still has enough energy to generate further reflections.

Reflection depends strongly on the angle of incidence. The same laws apply as in optics. If the boundary surface between two tissues is impinged perpendicularly, the reflected wave will fully return to the transducer. However, if the boundary surface is hit at an angle other than 90°, only a part of the wave will reach the transducer and can be used for imaging.

In this regard, the roughness of the boundary surface is very important since roughness leads to scattering (**Fig. 1.6**). The corresponding principle applies to all tissues.

Structures with dimensions about the size of the wavelength or smaller lead to scattering of the ultrasonic energy in all directions and therefore to attenuation in the direction of propagation. As a result of scattering, homogeneous soft tissue is displayed as an interference pattern, with the degree of fineness varying with frequency. Interferences of scattered echoes of adjacent structures are considered to be the cause of the "**speckle pattern**" displayed by soft tissue in ultrasound images.

If the sound wave velocities in the two parts of the tissue differ greatly, the sound waves will be refracted, as is well known from the corresponding situation in optics.

Thus, ultrasound is attenuated when passing through tissue. As well as reflection and refraction at boundary surfaces, that is on structures that are large compared with the wavelength λ, scattering and absorption are the key mechanisms.

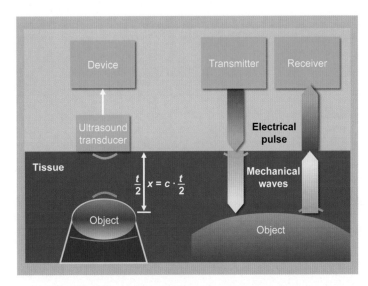

Fig. 1.4 Pulse-echo method of imaging. (Courtesy of Siemens AG.)

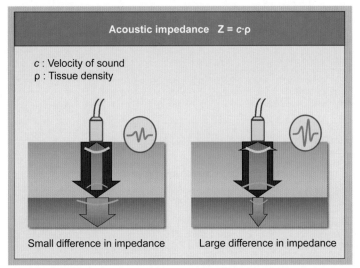

Fig. 1.5 Origin of reflection (echo). (Courtesy of Siemens AG.)

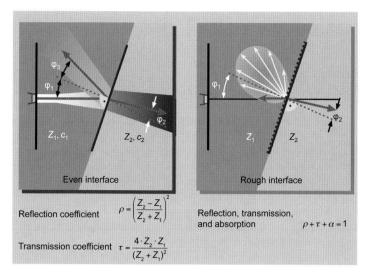

Fig. 1.6 Angle dependence of reflection, scattering, and refraction. (Courtesy of Siemens AG.)

Spatial Resolution

Spatial resolution is defined as the minimum distance between two points or dot-shaped objects that can still be distinguished from each other.

We differentiate between *axial* resolution (in the direction of sound propagation) and *lateral* resolution (transverse to the direction of sound propagation) (**Fig. 1.7**).

Axial resolution is mainly determined by the pulse length. Today's broadband transducers provide short excitation pulses and therefore excellent axial resolution. The axial resolution is superior to the lateral resolution.

Typical values for axial resolution are $\geq 1\lambda$. Short excitation pulses in connection with broadband sound transducers provide the best axial resolution.

Lateral resolution is one of the key parameters for ultrasound imaging quality and has the strongest influence on the diagnostic performance of the complete system (ultrasound unit plus transducer).

> The resolution characteristics of ultrasound transducers improve with increasing frequency.

Transmit Focusing

In transmission, the focus depth can be varied by *transmit focusing* (**Fig. 1.8**). Lateral resolution can be optimized throughout a larger range of depth via multistage transmit focusing. This means that each transmit pulse is focused on a certain depth and is used for creating a

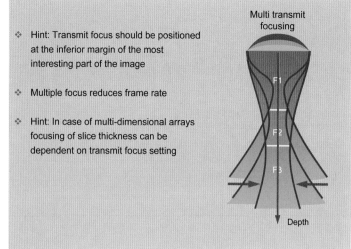

Fig. 1.8 Transmit focusing. (Courtesy of Siemens AG.)

part of the total image: for example, pulse 1 for area F1, pulse 2 for F2, and so on.

In contrast to the transmit technique, *receive focusing* is programmed dynamically, that is the electronic focus is always in the depth region from which the echoes are coming. This is achieved automatically in the system itself.

B-mode Image Acquisition; 2D Imaging

In B-mode imaging the amplitude of the demodulated echo is converted into a brightness value. The echoes received from one transmit pulse are allocated along a line corresponding to the time of their arrival from the depth of the tissue and form an ultrasound line.

A 2D (two-dimensional), sectional image (B-mode image) is created if several ultrasound lines are arranged side by side. The brightness-modulated signals derived from these ultrasound lines are buffered in a matrix. The content of this matrix is transferred to the screen and composed into a geometrically realistic sectional ultrasound image. In some countries the 2D image is called a B-mode image, where B stands for brightness.

In ultrasound diagnostics, **scan** means the periodic scanning of a sectional plane of the body region to be examined with ultrasound pulses in a certain scan format and in a defined temporal sequence.

When parallel line acquisition (as shown in **Fig. 1.9**) is used for imaging, we term it a **parallel scan**.

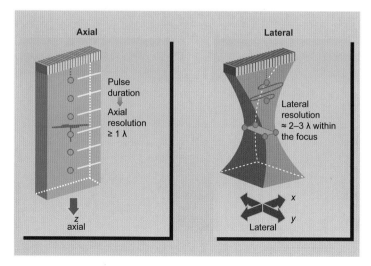

Fig. 1.7 Axial and lateral resolution. (Courtesy of Siemens AG.)

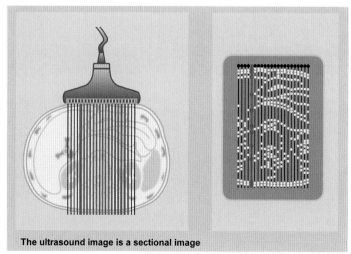

Fig. 1.9 B-mode image acquisition, parallel scan. (Courtesy of Siemens AG.)

An **array** is an arrangement of very small individual transducers or elements in a row.

Postprocessing

There are various **dynamic range** settings for adapting the contrast range of the 2D image to the diagnostic requirements (**Fig. 1.10a, b**). The dynamic range is the ratio of highest to the lowest level echo signal (e.g., 60 dB) that is to be displayed in the image, depending on the application. A large dynamic range (starting from 50 or 55 dB) is suitable for soft tissue display. A low dynamic range is suitable for high-contrast contour display.

Artifacts

Complex physical mechanisms such as reflection, refraction, absorption, and scattering lead to the generation of the echoes we see in an image.

The processing and display of echoes from the depth of the body are based on assumptions such as constant sound wave velocity and attenuation as well as the linearity of sound propagation. If the actual physical conditions deviate from these assumptions, artifacts may occur. Artifacts can, though do not necessarily, make diagnosis difficult. They frequently also provide additional information on the characteristics of tissue and liquids and can be of diagnostic use.

One of the most common artifacts is **shadowing by a strong reflector** on the distal side of the transducer (**Fig. 1.11a, b**). Strong reflectors may be bones, stones, calcifications, or air—the acoustic impedances of these substances differ strongly from that of soft tissue. They reflect the majority of the incident ultrasonic energy as echo signals.

If a strong reflector is hit perpendicularly, it will be shown as a strong, bright echo signal. The distal shadowing helps the user to identify the reflector as such and to define it.

However, if the reflector is **not hit perpendicularly in the scan plane**, but rather at a sufficiently large angle, the incident ultrasonic energy will again be largely reflected but this time out of the scanning plane (**Fig. 1.12a, b**). The echo will therefore not reach the transducer. Shadowing can be observed just as when incidence on a reflector is perpendicular, but the echo from the reflector will appear only weakly or not at all.

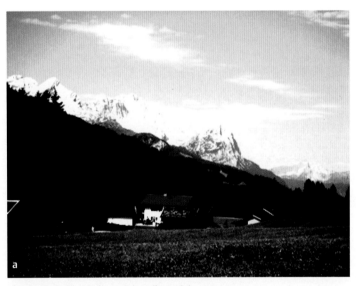

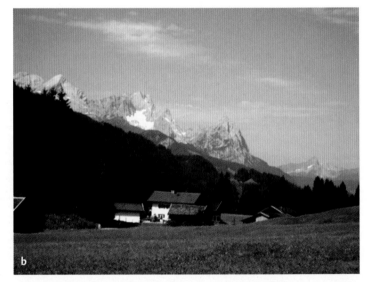

Fig. 1.10a,b Illustration of the effect of dynamic range.
a Low.
b High.

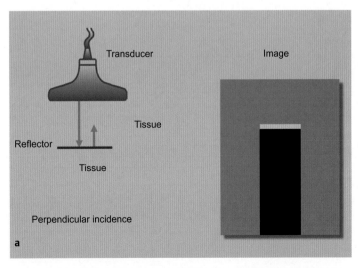

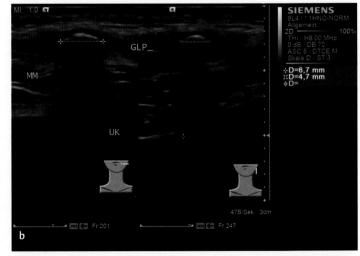

Fig. 1.11a,b Shadowing by a strong reflector. (Courtesy of Siemens AG.)
a Principle.
b Example. Salivary gland stone as strong reflector with distal shadowing. MM, mylohyoid muscle; GLP, parotid gland; UK, mandible.

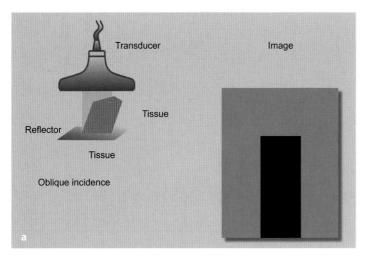

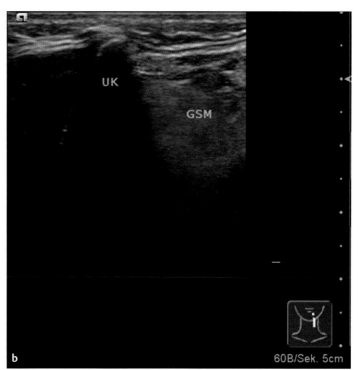

Fig. 1.12a,b Shadowing by an angled strong reflector. (Courtesy of Siemens AG.)
a Principle.
b Example. Longitudinal view of the submandibular gland (GSM). The plane of the mandible (UK) results in an angled shadowing.

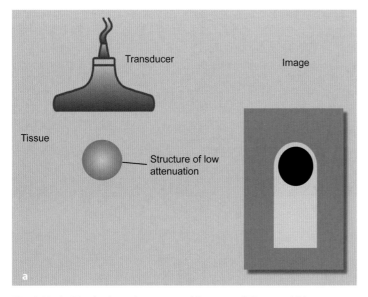

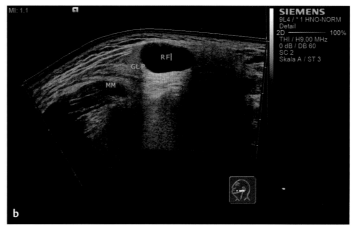

Fig. 1.13a,b Distal echo enhancement. (Courtesy of Siemens AG.)
a Principle.
b Example. A parotid lesion (RF) with distinct distal echo enhancement. GLP, parotid gland; MM, masseter muscle.

If ultrasound pulses travel through a region of limited lateral extension and of lower attenuation than that of the surrounding tissue, the echoes from the "shadow" behind this region appear enhanced (**Fig. 1.13a, b**). This artifact occurs because the user sets the depth-dependent gain control of the system to correspond to the attenuation in normal tissue. As this gain is actually too high for the less-attenuating region, the echoes originating from behind this region are displayed with too much gain and therefore appear brighter. The **echo enhancement** is of course not a real enhancement of the ultrasound energy but rather a weaker attenuation than is assumed. This artifact is used in diagnostics.

In cases of circular or elliptical boundary surfaces, total reflection may occur if the tissue is hit tangentially. In these regions the sound is deflected laterally and does not return to the transducer as an echo. The edge-forming structures therefore appear as not closed in the image, and **shadows** may be observed **distally from the tangentially hit edge structures** (**Fig. 1.14a, b**).

Edge structures of small echo-free objects may be projected into the echo-free area (**Fig. 1.15a**) and may give the **impression of a "sedimentary" structure**. This is caused by the lateral width of the ultrasound beam. A very similar artifact is observed even with good focusing in the scanning plane, owing to the limited resolution perpendicular to the scan plane (slice thickness, elevation plane) (**Fig. 1.15b**). It is known as slice thickness artifact or as "**partial volume effect**."

If a sound pulse hits the borders between two media having different acoustic properties, one portion will always be reflected whereas the other portion will cross the border's surface. If two strongly reflecting borders are hit perpendicularly, this may lead to internal reflections and therefore to **multiple echoes** of the same structure (**Fig. 1.16a, b**), colloquially called "**reverbs**" (for "reverberations"). If structures are located in front of a strong reflector, they will be "illuminated" by both the transmitted pulse and the echo pulse of this reflector, creating **mirror images** (**Fig. 1.17a, b**). This is also considered a type of multiple reflection.

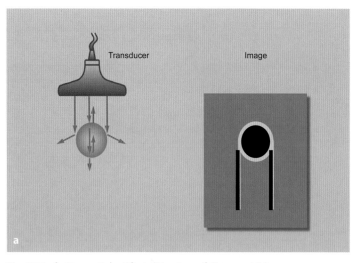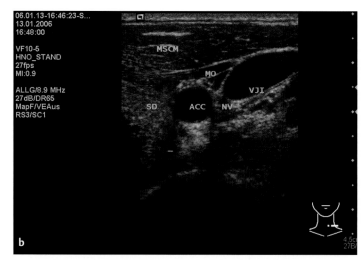

Fig. 1.14a,b Tangential artifact. (Courtesy of Siemens AG.)
a Principle.
b Example. Neck, left, with tangential artifact of the common carotid artery (ACC). VJI, internal jugular vein; SD, thyroid gland; MSCM, sternocleidomastoid muscle; MO omohyoid muscle; NV, vagal nerve.

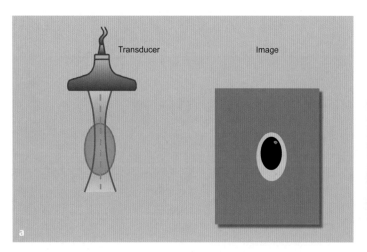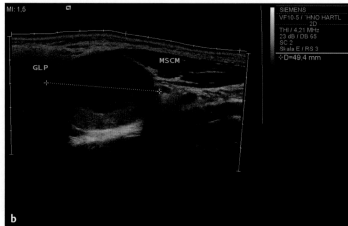

Fig. 1.15a,b Artifactual sedimentation and slice thickness. (Courtesy of Siemens AG.)
a Principle of tangential artifact.
b Example of slice thickness artifact, partial volume artifact. Panoramic view, neck, right. Between the sternocleidomastoid muscle (MSCM) and the parotid gland (GLP) lies a lateral cervical cyst.

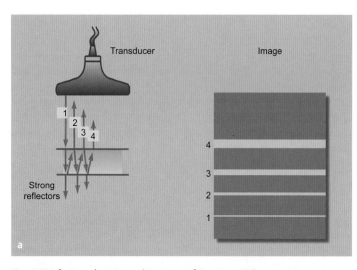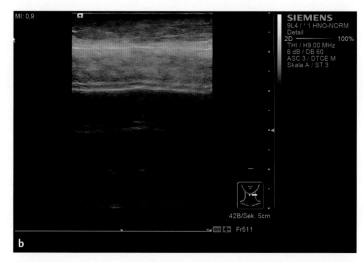

Fig. 1.16a,b Reverberations. (Courtesy of Siemens AG.)
a Principle.
b Example of reverberation artifacts, as shown here on the ventral wall of the left maxillary sinus.

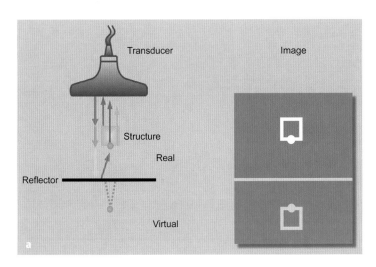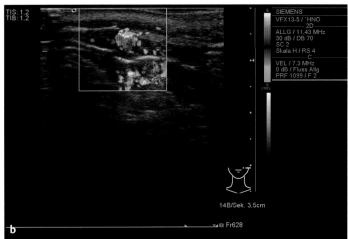

Fig. 1.17a,b Creation of a mirror image by a strong reflector. (Courtesy of Siemens AG.)
a Principle.
b Example. Anterior parotid region. The angled plane of the mandible, as a strong reflector, creates a virtual image beneath the bone.

2 Physical Principles of Doppler and Color Doppler Ultrasound

Gert Hetzel

Doppler Effect

The Doppler effect is named after the physicist Christian Doppler (1803–1853). Doppler observed that the light from stars moving toward the earth undergoes a blue shift (shorter wavelength, higher frequency) and the light from stars moving away from the earth undergoes a red shift (longer wavelength, lower frequency). He explained this observation physically and described it mathematically.

In a similar way, in blood flow the sound waves generated from erythrocytes and the echo signals returning to the transducer experience a slight frequency shift Δf with regard to the transmit frequency f (**Fig. 2.1**). The frequency shift Δf depends on the magnitude and direction of the blood flow velocity v.

The frequency shift Δf – generally referred to as the Doppler frequency in the following – is a direct measure for v. For a given value of v, Δf will be greater the higher the transmit frequency f. The Doppler frequency Δf also depends on the angle of incidence: Δf is at its maximum when the sound beam hits the blood vessel parallel to the vessel's axis. When the beam impinges perpendicularly ($\Theta=90°$), $\cos\Theta = 0$ and no Doppler signal will be registered.

Doppler Techniques

The different Doppler and color Doppler techniques are reviewed in **Table 2.1**.

Spectral Doppler Method: Pulsed-wave Doppler

Pulsed-wave Doppler (PW Doppler) meets the requirement for measuring flow in user-selected areas of interest (**Fig. 2.2a, b**). A group of array elements is activated for transmitting and receiving and (just as in B-mode) transmits sequences of short ultrasound sound pulses into the body. After the pulse has traveled to the selected sample and back (travel time T), the sample gate is opened for a short time, T_R, to receive the echoes. The size and depth of the sample volume in the B-mode

Table 2.1 Review of Doppler techniques

Doppler sonography (CW)	• Pencil probe examination; only spectral analysis
Duplex sonography	• Doppler information with B-mode • Spectral Doppler (CW/PW) and B-mode simultaneously, respectively time-displaced
Color duplex sonography	• Color Doppler with B-mode simultaneously • Power Doppler and B-mode simultaneously
Triplex mode	• Simultaneous display of B-mode, color Doppler, and spectral Doppler • Not (always) recommended

CW, continuous wave; PW, pulsed wave.

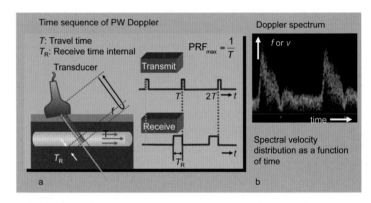

Fig. 2.2a,b Area of interest and temporal sequence of PW Doppler. (Courtesy of Siemens AG.)
a Principle.
b Example.

or the color Doppler image can be seen on the monitor and values are adjustable by the sonographer on the system.

Spectral Doppler in PW Doppler mode displays the temporal course of the frequency components, Δf, contained in the Doppler signal according to their magnitude, and their frequency of occurrence (amplitude), as a measure of the distribution of flow velocities v in the sample volume. This spectral analysis is based on the computational procedure known as the Fast Fourier Transform (FFT).

Aliasing and Nyquist Frequency

Both in PW Doppler and in color Doppler the aliasing effect (**Fig. 2.3**) determines the upper limit of the Doppler frequency that can be unambiguously displayed and calculated. The effect is familiar to movie and television viewers: the wheel spokes of a carriage that is moving forward seem to turn backward. Similarly, the movement performed by a trampolinist cannot be described unambiguously in a photographic sequence if the time between frames (sampling interval) is too long.

The FFT processor calculates the Doppler frequency from the Doppler signal values sampled at intervals $T = 1/\text{PRF}$ (PRF = pulse repetition frequency), assuming that this is the lowest frequency. If, for instance, the actual frequency was $^3/_2\,\text{PRF}$, it would be interpreted and displayed as an aliasing frequency of $\frac{1}{2}\text{PRF}$. The maximum frequency detectable without aliasing is $\pm\frac{1}{2}$ PRF (Nyquist limit) in both directions for bidirectional Doppler.

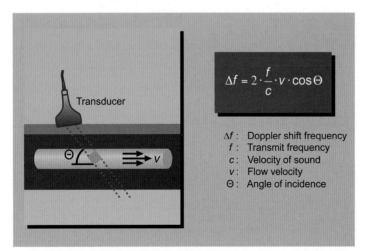

$$\Delta f = 2 \cdot \frac{f}{c} \cdot v \cdot \cos\Theta$$

Δf : Doppler shift frequency
f : Transmit frequency
c : Velocity of sound
v : Flow velocity
Θ : Angle of incidence

Fig. 2.1 The Doppler effect. (Courtesy of Siemens AG.)

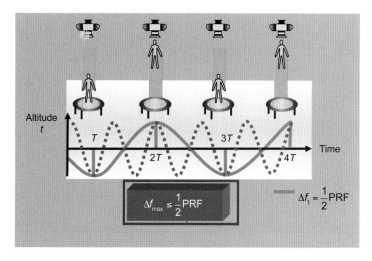

Fig. 2.3 Nyquist frequency and aliasing. (Courtesy of Siemens AG.)

In the Doppler spectrum, aliasing can be recognized by the fact that "positive" frequencies above the Nyquist limit reappear as "negative" frequencies at the bottom part of the spectral measuring range. Shifting the reference axis for the flow direction up or down (baseline shift) can extend the measuring range for one direction up to twice the Nyquist limit, that is up to the PRF. In that case, the opposite direction cannot be represented.

Angle Correction and Accuracy of Angle Correction (Spectral Doppler)

By means of the Doppler formula (**Fig. 2.1**) the velocity distribution can be calculated from the spectral Doppler frequencies. This requires the user to measure the angle of incidence Θ toward the vessel axis in the B-mode, color Doppler, or power Doppler image. This is done by placing a reference line (cursor) in the measuring gate and aligning it along the vessel axis (**Fig. 2.4**).

The accuracy of the angle correction depends strongly on the adjustment of the angle of incidence. Assuming an accuracy of estimate of, say, ±3° for the angle measurement, its influence on the angle-corrected velocity is low for small angles Θ, but significant for large angles. This can be explained by the cosine curve, which is very flat for small angles (0° to 30°), but much steeper for angles above 45°.

Table 2.2 shows some values for correction factor and correction error depending on the adjusted angle, with an assumed estimated accuracy of ±3° for the angle determination in the B-mode image.

The flow rate can be reliably calculated only for small angles of incidence (e.g., <60°). In many standard situations, however, the vessels are accessible only with larger angles of incidence. In these cases the ratios of Doppler frequencies or velocities (indices such as the pulsatility index [PI] and resistance index [RI]) are helpful for analyzing the hemodynamic situation, as they are independent of the angle measurement and the associated potential errors.

> Direct quantitative evaluation of flow rates should be attempted with an angle of incidence <60°, but the calculation of angle-independent indices (e.g., RI or PI) may be possible.

Doppler Sampling Locations

For **PW Doppler** and **CW** (continuous-wave) **Doppler** the measurement is limited to a fixed ultrasound line (**Fig. 2.5a**). For PW Doppler the **location and size of the sampling gate**, the "**Doppler gate**," can be adjusted along this line. For CW Doppler the gate size extends throughout the entire line.

For **color Doppler** and **power Doppler** the flow is analyzed in numerous sampling gates that are distributed over the entire sectional image or a part of it—the **color window** (flow mapping) (**Fig. 2.5b**). The color Doppler image is reconstructed in a similar way as the B-mode image, line by line. However, Doppler and B-mode image lines are registered in alternation rather than simultaneously. The number of measuring points along a line (e.g., up to 512) and the line density define the pixel resolution in the color image.

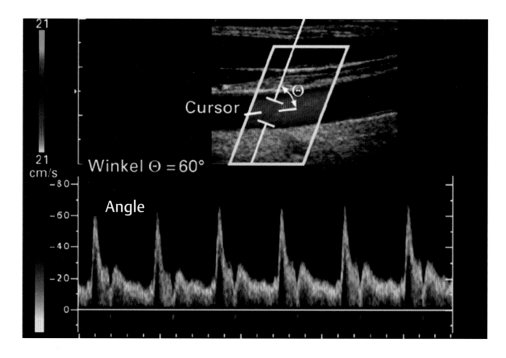

Fig. 2.4 Angle correction measured in the common carotid artery. (Courtesy of Siemens AG.)

Table 2.2 Accuracy of angle correction

Angle Θ	Correction factor	
	$1/\cos\Theta$	Correction error[a]
30°	1.15	+3%
45°	1.41	+6%
60°	2.00	+9%
72°	3.24	+15%
75°	3.86	+21%
92°	5.76	+30%

$$v \approx \frac{\Delta f}{\cos\theta}$$

[a] For Θ measured with an assumed accuracy of ±3°.

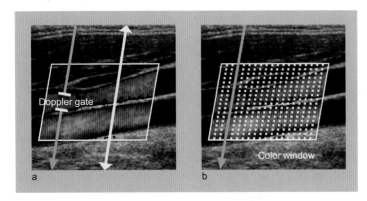

Fig. 2.5a,b Doppler sampling locations in the internal jugular vein (blue) and common carotid artery (red). (Courtesy of Siemens AG.)
a PW and CW Doppler.
b Color and power Doppler.

Color-coded Duplex Sonography, Color Doppler

As an addition to the anatomical information in the B-mode image, color-coded duplex sonography (CCDS) provides the possibility of displaying the blood flow using color Doppler or power Doppler.

The blood flow information is acquired by means of an **autocorrelation processor**. The color output signals correspond to the **mean velocity** in the sampling gate (color pixel) and are encoded to color values characterizing velocity and direction of flow.

Different types of color coding are commonly used. In vascular diagnostics, a **red–yellow** or **blue–cyan** color map is selected in most cases; red–yellow mostly designating the flow direction toward the transducer and blue–cyan designating the flow direction away from the transducer. This might be inverted by the user so that red–yellow shows flow away from transducer and blue–cyan that toward the transducer. Other **color maps** are available. If the Nyquist frequency is exceeded, aliasing will occur in the form of color changes.

Color Doppler yields information on the direction of flow in relation to the incident direction of the ultrasound (encoded in red or blue), on the flow amplitude (color brightness), and on flow dynamics. As an example, color Doppler is utilized to recognize and localize vessels and vascular blockages, to evaluate hemodynamic situations by viewing flow patterns and flow dynamics, and to rule out vascular occlusions.

Power Doppler

Power Doppler information is also gained from the autocorrelation processor. Power Doppler is named after the term "Power P," which is the sum of the amplitudes squared (Doppler signal intensities) of the individual Doppler frequencies at the point of measurement.

Power Doppler is largely independent of the direction and has no aliasing.

With power Doppler, the color maps are mostly monochrome—yellow, yellow–orange, green, blue, or white. Power Doppler can also be combined with the color Doppler directional information and is then referred to as **direction-coded power mode**.

In power Doppler-mode, information on the existence of blood flow in vessels is gathered and superimposed on the B-mode image, in a single color, as a spatial distribution of flow. The original power Doppler image does not contain information on flow direction. It provides a complete and clear view of even very small vascular structures and pathological changes. It also enables the physician to rule out vascular occlusions and to differentiate between blood-carrying vessels and other fluid features. The evaluation of hemodynamic properties, such as the pulsation of flow, is limited, since, most often, the image frame rate is too low.

Wall Filter

A motion detector (clutter canceller) connected upstream from the color Doppler processor is used for clear separation of stationary tissue echoes such as vascular wall echoes in the B-mode image and the color-coded flow information, as well as for the prevention of motion artifacts (**Fig. 2.6**).

The echo signals of one ultrasound line are stored for a period of time T between two consecutive transmit pulses and subtracted from the echo signals of the next transmit pulse. At high velocity the phase difference between the two signals at one measuring point, and thus also the signal difference, is significant and the echo signals are accepted as flow signals and forwarded to the phase detector. At low velocity the phase shift is minor and, consequently, the subtraction signal will be so small that the echoes are not recognized as flow signals and will be further processed as tissue echoes.

As a result of this technique, wall filters for color Doppler and power Doppler influence the PRF setting.

Aliasing with Color Doppler

The flow rate within a vessel can vary greatly. This may have pathological causes, such as stenosis. If the course of flow is constricted, the flow velocity will increase substantially and the rendered color will become lighter. If the flow velocity exceeds the measuring range defined by the Nyquist frequency of ±PRF/2, aliasing will occur and color reversals will

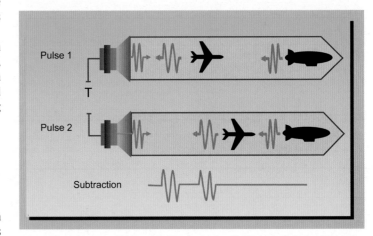

Fig. 2.6 Wall filter for color Doppler and power Doppler. (Courtesy of Siemens AG.)

occur. In contrast to reversals due to changes in direction, the color reversal of aliasing always causes the lighter colors representing high flow velocities to change, for example from light yellow to light blue without displaying a dark-colored seam (**Fig. 2.7a, b**).

Influence of Angle in Color Doppler

For curved vessels, color coding in the image is not always a measure of flow direction and velocity of flow but rather depends on the angle of incidence to the changing flow direction. **Figure 2.8**, acquired with a linear array, shows that the color brightness increases as the angle becomes smaller. The coloring becomes darker as the angle becomes steeper.

When changing from <90° to >90° the color is interrupted by a dark seam and a color change from dark red to dark blue is observed, without a reversion of flow actually having occurred. In contrast to aliasing, this color reversal is always characterized by a dark-colored seam.

A change of angle in the course of the vessel with reference to the direction of sound propagation leads to apparently higher or lower flow rates (**Fig. 2.9**).

The change of the angle of incidence for vascular visualization in color Doppler flow mode (but not in power Doppler mode) across the color window finds expression in two artifacts: "**flow acceleration artifact**" or "**pseudo flow acceleration**" (**Fig 2.9**) and "**flow reversal artifact**" (**Fig. 2.10a, b**). If the change of angle alters the flow direction from *toward* to *away from* the transducer, we speak of "flow reversal artifact."

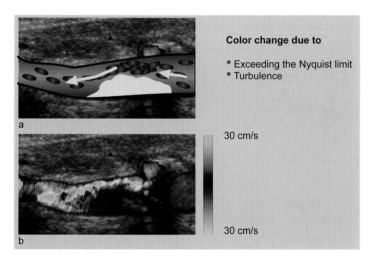

Color change due to

* Exceeding the Nyquist limit
* Turbulence

30 cm/s

30 cm/s

Fig. 2.7a,b Aliasing with color Doppler. (Courtesy of Siemens AG.)
a Principle.
b Example.

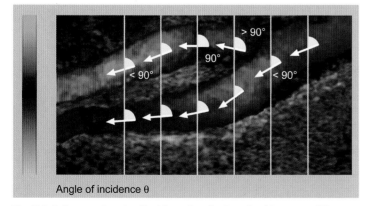

Angle of incidence θ

Fig. 2.8 Influence of angle of incidence in color Doppler. (Courtesy of Siemens AG.)

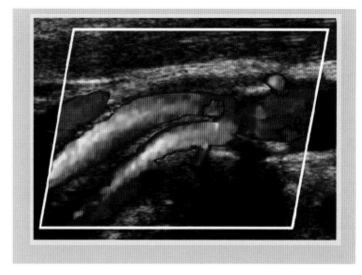

Fig. 2.9 "Pseudo flow acceleration" or "flow acceleration artifact." A change of angle leads to seemingly higher or lower flow velocities in the external and internal carotid arteries. (Courtesy of Siemens AG.)

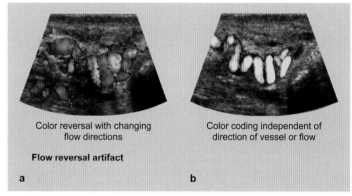

Color reversal with changing flow directions

Color coding independent of direction of vessel or flow

Flow reversal artifact

a   b

Fig. 2.10a,b Behavior of color Doppler and power Doppler in the event of direction changes. (Courtesy of Siemens AG.)
a Color Doppler "flow reversal artifact."
b Power Doppler.

While changes of flow direction (toward or away from the transducer) lead to a color change in color flow imaging, visualization in power Doppler mode is independent of the direction of the vessel or the blood flow. For this reason, more complex vascular structures can be identified more easily in power Doppler mode (**Fig. 2.11a, b**).

Spectral Doppler Parameters for Optimizing Spectral Doppler Recording

PRF (Pulse Repetition Frequency)

PRF allows control of the velocity measure range for spectral Doppler.
   Optimal PRF setting:
   • **High** for avoiding aliasing with high flow rates
   • **Low** for detecting low flow rates (format-filling spectrum display)

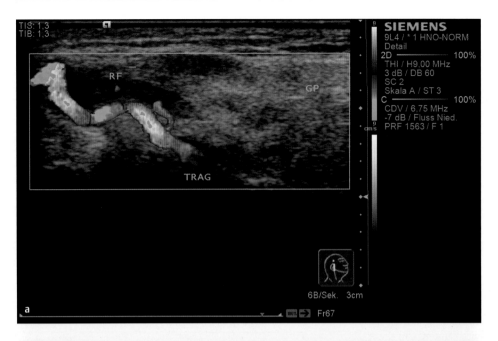

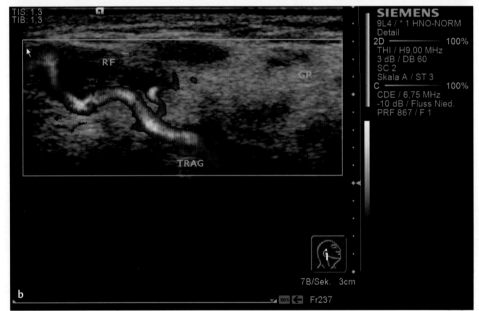

Fig. 2.11a,b Angle dependence of color Doppler and power Doppler in visualization of the preauricular region, longitudinal, with infected preauricular fistula (RF). TRAG, tragus.
a Color Doppler. Color reversal with changing flow directions.
b Power Doppler. Color coding independant of direction of vessel or flow.

> The maximum pulse repetition frequency PRF_{max} for spectral Doppler depends on the position of the (lower) limit of the Doppler gate (in the depth of the tissue).

D-Gain (Gain for Spectral Doppler)

> Gain should be adjusted to be just sufficiently high that no noise can be seen.

Wall Filter

The wall filter is a high-pass filter that suppresses frequencies around the baseline.

The wall filter frequency should be set so that low frequencies are not suppressed but tissue movements do not interfere.

Wall filter reference values:
- Arteries: 100 Hz
- Veins: 50 Hz

Color Flow and Power Doppler Parameters

Parameters to be set for optimizing color flow and power Doppler images are shown in **Fig. 2.12** and are discussed below.

Optimal PRF (Pulse Repetition Frequency) Setting

- **High** for avoiding aliasing with high flow velocities
- **Low** for detecting low flow velocities (improved color filling)

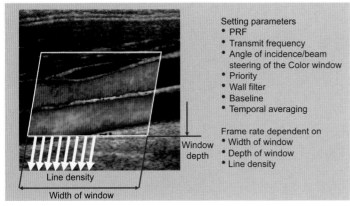

Fig. 2.12 Color flow and power Doppler setting parameters. (Courtesy of Siemens AG.)

If possible, the PRF should be so set that the vessel is sufficiently filled with color but no reverse color due to aliasing is visible.

If flow velocities exceed the PRF, aliasing will occur with color Doppler, but not with power Doppler.

Beam Steering of the Color Window

High **flow detection sensitivity** is achieved by setting the **angle of incidence** to the flow direction **as low as possible**. Accordingly it is sometimes helpful if the color window can be steered electronically in both directions.

Color Gain

Color gain should be set just so that no noise artifacts are visible.

Wall Filter

The wall filter is a high-pass filter to suppress wall motion and tissue motion artifacts, influencing the PRF setting.
  Setting the wall filter:
  - "Type of flow" (e.g., "High-flow" or "Low-flow") must be selected first, then PRF, then the filter.
  - The wall filter setting is connected with the pulse repetition frequency (PRF).
  - Settings that are too high will reduce sensitivity for slow blood flows.

Temporal Averaging

Sensitivity and **signal-to-noise ratio** can be optimized, but at the expense of the frame rate, by setting a high **temporal averaging**. This is the **number of transmit pulses (samplings) per color line that can be used to calculate autocorrelation**. For power Doppler the flow detection sensitivity can be further increased by setting high correlation ("persistence").

The Color Flow Line Density

This concerns the number of color lines (within the color window, spread in the lateral direction) and influences the lateral color Doppler resolution and the frame rate.
  Low line density:
  - Poor lateral resolution of the color Doppler flow

  but causes

  - High color frame rate

  High line density:
  - Improved lateral resolution of the color Doppler flow

  but causes

  - Lower color frame rate

A compromise has to be found between line density and color frame rate.

Summary: Guide for Doppler Parameter Setting

Table 2.3 shows the procedure of parameter setting for color Doppler and spectral Doppler.

Table 2.3 Procedure in color Doppler and spectral Doppler

Color Doppler	Spectral Doppler
1. Selection of color Doppler (e.g., button C)	1. Selection of spectral Doppler
2. Flow state (high-flow, low-flow if existing) or application preset	2. Position/angle and size of Doppler gate in B-image
3. Position and size of window	3. Selection of spectral Doppler
4. Angle/steering of color window	4. PRF
5. Color gain (receive gain)	5. Doppler gain (receive Doppler gain)
6. PRF scale (measured velocity range)	6. Baseline
7. Temporal averaging (if existing)	7. Freeze
8. Color invert	8. Measuring: Manual or automatic measurement of RI and PI

Summary: Guide to Understanding an Ultrasound Image

Fig. 2.13 explains the key configuration and setup of an ultrasound image.

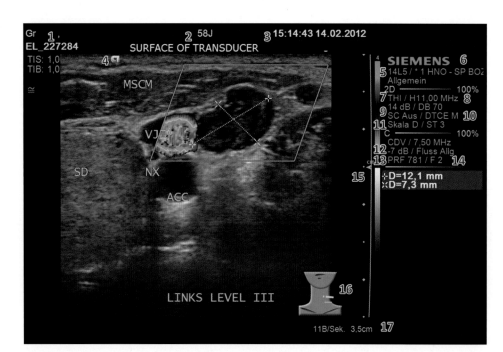

Fig. 2.13 Neck, level III, left, transverse.

(1) Name of patient.
(2) Age or date of birth.
(3) Date of examination.
(4) Golden symbol indicates the left-hand side of the image, corresponding to a marking found on the transducer.
(5) Selected transducer.
(6) Selected examination protocol.
(7) Tissue harmonic imaging (THI) function is activated; (8) selected insonation frequency (11 MHz).
(9) Overall enhancement "Gain" measured in decibels (14 dB).
(10) Compound image-activated medium setting (DTCE M).
(11) Color scale selected in B mode; (12) color gain (–7 dB), preset medium low velocity (Fluss Allg); (13) selected PRF (PRF).
(14) Set wall filter (F2).
(15) Focus region at 1.5 cm (white triangle).
(16) Pictogram indicating anatomic region, the point at the end corresponds to the upper left image margin (golden "a" symbol).
(17) Number of frames per second that are used for image formation (11).

A high number enables a fluent dynamic visualization. Depth setting scale (in this case selected from 0 to 3.5 cm), the most inferior point is indicated (3.5 cm). SD, thyroid gland; MSCM, sternocleidomastoid muscle; NX, vagal nerve; ACC, common carotid artery; VJI, internal jugular vein.

3 Practical Tips on Ultrasound Examination Technique

The patient is positioned in a dimmed room in supine position, with the head tilted. The examiner usually sits to the right side of the patient.

The basic system setting should be stored in a standardized way, individually or by department. The user "adjusts" the system and the brightness of the monitor individually for each patient, depending on the acoustic tissue type of the patient, e.g., obese or slim.

Today's ultrasound systems provide various setting options for obtaining an optimal B-scan image; further modifications apply to color duplex sonography or color-coded duplex sonography (CCDS). It is good practice to define the parameter setting characteristic for certain examination scenarios (e.g., vessels, surface rendering, deep structures; see Table 2.3) in the presets.

Resolution and Penetration

The transmit frequency and the resulting diagnostic capabilities are correlated: the higher the frequency, the better the resolution will be, while the depth of penetration will be lower (**Figs. 3.1, 3.2**).

This relationship must be taken into account when selecting the transducer for a particular examination. For slim patients, a depth setting of 45 mm will certainly be sufficient. As a reliable landmark, the echo-dense contour of the vertebral body should be visible in the lower end of the image. From our experience, for the complete obligatory display of tongue and oropharynx, the depth setting will always have to be increased to 60–70 mm (**Figs. 3.3, 3.4**).

Sound Field Characteristics

In contrast to the ideal case of truly linear sound wave propagation, there is in practice a spatial spreading (producing a "sound beam") that is represented by the term "sound field characteristics." Perpendicular to the direction of propagation, the width of the sound beam changes substantially and three areas (near field, focus region, and far field) are distinguished:

1. Because of different run times, strong interferences occur close to the transducer, such that different pulses may even cancel each other out. Objects located in this near field can be displayed more clearly if the width of the transducer (aperture) and the transmit frequency are increased. In practice this important issue can be avoided by using a standoff in which the near field is virtually "hidden."
2. With growing distance from the transducer, the optimal resolution can be found in the focus region, the aperture being inversely proportional to the focus width. Ultrasound systems frequently provide the option to change the focus depth or to achieve focusing of the sound beam at multiple depths through a multiple focus.
3. In the far field, the ultrasound beam becomes increasingly wider, the opening angle being smaller the higher the transducer frequency.

Figures 3.5 and 3.6 show different depths of focus of the same region.

Gain and Time Gain Compensation

On their way through the tissue the sound waves are attenuated through "internal friction," so that echoes of deeper objects are attenuated on their way back to the transducer to a greater extent than echoes of objects close to the transducer. To compensate for this depth-dependent attenuation and generate a homogeneous image the overall enhancement is regulated via a control usually called "Gain." It is the task of the time-dependent depth compensation, known as time gain compensation (TGC), to additionally compensate this amplification in a depth-dependent way; in practice TGC provides for the adjustment of the gain to individual examination requirements (**Figs. 3.7, 3.8**).

For orientation, the following "four-button rule" should be used for B-mode image optimization, since this usually enables optimized settings.

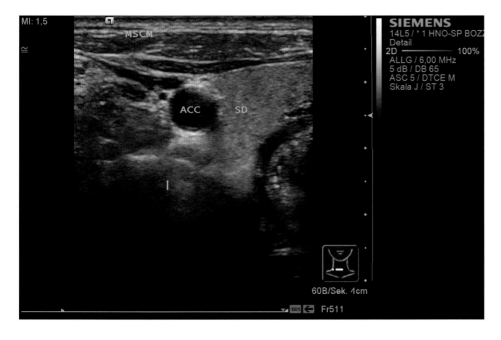

Fig. 3.1 Neck, right, transverse. The transmit frequency is 6 MHz. All cervical soft tissue structures are clearly visible. The green cursor marks the echodense contour of the vertebral body. ACC, common carotid artery; MSCM, sternocleidomastoid muscle; SD, thyroid gland.

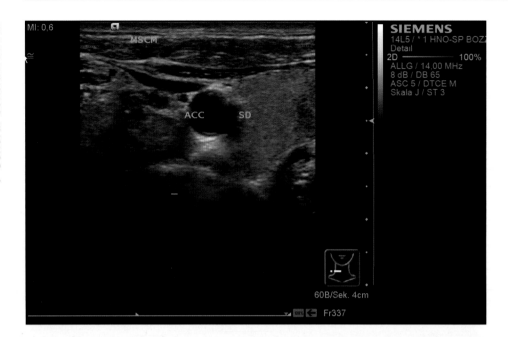

Fig. 3.2 Neck, right, transverse. If the transmit frequency is increased to 14 MHz, the tissue elements such as vascular walls and internal texture of the visible tissues are more clearly demarcated. The loss of deep structures in this "near field" of 35 mm is marginal. ACC, common carotid artery; MSCM, sternocleidomastoid muscle; SD, thyroid gland.

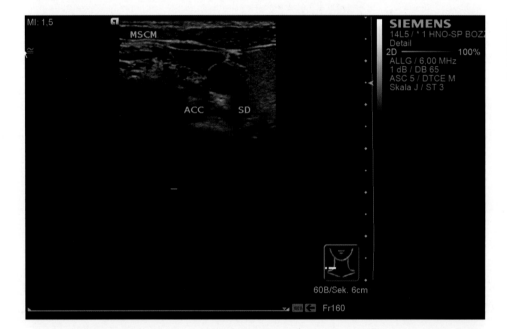

Fig. 3.3 Neck, right, transverse. With a penetration depth of 60 mm, half of the usable field of view is not utilized in this slim patient. ACC, common carotid artery; MSCM, sternocleidomastoid muscle; SD, thyroid gland.

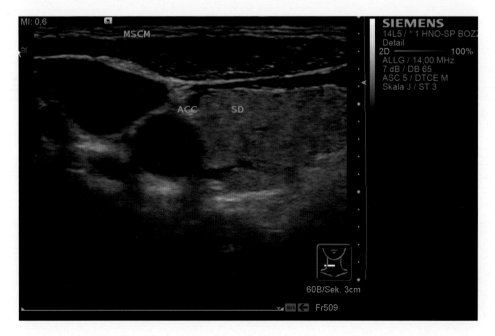

Fig. 3.4 Neck, right, transverse. After adjustment of the penetration depth from 60 mm to 30 mm, a substantial advantage in viewing the details is observed. For routine examinations, the depth border should be the hyperechoic reflection of the ventral surface of the vertebral body. ACC, common carotid artery; MSCM, sternocleidomastoid muscle; SD, thyroid gland.

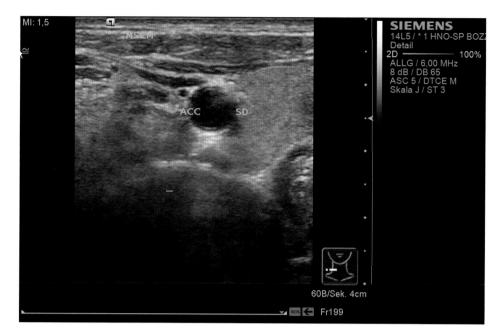

Fig. 3.5 Neck, right, transverse. The monofocus as a triangle on the left image edge at the depth scaling (at 15 mm) is set to the center of the displayed image section and therefore on the level of the common carotid artery (ACC) and in the center of the thyroid gland (SD). MSCM, sternocleidomastoid muscle.

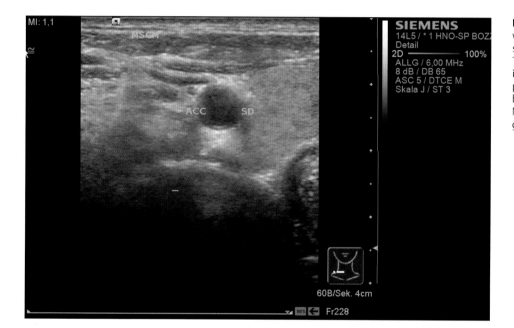

Fig. 3.6 Neck, right, transverse. The monofocus was shifted deeper (35 mm), so that now the structures of this region can be seen more clearly. The contour of the vertebral body front surface is demarcated more clearly, and the apex of the piriform sinus deep inside the thyroid gland becomes visible. ACC, common carotid artery; MSCM, sternocleidomastoid muscle; SD, thyroid gland.

Pearls and Pitfalls

"Four-button rule":

1. Set the depth (typically 45 mm for the neck and 60 mm for the tongue and oropharynx).
2. Adjust the transmit frequency.
3. Position the focal zone (typically 25–30 mm).
4. Adapt gain and TGC.

For color-coded Doppler sonography, other parameters and image setting modalities are necessary and are further explained in Chapter 2, Table 2.3.

Nevertheless, two further parameters are relevant here for the basic image settings: the pulse repetition frequency (PRF) and the color gain. The PRF should be adapted to the expected flow rate of the organ system currently under examination. A PRF of 2000 for evaluating the carotid arteries is suggested. For the evaluation of the lymphonodular angioarchitecture and with it the detection of even the smallest flow signals, the aim should be ~500. The color gain should always be increased to the extent that some artifacts are just visible in the systole.

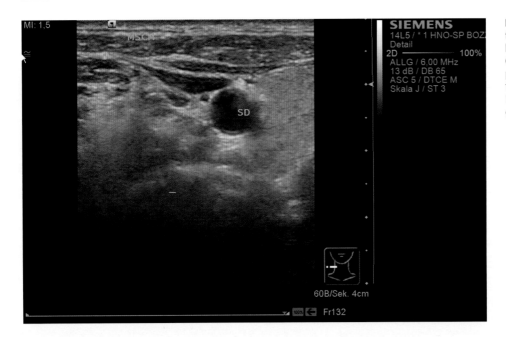

Fig. 3.7 Neck, right, transverse. The gain (13 dB at the upper left) was intentionally set to a high value here and gives a very bright image impression. Optical tissue differentiation is therefore not possible in an optimal way. All structures appear to be hyperechoic. ACC, common carotid artery; MSCM, sternocleidomastoid muscle; SD, thyroid gland.

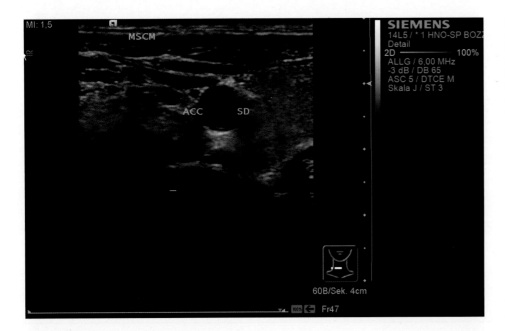

Fig. 3.8 Neck, right, transverse. With a low gain setting (−3 dB at the upper left) the image impression is too dark. The contrast between muscle and thyroid gland appears clearer, but intrastructural echoes such as the alignment of muscle fibers cannot be seen clearly. ACC, common carotid artery; MSCM, sternocleidomastoid muscle; SD, thyroid gland.

Clinical Examination of Neck Levels

The topographic classification of the cervical lymph node compartments according to the current version of the American Academy of Otolaryngology–Head and Neck Surgery will be presented in brief, before the actual examination procedure is described.

The level system describes the topographic position of neck lymph nodes (**Fig. 3.9**):

- Level I   submental and submandibular
- Level II   superior jugular
- Level III   middle jugular
- Level IV   inferior jugular
- Level V   posterior triangle
- Level VI   anterior compartment

Level IA: Submental Group

These lymph nodes are found within the triangular boundary of the anterior belly of both digastric muscles and the hyoid bone (**Figs. 3.9, 3.10, 3.11, 3.12**).

Level IB: Submandibular Group

Lymph nodes within the boundaries of the anterior and posterior bellies of the digastric muscles, the stylohyoid muscle, and the body of the mandible (**Figs. 3.9, 3.13, 3.14**). In ultrasound, the vertical plane defined by the posterior end of the submandibular gland demarcates the posterior aspect of level IB from IIA. The group includes the pre- and postglandular nodes, and the pre- and postvascular nodes.

Pearls and Pitfalls

These nodes are prone to harbor metastases from the floor of the mouth, the anterior oral tongue, the anterior mandibular alveolar ridge (level IA), the oral cavity, the anterior nasal cavity, the soft tissue structures of the mid-face, and the submandibular gland and lower lip (level IB) (**Fig. 3.12**).

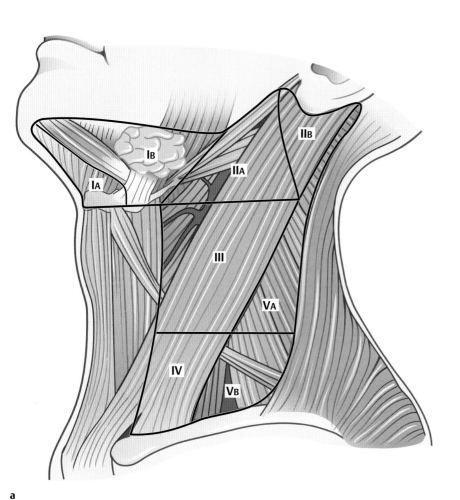

a

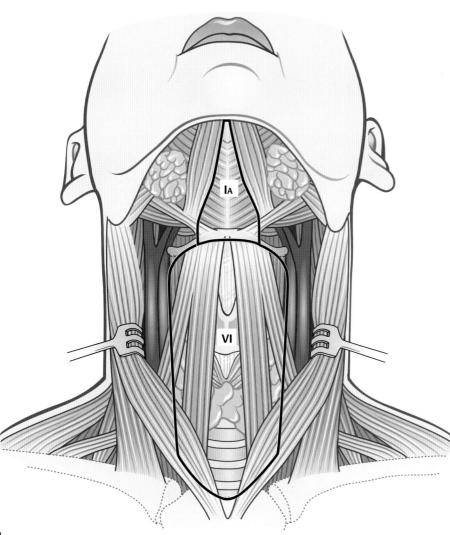

b

Fig. 3.9a,b Classification of the cervical lymph node compartments according to the current version of the American Academy of Otolaryngology–Head and Neck Surgery.
a Lateral view.
b Anterior view.
IA submental nodes
IB submandibular nodes
IIA upper jugular nodes anterior to the eleventh nerve
IIB upper jugular nodes posterior to the eleventh nerve
III middle jugular nodes around the middle part of the jugular vein and carotid bifurcation
IV lower jugular group caudal to the omohyoid muscle
VA lymph nodes in the posterior triangle located above the level of the inferior border of the cricoid cartilage
VB lymph nodes in the posterior triangle located below the level of the inferior border of the cricoid cartilage
VI anterior compartment

Adapted from Gavilán J, Herranz J, DeSanto LW, Gavilán C. Functional and Selective Neck Dissection. New York: Thieme; 2002:31.

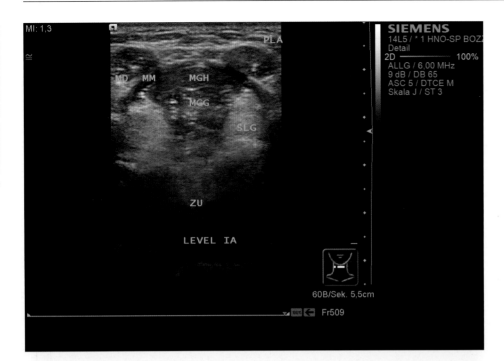

Fig. 3.10 Floor of the mouth, transverse. Level IA. SLG, sublingual gland; PLA, platysma; ZU, tongue; MD, digastric muscle; MM, mylohyoid muscle; MGG; genioglossus muscle; MGH, geniohyoid muscle.

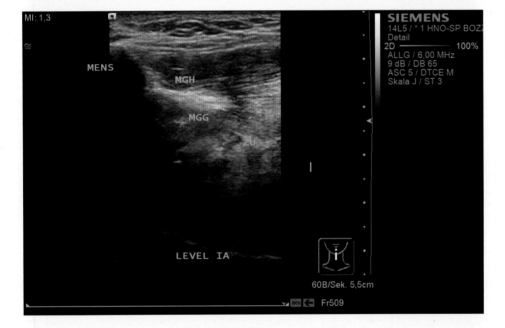

Fig. 3.11 Floor of the mouth, longitudinal plane. Level IA. MENS, point of the chin; MGG, genioglossus muscle; MGH, geniohyoid muscle; ZU, tongue.

Levels IIA and IIB: Superior Jugular Group

Lymph nodes located around the upper third of the internal jugular vein and adjacent spinal accessory nerve extending from the level of the skull base (superior) to the level of the inferior border of the hyoid bone (inferior). The anterior (medial) boundary is the lateral border of the sternohyoid muscle and posterior aspect of the submandibular gland, and the posterior (lateral) boundary is the posterior border of the sternocleidomastoid muscle. Sublevel IIA nodes are located anterior (medial) to the vertical plane defined by the spinal accessory nerve; those in level IIB are located posteriorly (**Figs. 3.9, 3.15**).

The surgical landmark that defines the lateral boundary of levels II, III, and IV and the corresponding medial boundary of the posterior triangle (level V) is the plane that parallels the sensory branches of the cervical plexus.

Pearls and Pitfalls

The superior jugular nodes are affected in cancers from the oral cavity, nasal cavity, nasopharynx, oropharynx, hypopharynx, larynx, and parotid gland (**Fig. 3.12**).

Level III: Middle Jugular Group

This lymph node compartment is located around the middle third of the internal jugular vein. It extends from the inferior border of the hyoid bone (superior) to the inferior border of the cricoid cartilage (inferior). The anterior/medial border is the lateral aspect of the sternohyoid muscle, and the posterior/lateral boundary is the posterior border of the sternocleidomastoid muscle (**Figs. 3.9, 3.16, 3.17**).

Pearls and Pitfalls

Metastases from cancers arising from the oral cavity, nasopharynx, oropharynx, hypopharynx, and larynx frequently become apparent in this compartment.

Level IV: Lower Jugular Group

This group comprises lymph nodes located around the lower third of the internal jugular vein extending from the inferior border of the cricoid cartilage (superior) to the clavicle (inferior) (**Figs. 3.9, 3.17, 3.18**).

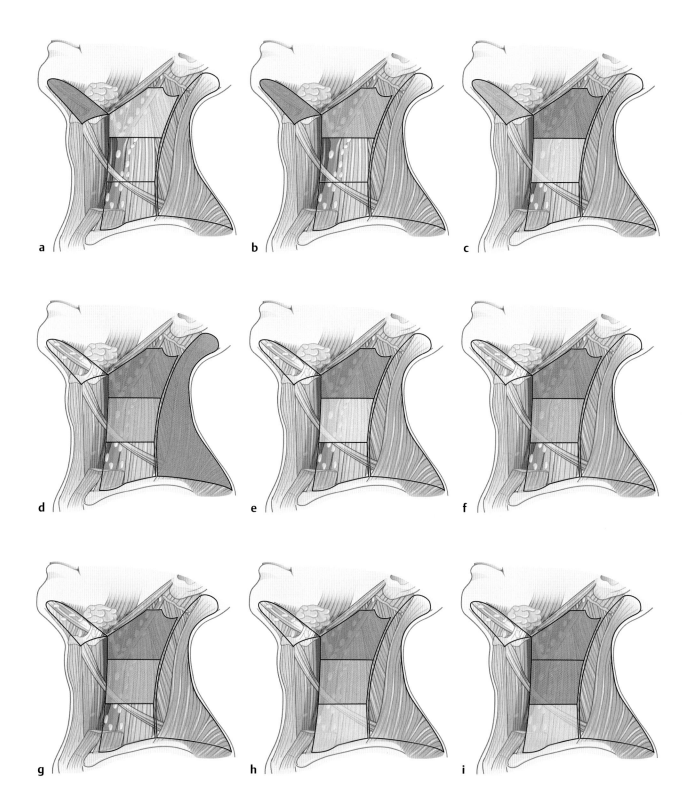

Fig. 3.12a–i Schematic drawings of predominant initial lymphatic metastatic spread of head and neck tumors depending on the primary tumor site. Darker shading depicts increasing probability of initially affected neck region.

a Lower lip.
b Floor of the mouth.
c Anterior two-thirds of the tongue.

d Nasopharynx.
e Tonsils.
f Base of the tongue.

g Supraglottis.
h Glottis.
i Hypopharynx.

Adapted from Strutz J, Mann W. Praxis der HNO-Heilkunde, Kopf- und Halschirurgie. 2nd ed. Stuttgart: Thieme; 2010.

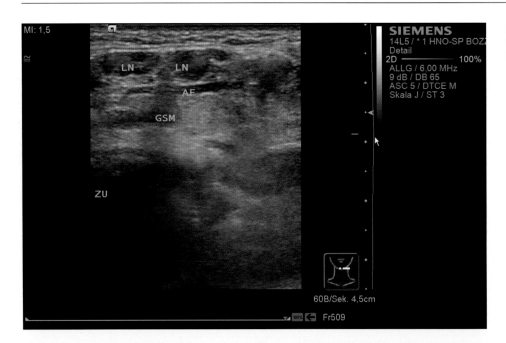

Fig. 3.13 Neck, left, transverse, level IB. GSM, submandibular gland; AF, facial artery; ZU, tongue; LN, lymph node.

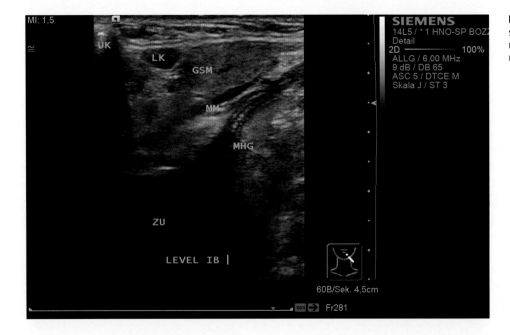

Fig. 3.14 Neck, left, longitudinal, level IB. GSM, submandibular gland; ZU, tongue; LK, lymph node; MM, mylohyoid muscle; MHG, hyoglossus muscle; UK, mandible.

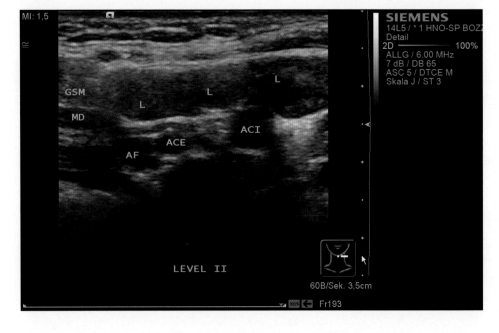

Fig. 3.15 Neck, left, transverse, level II. GSM, submandibular gland; AF, facial artery; ACE, external carotid artery; ACI, internal carotid artery; L, lymph node; MD, digastric muscle.

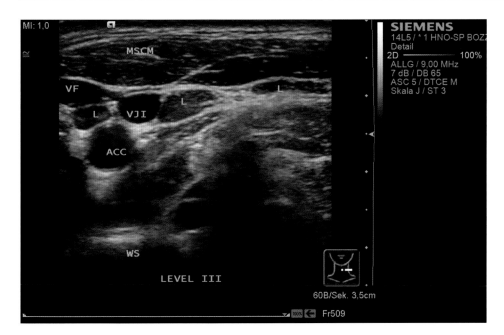

Fig. 3.16 Neck, left, transverse, level III. MSCM, sternocleidomastoid muscle; VF, facial vein; VJI, internal jugular vein; ACC, common carotid artery; L, lymph node; WS, spine.

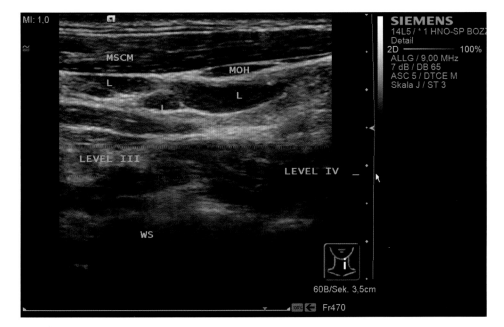

Fig. 3.17 Neck, left, longitudinal, levels III and IV. MSCM, sternocleidomastoid muscle; VF, facial vein; MOH, omohyoid muscle; L, lymph node; WS, spine.

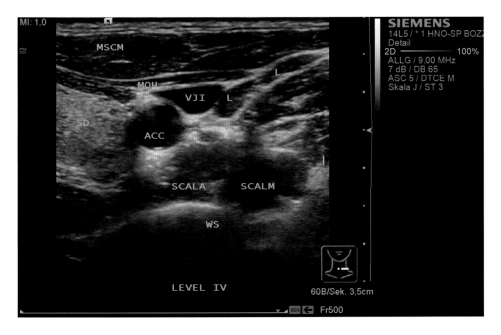

Fig. 3.18 Neck, left, transverse, level IV. MSCM, sternocleidomastoid muscle; SCALA, anterior scalenus muscle; SCALM, medium scalenus muscle; VJI, internal jugular vein; MOH, omohyoid muscle; ACC, common carotid artery; L, lymph node; WS, spine.

The anterior boundary is the lateral border of the sternohyoid muscle, and the posterior (lateral) boundary is the posterior border of the sternocleidomastoid muscle.

Levels VA and VB: Posterior Triangle Group

This group comprises predominantly the lymph nodes located along the lower half of the spinal accessory nerve and the transverse cervical artery. The supraclavicular nodes are also included in the posterior triangle group. The superior boundary is formed by the converging sternocleidomastoid and trapezius muscles. The inferior boundary is the clavicle, the anterior (medial) boundary is the posterior border of the sternocleidomastoid muscle, and the posterior boundary is the anterior border of the trapezius muscle. Sublevel VA is separated from sublevel VB by a horizontal plane marking the inferior border of the arch of the cricoid cartilage (**Figs. 3.9, 3.19**).

> **Pearls and Pitfalls**
>
> Metastases from cancers arising from the hypopharynx, cervical esophagus, and larynx are tributary to this compartment (**Fig. 3.12**).

> **Pearls and Pitfalls**
>
> The posterior triangle nodes are at greatest risk for harboring metastases from cancers arising from the nasopharynx and oropharynx (sublevel VA) and the thyroid gland (**Fig. 3.12**).

Level VI: Anterior Compartment Group

The lymph nodes in this section include the pre-and paratracheal nodes, the precricoid node (also called the Delphian node), and the perithyroidal nodes, including the lymph nodes along the recurrent laryngeal nerves (**Figs. 3.9 and 3.20**). The superior border is the hyoid bone, the inferior boundary is the suprasternal notch, and the lateral boundaries are given by the common carotid arteries.

> **Pearls and Pitfalls**
>
> These nodes are at greatest risk for harboring metastases from cancers arising from the thyroid gland, the glottic and subglottic larynx, the apex of the piriform sinus, and the cervical esophagus (**Fig. 3.12**).

Examination Sequence

After application of an adequate amount of ultrasound gel, the actual examination starts. The patient is requested to tilt his or her head backward and rotate it to the opposite side. The transducer is placed on the right supraclavicular region and the hyperechoic parenchyma of the thyroid gland is identified as the first landmark.

Since all echogenicities are present here, this starting point is suggested for adjusting the system settings for the beginning of the examination (**Fig. 3.21**).

> **Pearls and Pitfalls**
>
> A typical mistake in this situation is to concentrate directly on the clinically apparent finding. Here, there is a particularly high risk of missing a subsequent abnormality within the scope of an incomplete examination (**Fig. 3.12**). So, don't forget to do a complete examination.

After evaluation of level V and the thyroid gland pouch, the transducer is moved in the cranial direction and levels V, IV, III, and II are examined (▶ Videos 3.1, 3.2).

Now the transducer, having arrived at the angle of the mandible, can be directed either cranially to the lobulus to further examine the parotid and buccal region or parallel to the horizontal mandibular ramus to examine level IB. When viewing the submandibular region (level IB) the transducer, after change of the grip of the transducer, should be brought around the mandible medially to access the space between the medial side of the mandible and submandibular gland. Identification of the tongue and the submandibular gland in one image

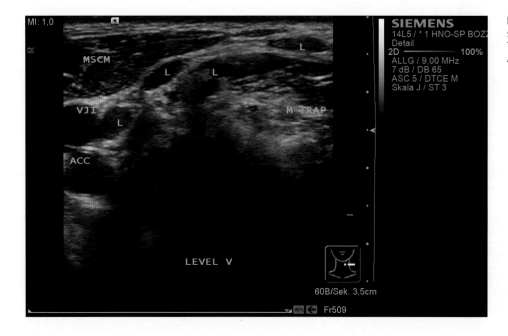

Fig. 3.19 Neck, transverse, level V. MSCM, sternocleidomastoid muscle; L, lymph node; M TRAP, trapezius muscle; VJI, internal jugular vein; ACC, common carotid artery.

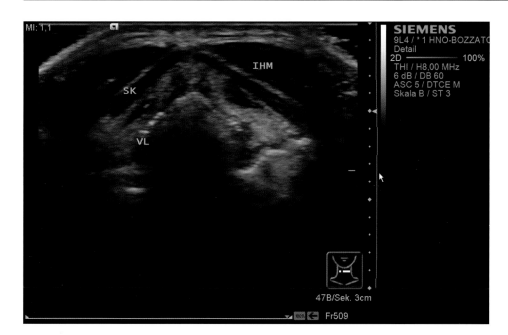

Fig. 3.20 Larynx, transverse, level VI. VL, laryngeal ventricle; SK, thyroid cartilage; IHM, infrahyoid muscles.

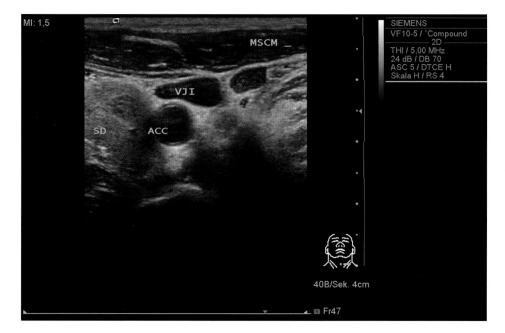

Fig. 3.21 Neck, left, transverse. The cervical paramedian section at thyroid level is suitable for starting an examination. It is recommended to set the system parameters in the following order: depth, frequency, focus, and gain. The sternocleidomastoid muscle can be considered hypoechoic; the healthy thyroid gland is hyperechoic. The vascular lumina of the carotid artery and internal jugular vein interna are anechoic. The thyroid gland (SD) shows a homogeneous, hyperechoic internal pattern. The sternocleidomastoid muscle (MSCM) constitutes the representative hypoechoic structure. ACC, common carotid artery; VJI, internal jugular vein.

is a suitable setting for visualization of the palatine tonsil lying in a triangle between these two landmarks (▶ Video 3.3).

Finally the transducer is moved far lateral of levels II, III, and IV back to a caudal direction in order not to miss lateral changes of level V and the nuchal area.

After the patient's head is tilted backwards in a median direction, the transducer is placed on the point of the chin and moved axially in caudal direction to evaluate level IA, the tongue, the base of the tongue, and the larynx. The end of this stage is again the thyroid gland pouch. With sliding laterally to the contralateral side, the examination is repeated (▶ Video 3.4).

Depending on the clinical indication, the soft or bony tissues of the face or the paranasal sinuses areas are examined separately, as explained in the individual chapters.

Although the sequence of examination of the cervical areas can be changed, the procedure described above has proved itself in our opinion.

Pearls and Pitfalls

A consistent and standardized procedure is very important. It is mandatory to examine structures that appear even only rudimentarily abnormal always in both planes.

4   Documentation and Terminology

The diagnostic quality of head and neck ultrasonography depends greatly on a precise description of the findings and written documentation. As well as hard copies of reports, digital documentation and archiving systems are now increasingly being used.

For the documentation, care is taken to ensure that the representation of the results is specific with respect to the particular organ concerned and the findings. All descriptions and any conclusions have to be understandable for subsequent investigations and different examiners. Only in this way is it possible to recognize any dynamic developments in the findings at follow-up and to assess the clinical situation correctly. Digital documentation usually involves basic text elements that make it easier to maintain the uniformity of the descriptors.

In addition to recording the images themselves, all findings have to be documented in such a way as to allow quality control by a third party at any time.

A logical terminology is needed for a precise and generally understandable description in the written report. This terminology must be based on basic physical principles while at the same time being relevant to the conditions under investigation. It must take account of both practical and clinical concerns.

The written documentation of an ultrasound examination should include:

1. Patient identification (name and age)
2. Identity of the examiner
3. Examination date
4. Question posed and/or indication for the examination
5. Any conditions limiting the examination or its assessment
6. Organ-specific description of the findings, except when no abnormality is detected
7. (Provisional) diagnosis
8. Any conclusions about diagnostic and/or therapeutic consequences and/or further action

Documentation of the images should cover:

1. Images recorded in a digital or analog medium appropriate to the archiving modality including: B-scan image with distance scale; measured values; caliper; transmission frequency or frequency range; focus position; patient identity; date of examination; description of transducer; details of the institute; pictogram showing the positioning and orientation of the transducer.
2. Normal findings: provide one or more appropriate section planes to confirm normal findings in relation to the indication for the scan (B-mode only).
3. Pathological findings: images in two section planes or—if this is not possible—in one plane (B-mode only). Details of perfusion should be given whenever color-coded duplex sonography (CCDS) and Doppler scanning are performed.

Standard Sonographic Descriptors

Localization

Position in relation to major anatomical structures:
- Major vessels of the neck (**Fig. 4.1**)
- Sternocleidomastoid muscle (**Figs. 4.2, 4.3**)
- Glands of the head and their ducts (**Fig. 4.4**)
- Bony and cartilaginous structures (**Fig. 4.5**)
- Midline (**Fig. 4.6**)

Structure (Echogenicity)

- Hyperechoic (**Fig. 4.7**)
- Echogenic (**Fig. 4.8**)
- Hypoechoic (**Fig. 4.9**)
- Isoechoic (**Fig. 4.10**)
- Anechoic (**Fig. 4.10**)
- Homogeneous (**Fig. 4.11**)
- Inhomogeneous (**Fig. 4.12**)

Shape

- Round (**Fig. 4.13**)
- Oval (**Fig. 4.14**)
- Polycyclic/lobulated (**Fig. 4.15**)
- Spindle-shaped (**Fig. 4.16**)

Contour

- Smooth (**Fig. 4.17**)
- Irregular (**Fig. 4.18**)

Margins

- Distinct/sharp (**Fig. 4.19**)
- Ill-defined (**Figs. 4.20, 4.21**)

Distal Phenomena

- Distal acoustic enhancement (**Fig. 4.22**)
- Distal acoustic shadowing (attenuation) (**Fig. 4.23**)
- Total distal acoustic shadow (**Fig. 4.24**)

Sonographic Palpation

The compressibility of structures can be examined by applying pressure with the ultrasound probe, and the movement of one structure against another provides useful additional evidence in the assessment of the findings; these aspects improve the quality of the results. Movement due to the arterial blood pressure opposing the transducer pressure reveals planes of movement between an artery and a metastasis, for example (▶ Videos 4.1, 4.2).

Pressure over a cyst causes flattening of the liquid or viscous contents parallel to the direction in which the pressure is applied (▶ Video 4.3). Pulsations transmitted by or generated in a space-occupying lesion also provide haptic records.

Pearls and Pitfalls

The paramedian transverse cervical slice at the level of the thyroid gland is the best place to start the examination. Adjustments to scanner settings are best made in the following order: depth, frequency, focus, and gain. The sternocleidomastoid muscle is a hypoechoic structure, while the healthy thyroid gland is echogenic (**Fig. 4.25**). The lumina of the carotid artery and the internal jugular vein are anechoic.

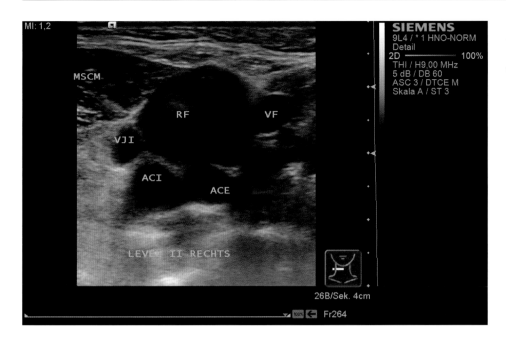

Fig. 4.1 Neck, right, transverse. This space-occupying lesion (RF) lies anterior to the carotid bifurcation (ACI/ACE) and between the internal jugular vein (VJI) and the facial vein (VF). MSCM, sternocleidomastoid muscle. Diagnosis: **Regional metastasis of oropharyngeal carcinoma**.

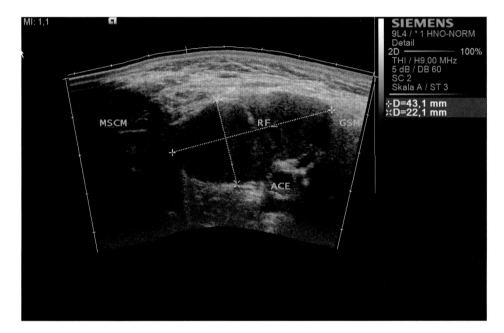

Fig. 4.2 Neck, right, transverse. A space-occupying lesion (RF) lies at the anterior border of the sternocleidomastoid muscle (MSCM). ACE, external carotid artery; GSM, submandibular gland. Diagnosis: **Regional metastasis of oral cavity carcinoma**.

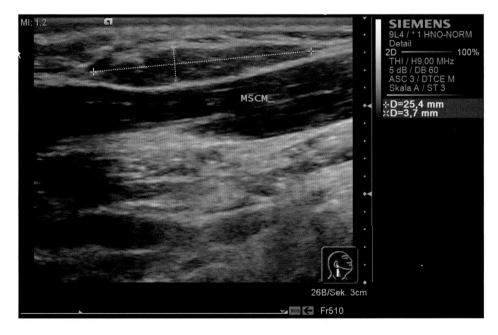

Fig. 4.3 Neck, right, longitudinal. A neck lesion with a spindle-shaped configuration lies at the anterior border of the sternocleidomastoid muscle (MSCM), and is clearly demarcated from the edge of the muscle. Diagnosis: **Lymphadenitis**.

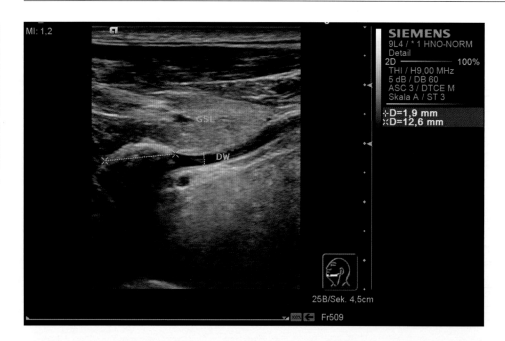

Fig. 4.4 Floor of the mouth, longitudinal, anterior. A hyperechoic **salivary stone** (caliper) lies directly on the sublingual gland (GSL) and is causing stasis proximally in the Wharton duct (DW).

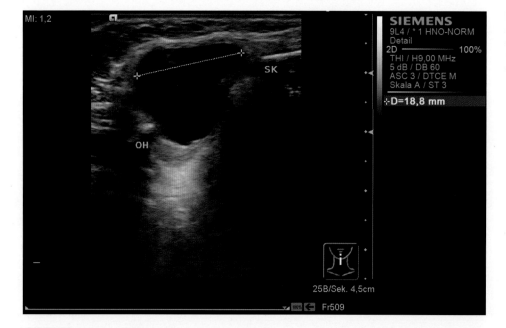

Fig. 4.5 Neck, longitudinal, paramedian. An anechoic space-occupying lesion (median neck cyst) between the hyoid bone (OH) and the upper edge of the thyroid cartilage (SK) extends anteriorly into the subcutaneous tissue.

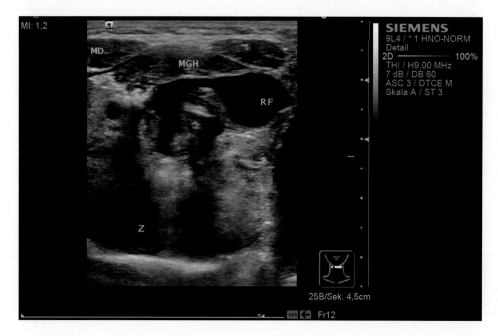

Fig. 4.6 Tongue, median, transverse. A dumbbell-shaped anechoic change (RF) can be seen on the left side of the floor of the mouth (MGH), extending into the median plane of the intrinsic muscles of the tongue (Z). MD, digastric muscle. Diagnosis: **Ranula**.

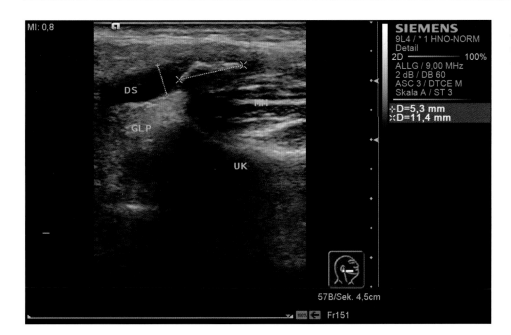

Fig. 4.7 Parotid gland, right, transverse. A **salivary stone** (right caliper) in the Stensen duct (DS) with a hyperechoic surface structure. GLP, parotid gland; MM masseter muscle; UK, mandible.

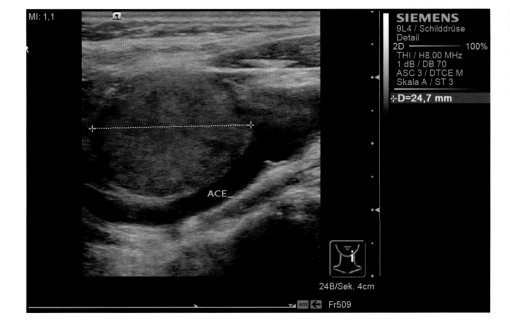

Fig. 4.8 Neck, left, longitudinal. An echogenic **metastatic lymph node** with clearly defined margins. The parenchyma of the thyroid, parotid, submandibular, and sublingual glands is also usually echogenic. The lumina of blood vessels, such as the external carotid artery (ACE), are usually hypoechoic or anechoic.

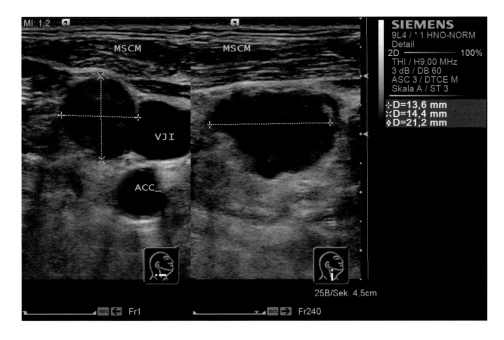

Fig. 4.9 Split screen of neck, right, transverse. A **lymph node metastasis** with a hypoechoic texture, lying lateral to the internal jugular vein (VJI), which is anechoic. ACC, common carotid artery; MSCM, sternocleidomastoid muscle.

I General Considerations

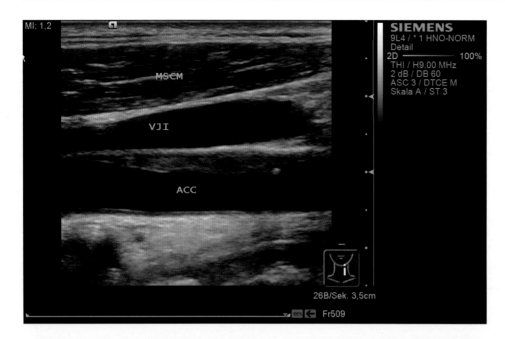

Fig. 4.10 Neck, left, longitudinal. The lumina of the common carotid artery (ACC) and internal jugular vein (VJI) are both anechoic and, therefore, in mutual comparison are said to be isoechoic. In contrast, the sternocleidomastoid muscle (MSCM) can be seen to be hypoechoic. Diagnosis: **Hypoechoic thickening of the carotid wall**.

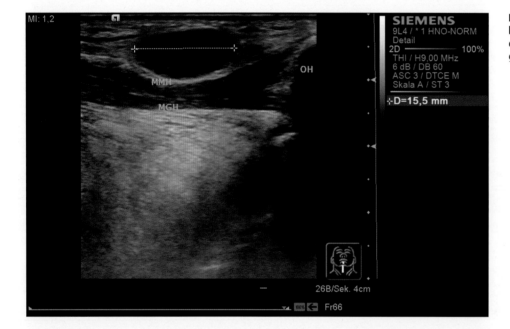

Fig. 4.11 Floor of the mouth, longitudinal. An oval **lymph node** shows a homogeneous hypoechoic echotexture. MMH, mylohyoid muscle; MGH, geniohyoid muscle; OH, hyoid bone.

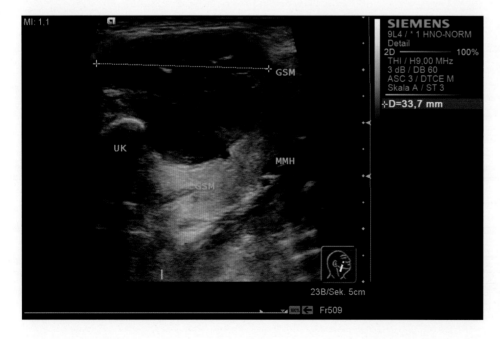

Fig. 4.12 Neck, right, longitudinal. A space-occupying lesion with an inhomogeneous and hypoechoic echo pattern lies in the bed of the submandibular gland. GSM, submandibular gland; MMH, mylohyoid muscle; UK, mandible. Diagnosis: **Metastasis of an oral cavity carcinoma**.

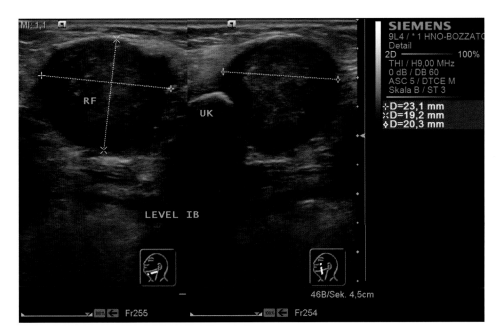

Fig. 4.13 Split screen of neck, left, submandibular. A space-occupying lesion (RF) with inhomogeneous and hypoechoic echo pattern can be seen in both the longitudinal and the transverse views as a round, poorly defined shape in the bed of the submandibular gland. The lesion is directly situated at the mandible. The risk for a facial nerve affection during surgery increased. GSM, submandibular gland; UK, mandible. Diagnosis: **Metastasis of a malignant melanoma**.

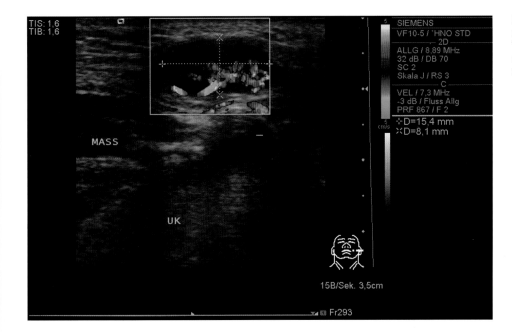

Fig. 4.14 Parotid gland, left, transverse. A **lymph node** shows an oval, clearly defined configuration. The sagittal diameter is just about half of the axial diameter in the view shown. MASS, masseter muscle; UK, mandible. Diagnosis: **Lymphadenitis**.

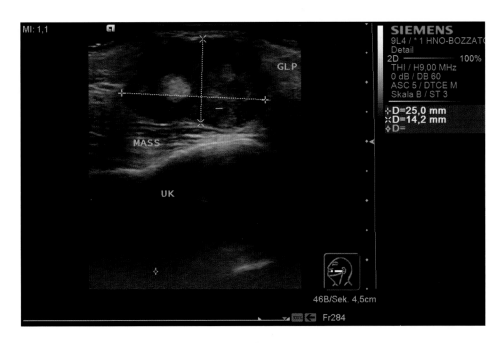

Fig. 4.15 Parotid gland, left, transverse. A tumor **(mucoepidermoid carcinoma)** shows an oval, clearly defined polycyclic configuration and has a nodular echogenic texture as a distinctive feature. GLP, parotid gland; MASS, masseter muscle; UK, mandible.

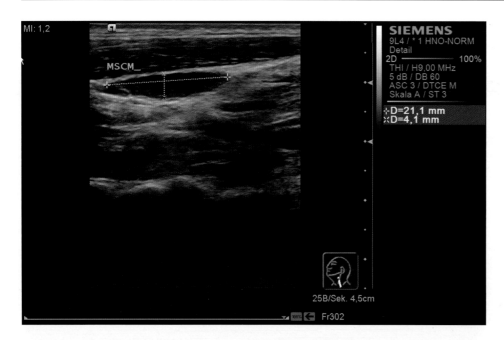

Fig. 4.16 Neck left, longitudinal oblique. A **lymph node** in level V with a spindle-shaped configuration lies beneath the sternocleidomastoid muscle (MSCM) but is clearly separated from the muscle border. The architecture of the scalene muscles and the echogenic outline of the spine can be recognized deeper in the view.

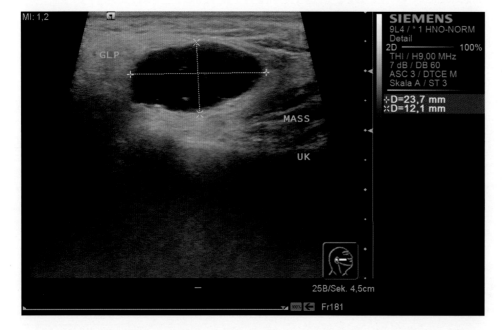

Fig. 4.17 Parotid gland, right, transverse. The hypoechoic inhomogeneous solid tumor exhibits a smooth outline. GLP, parotid gland; MASS, masseter muscle; UK, mandible. Diagnosis: **Adenoma**.

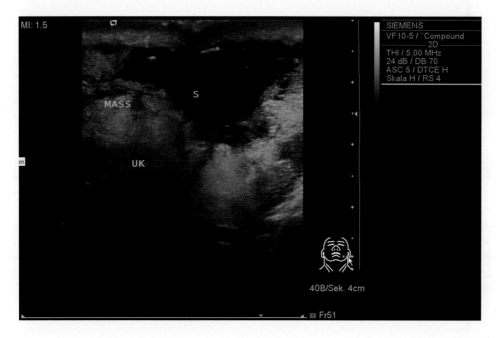

Fig. 4.18 Bed of the parotid gland, left, transverse, after partial parotidectomy. Depending on its echogenicity, a hypoechoic formation with irregular contours in the region of a wound is consistent with a **seroma (S) or hematoma**. The more echogenic the internal structure, the more viscous is the secretion it contains and the more organized is the hematoma. MASS, masseter muscle; UK, mandible.

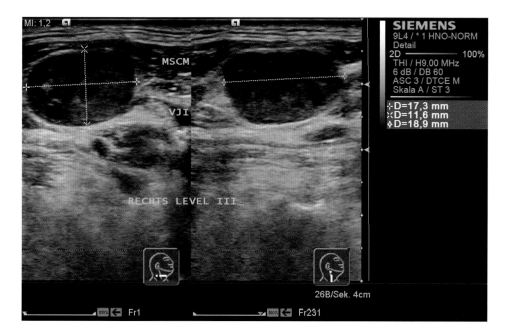

Fig. 4.19 Split screen of neck, right. A **lymph node metastasis** with inhomogeneous echotexture can be distinguished from the surrounding tissues by its clearly defined margins. MSCM, sternocleidomastoid muscle; VJI, internal jugular vein.

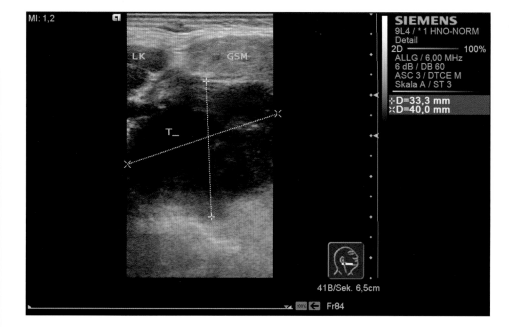

Fig. 4.20 Neck, right, transverse, submandibular. The **abscess formation** in the right tonsillar bed is difficult to distinguish from neighboring structures because of the surrounding diffuse inflammatory reaction. GSM, submandibular gland; LK, lymph node; T, tonsilar region.

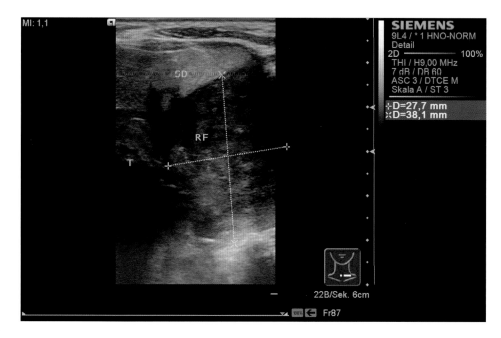

Fig. 4.21 Neck, left, transverse. The **malignant mass (RF)** adjacent to the thyroid gland (SD) and the trachea (T) has poorly defined margins due to infiltration.

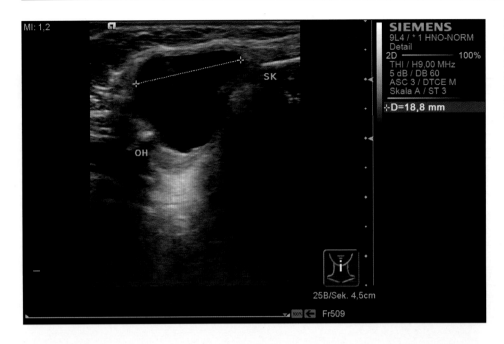

Fig. 4.22 Neck, longitudinal, paramedian. An anechoic space-occupying lesion (median neck cyst) lies between the hyoid bone (OH) and the upper edge of the thyroid cartilage (SK). The echo from areas behind less-attenuating tissue is referred to as distal acoustic enhancement (e.g., dorsal enhancement behind cysts or lymphomas). Diagnosis: **Medial cervical cyst**.

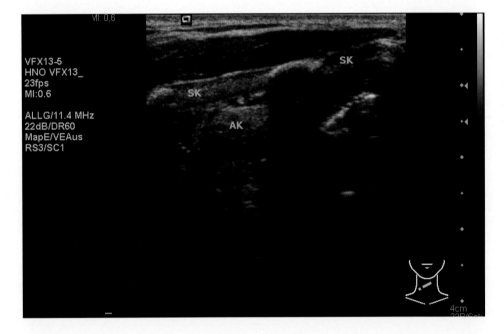

Fig. 4.23 Larynx, right, transverse. Distal acoustic shadowing may be caused by reflection, absorption, scattering, and refraction, in the medium being examined and at the interfaces. It must be compensated for by an appropriate adjustment of depth. The **ossification of the right lamina of the thyroid cartilage** (SK) attenuates the demonstration of endolaryngeal structures. AK, arytenoid cartilage.

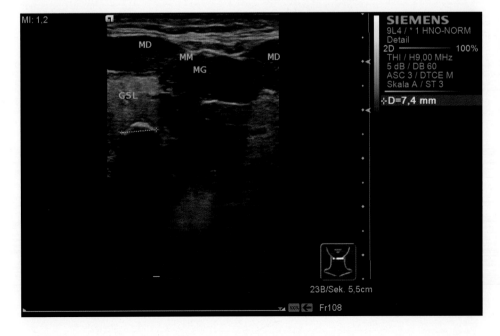

Fig. 4.24 Floor of the mouth, transverse. Weakly reflective or anechoic areas behind attenuating tissue are seen as complete shadows (e.g., behind the mandible). An echogenic **salivary stone** (between calipers) shows a complete distal shadow—picturesquely known as a comet-tail artifact. MD, digastric muscle; MM, mylohyoid muscle; MG, genioglossus muscle; GSL, sublingual gland.

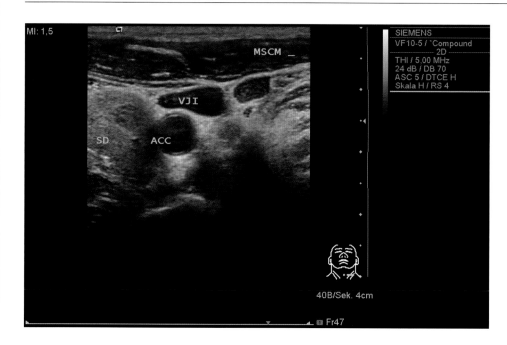

Fig. 4.25 Neck, left transverse. The thyroid gland (SD) has a homogeneous, echogenic internal structure. The sternocleidomastoid muscle (MSCM) is representative of a hypoechoic structure, while the lumina of the common carotid artery (ACC) and the internal jugular vein (VJI) are anechoic. Diagnosis: **Non-neoplastic lymph node lateral to the VJI.**

II Sonographic Anatomy and Pathology

5 Thyroid Gland
Deike Strobel

Diseases of the thyroid gland are common. One epidemiological study (Schilddrüsen-Initiative Papillon) showed that 37.6% of women and 40.3% of men in Germany had a goiter and/or thyroid nodules. Given the high prevalence of thyroid disease a rational approach to the various diagnostic tools (laboratory tests, ultrasonography, and scintigraphy) is essential (**Table 5.1**). Ultrasonography of the thyroid gland is simple and inexpensive, does not involve exposure to ionizing radiation, and provides valuable information.

Ultrasonography is the mainstay of diagnostic imaging of the thyroid gland: the superficial lie of the gland means that its size, shape, fine structure, and vascularity can be demonstrated using high-frequency probes (linear array transducer, 7.5–15 MHz) with excellent and unique axial and lateral image resolution (<1 mm). At present, MRI and CT scans do not achieve such high resolution and are usually omitted in the diagnostic work-up (except for retrosternal goiter). In addition to B-scan, color Doppler imaging provides useful information on thyroid perfusion, which is helpful in the differential diagnosis of inflammatory diseases of the thyroid gland and thyroid nodules.

Basic diagnostic work-up of suspected thyroid disease includes hormone testing (basal TSH, T_3, and T_4) and high-frequency ultrasound (B-scan, color Doppler).

New ultrasound techniques:
- Contrast-enhanced ultrasound has evolved over the last 10 years to become a keystone technique in abdominal ultrasound (e.g., in the differential diagnosis of liver lesions). The use of contrast agents with high-frequency probes was a technical challenge until recently, so that studies on the clinical value of contrast-enhanced ultrasound in thyroid disease are still limited. Compared with color Doppler imaging, contrast-enhanced ultrasound can visualize microperfusion of thyroid parenchyma and nodules in real time with very high resolution. Apart from scientific research questions, contrast-enhanced ultrasound of the thyroid gland might be of practical relevance in individual cases, for example in assessing the success of percutaneous ethanol injection therapy (PEIT) for autonomous thyroid nodules.
- Elastography provides additional information on tissue elasticity during the ultrasound examination. Although elastography has gained clinical relevance in the diagnosis of parenchymal liver diseases (noninvasive diagnosis of hepatic cirrhosis) and the differential diagnosis of tumors (breast, prostate), its value in the diagnostic investigation of the thyroid has not been sufficiently evaluated. Preliminary studies show that the hardness of thyroid nodules can be measured with elastography, which may be helpful in differentiating benign from malignant nodules. Malignant thyroid nodules are usually hard (with the exception of follicular cancer), although this measurement has its limitations with false-positive elastographic results from calcified benign nodules.

Table 5.1 Diagnostic work-up of thyroid disease

• Palpation
• Hormone tests including thyroid antibodies
• Ultrasonography (B-scan, color Doppler, fine-needle aspiration biopsy)
• Scintigraphy
• Rarely: radiography— thoracic inlet views and barium swallow
• Rarely: CT and MRI

Topographic Anatomy

The thyroid gland, which weighs 14–18 g, is located superficially in the anterior lower neck. Its two lobes lie on either side of the trachea and are joined by a thin bridge of parenchymal tissue (the isthmus), giving the gland a butterfly shape. Children and adolescents, and ~10% of adults, may also have a pyramidal lobe (a remnant of the thyroglossal duct left after the embryonic development of the thyroid gland from the base of the tongue), which extends in a cranial direction from the isthmus. The thyroid gland is surrounded by muscles. The sternothyroid and sternohyoid muscles lie anterior to the thyroid, the sternocleidomastoid muscle is anteromedial to the gland. The longus colli muscle is located posterior and the scalene group posterolateral to the thyroid gland. The esophagus runs behind the trachea and the left lobe of the thyroid gland. The internal jugular vein and common carotid artery are located lateral to the gland. Blood supply of the thyroid gland is provided by two thyroid arteries (branches of the external carotid artery), which run to the upper and lower pole of the thyroid (superior thyroid artery and inferior thyroid artery). Venous drainage is via the capsular venous plexus and superior, middle, and inferior thyroid veins into the internal jugular vein.

Ultrasound Examination

The examination is best performed with the patient reclining the neck to give a better view of the retrosternal parts of the thyroid and of the region of the inferior parathyroid glands. Systematic examination of the thyroid gland starts in the transverse plane anteriorly in the lower third of the neck. Imaging in the transverse plane provides an axial view of the thyroid gland and the thyroid compartment.

Figure 5.1 is a panoramic view of both lobes and the isthmus of the thyroid gland in the transverse plane, showing their positional relationship to the muscles and vessels. The central acoustic shadow, which is caused by the tracheal cartilage, serves for orientation and to identify the lobes of the thyroid lying lateral.

The curve of the neck usually makes it impossible to see both lobes of the gland completely at the same time in the anterior transverse view. The ultrasound probe therefore has to be moved lateral to the right and the left part, and the two lobes are scanned separately in transverse and longitudinal images. Care should be taken in this to adjust the B-mode gain correctly. Subcutaneous fat appears hypoechoic. The echogenic texture of the normal thyroid parenchyma should be hyperechoic relative to the muscles, and the vessels appear anechoic when the scanner settings are correct.

Normal Sonographic Findings

The normal thyroid gland has a smooth contour; the echo pattern of the parenchyma is homogeneous and hyperechoic compared with the surrounding muscles.

In the longitudinal plane, the craniocaudal longitudinal diameter is measured from the upper to the lower pole; in the transverse plane, the maximum width and depth diameters are determined (**Figs. 5.2, 5.3**).

The two thyroid lobes are measured separately. Their volumes are calculated and added together. The normal range for the total thyroid volume in adults is 8–18 mL for women and 9–25 mL for men (**Table 5.2**). Although the isthmus is not taken into consideration when calculating the volume, it must be examined just as carefully as the rest of

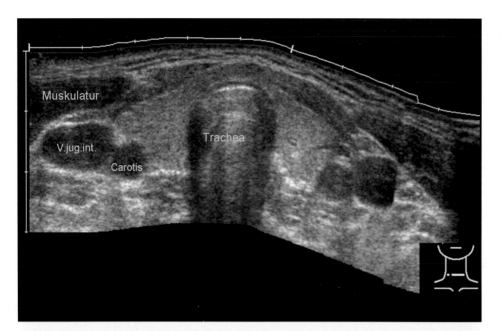

Fig. 5.1 Axial view of the thyroid gland and the thyroid compartment.

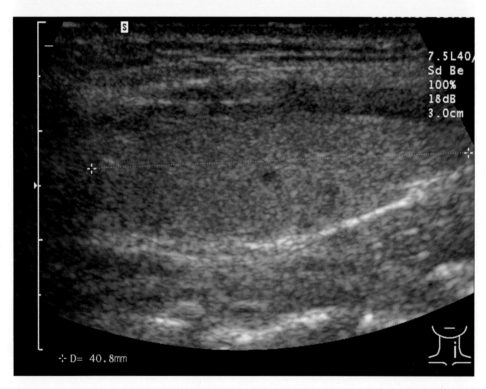

Fig. 5.2 Measurement of the craniocaudal longitudinal diameter in the longitudinal plane.

Table 5.2 Reference ranges of thyroid volumes; normal values

Age	Volume
1–4 years	<4 mL
6–10 years	5–9 mL
11–14 years	10–15 mL
15–16 years	<16 mL
Women	<18 mL
Men	<25 mL

the thyroid parenchyma. A thyroid volume of less than 6 mL in an adult may be associated with reduced function. Hormone status has to be assessed, and in case of low levels of T_3/T_4 replacement therapy might be necessary.

> **Sonographic measurement of the thyroid volume:**
>
> Mathematical formula of an ellipsoid (Brunn's rotational ellipsoid):
>
> length (cm) × width (cm) × depth (cm) × 0.479 = volume (mL)

In addition to the size of the gland, the systematic ultrasound examination includes shape (horseshoe-shaped in cross-section), contours (smooth), echogenic texture (fine, homogeneous individual echoes, hyperechoic in relation to the surrounding muscles), and movement on swallowing. Color Doppler sonography complements the B-mode real-time assessment of the thyroid. In the longitudinal view, the superior and inferior thyroid arteries can usually be found at the cranial and caudal poles of the thyroid gland. Color Doppler scans also reveal regular small vascular segments within the gland itself. Inflammatory changes in the gland may cause a marked increase in vascularity, particularly in Graves disease (as described below). Intrinsic vascularity of autonomous adenomas is an indicator of increased functional activity, while regressive nodules usually show only perinodular flow.

> **Pearls and Pitfalls**
>
> If the ultrasound findings are normal and the TSH is in the normal range, clinically relevant thyroid disease can almost certainly be ruled out.

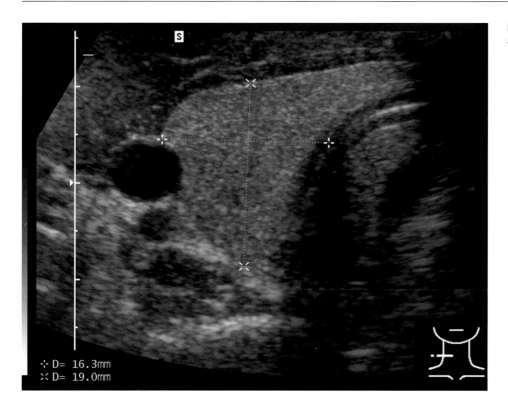

Fig. 5.3 Measurement of the maximum width and depth dimensions in the transverse plane.

÷ D= 16.3mm
✕ D= 19.0mm

Ultrasound Pathology of Diffuse Thyroid Disease

Congenital Malformations

In the case of congenital hypothyroidism, ultrasound scanning can differentiate a malformation (agenesis or hypoplasia) from a diffusely enlarged thyroid gland. If there is congenital hypoplasia or aplasia of one lobe of the thyroid, the contralateral lobe is hypertrophied. Thyroid gland scintigraphy is the method of choice to demonstrate ectopic thyroid tissue (lingual goiter, intrathoracic goiter).

Goiter (Diffuse, Nodular)

A goiter is defined as an enlargement of the gland. Goiter is a common disease with a prevalence of 20%–30% in Germany. The main cause is a dietary iodine deficiency, although rare causes include inflammation and tumors. A diffuse goiter is a globally enlarged thyroid gland with smooth contours (**Fig. 5.4**).

If nodules can be demonstrated in the enlarged thyroid gland, it is referred to as a nodular goiter. There is a spectrum from a single nodule in an enlarged gland (uninodular goiter) through to a goiter with multiple nodules (multinodular goiter). The increasing replacement of normal tissue by nodules gives rise to irregular contours and a fuller shape (**Fig. 5.5**).

The lower pole of an extremely enlarged thyroid might no longer be depicted. Parts of the thyroid gland behind the clavicles or sternum cannot be assessed with ultrasound (retrosternal goiter). As a precise determination of the volume is no longer possible in this situation, the examiner has to be content with describing the findings and measuring the maximum sagittal diameters of the right and left lobes. Thyroid function cannot really be deduced from the size of the gland. Even with a small gland the patient may be euthyroid if sufficient hormone is being produced by ectopic tissue (e.g., lingual goiter). On the other hand, a patient with a greatly enlarged thyroid gland may be hypothyroid.

Tables 5.3 and 5.4 summarize the differential diagnosis of thyroid gland enlargement and clinical work-up of goiter.

Thyroiditis

> **Pearls and Pitfalls**
>
> The finding of a hypoechoic thyroid gland on ultrasonography is common to all inflammatory thyroid diseases.

During inflammation the thyroid gland's normal hyperechoic echotexture (in comparison with muscle) becomes diffuse hypoechoic (**Fig. 5.6**). The internal echoes of the thyroid gland with inflammatory changes may be homogeneous or inhomogeneous—the ill-defined hypoechoic areas correspond to the inflammatory foci (**Fig. 5.7**).

The finding of a hypoechoic gland may be due to several different inflammatory conditions; the most common are Hashimoto thyroiditis, Graves disease, de Quervain thyroiditis, and postpartum thyroiditis (**Table 5.5**). Thyroiditis due to medication or irradiation is also possible. Acute thyroiditis occurs very rarely in immunosuppressed patients or by hematogenous spread in sepsis.

A distinction between these inflammatory conditions is not possible on the basis of B-mode scans alone. Color Doppler imaging may provide additional information on the differential diagnosis, as extreme hypervascularity of a greatly enlarged thyroid gland (vascular inferno) is usually seen in Graves disease (**Fig. 5.8**).

Hashimoto thyroiditis (**Fig. 5.9**) and de Quervain thyroiditis are less markedly hypervascular. With de Quervain thyroiditis there is local tenderness, and the hypoechoic areas are less rounded and tend to be confluent. Differentiation between Hashimoto thyroiditis, Graves disease, and de Quervain thyroiditis is based primarily on the clinical picture and laboratory tests with the determination of antibodies. Scintigraphy in the diagnosis or differential diagnosis of thyroiditis is now considered obsolete.

Graves disease is an autoimmune thyroiditis with hyperthyroidism. Clinically, exophthalmos caused by endocrine orbitopathy may be identifiable. Laboratory tests show hyperthyroidism with an increase in free T_3 and T_4 levels with low suppressed TSH levels. TSH receptor antibodies (TSH-R Ab) may also lead to thyroid enlargement (goiter)

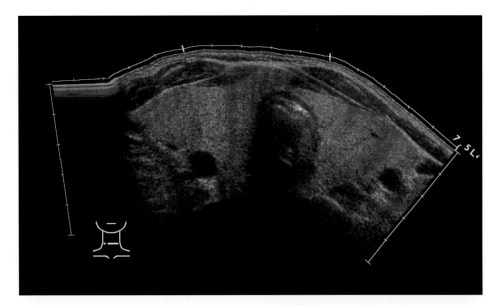

Fig. 5.4 Diffuse goiter.

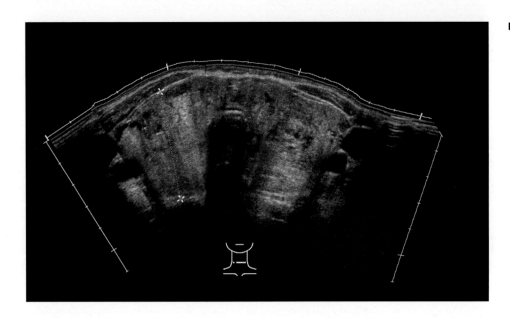

Fig. 5.5 Nodular goiter.

Table 5.3 Differential diagnosis of thyroid gland enlargement

- Goiter with or without nodules
- Thyroiditis (autoimmune, postpartum, subacute thyroiditis, de Quervain)
- Amyloidosis
- Circumscribed enlargement. Differential diagnosis: tumor

Table 5.4 Clinical work-up of goiter

- History and clinical examination
- Laboratory tests (basal TSH, CRP)
- Ultrasonography (B-mode/CDS)

through a TSH-like effect, and can be detected in 90% of patients with Graves disease. Besides the increased parenchymal hypervascularity of Graves disease (**Fig. 5.8**), color Doppler sonography also shows an increased peak flow rate in the superior and inferior thyroid arteries.

Subacute de Quervain thyroiditis is probably triggered by a viral infection of the thyroid gland and characterized clinically by the symptoms of a viral infection (fever) with localized pain and local tenderness. In addition to the standard inflammatory markers (raised erythrocyte sedimentation rates [ESR], elevated C-reactive protein [CRP]), transient hyper- or hypothyroidism is found in 50% of those affected. The ultrasound images usually show an enlarged, ill-defined thyroid gland with well-demarcated hypoechoic areas that may be confluent (**Fig. 5.10**).

The diagnosis is usually made on a clinical basis and confirmed with B-mode scans. In cases that are not absolutely clear, ultrasound-guided fine-needle aspiration may provide the evidence of giant cells and histiocytes that is needed to diagnose de Quervain thyroiditis.

The most common type of thyroiditis (and the most common cause of hypothyroidism in both adults and children) is lymphocytic Hashimoto thyroiditis. The early stage of the disease (primary transient hyperthyroidism and an enlarged hypervascular thyroid gland, which is visible on color Doppler imaging; **Figs. 5.11, 5.12**) is less often diagnosed.

Most female patients are asymptomatic for years. The chronic inflammatory process over many years causes atrophy of the gland and the diagnosis is made at the hypothyroid stage. Ultrasound scans then show a shrunken (atrophic) gland with an inhomogeneous hypoechogenicity and reduced vascularity on color Doppler sonography (**Fig. 5.13**).

The increasing use of basal TSH (bTSH) measurements leads to a more frequent diagnosis of Hashimoto thyroiditis at an earlier stage of latent hypothyroidism (bTSH elevated, T_3/T_4 within normal limits). These patients may have a normal-sized thyroid gland with multiple small (<1–1.5 cm) hypoechoic areas scattered diffusely throughout the

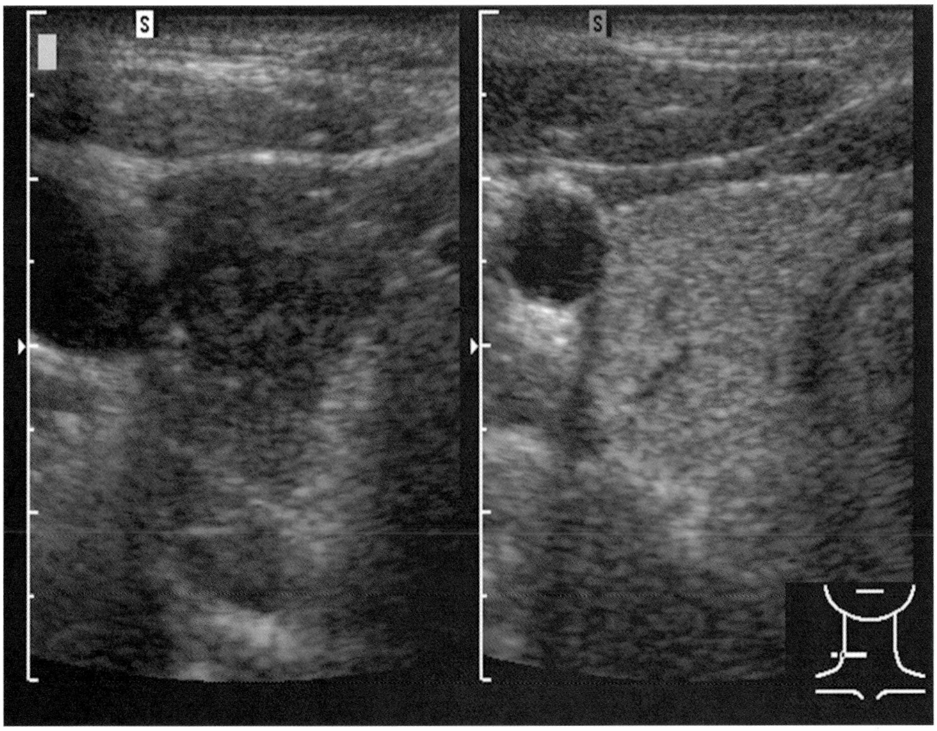

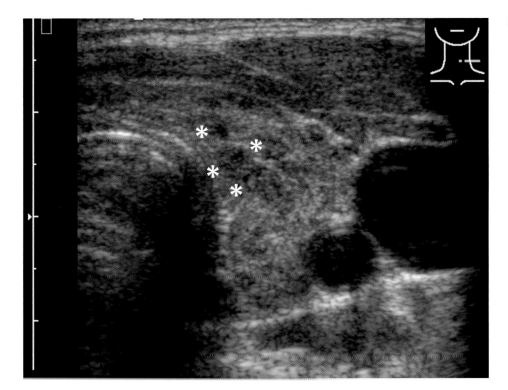

Fig. 5.6 Thyroiditis. Hypoechoic echotexture (left panel), normal echotexture (right panel).

Fig. 5.7 Thyroiditis. Inflammatory foci.

Table 5.5 Differential diagnosis of hypoechoic thyroid gland

| | Vascularization on | |
	CDS	Size enlargement
Autoimmune thyroiditis (Hashimoto thyroiditis)	+	–
Graves disease	+++	+++
Postpartum thyroiditis (history)	+	+
de Quervain thyroiditis (painful, history of infection)	–/+	++
Drug-induced thyroiditis	+	+

–, none; –/+, low; +, minor; ++, moderate; +++, intense.

two lobes. The vascularity is normal in lymphocytic Hashimoto thyroiditis. The presence of antibodies to thyroid peroxidase (TPO Ab) and the characteristic ultrasound findings are typical diagnostic criteria for Hashimoto thyroiditis. Fine-needle aspiration (lymphocytic infiltration) is seldom needed in unclear cases of thyroiditis.

Postpartum thyroiditis (incidence: 5% of all pregnancies) develops 1–3 months after delivery with transient hyperthyroidism, followed by hypothyroidism (4–10 months), and then a return to the euthyroid state. Ultrasonography shows diffuse hypoechogenicity with no (or only very slight) increase in vascularity. The condition is usually self-limiting and resolves within a year.

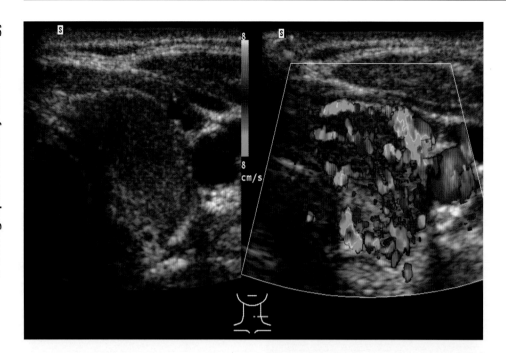

Fig. 5.8 Graves disease. Homogeneous hypo-echoic thyroid gland (left image, B-scan) with markedly increased vascularization (right image, color Doppler).

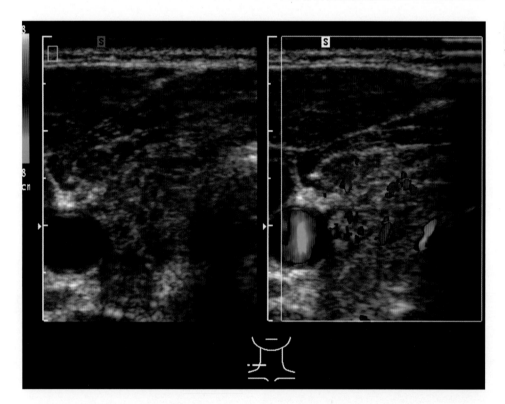

Fig. 5.9 Hashimoto thyroiditis. Hypoechoic inhomogeneous thyroid gland (left image, B-scan) with no increased vascularization (right image, color Doppler).

The Thyroid Gland after Surgery

In surgical resection of a goiter, the goiter is removed to leave a residual parenchyma measuring up to 2–4 cm × 2 cm × 2 cm (length × width × depth). Nodular parts of the gland are resected. Owing to the small size of the residual gland and the change in shape after subtotal resection, a precise volumetric calculation using the ellipsoid formula is no longer possible. According to the postoperative findings, the sagittal diameters of the right and left lobes are measured and any recurrent nodules are reported. In the case of thyroid cancer, total thyroidectomy requires the removal of the entire thyroid gland. No glandular tissue should be visible on postoperative ultrasonography except in local recurrence.

Thyroid Nodules

Cysts

Ultrasound scans detect cysts measuring 2 mm and more. As in all other organs, uncomplicated serous cysts can be seen as round or polygonal anechoic lesions with smooth, well-demarcated margins, with no wall enhancement but with distal acoustic enhancement (**Table 5.6**). Color Doppler sonography shows that cysts are avascular.

True cysts are less common in the thyroid gland than in other organs, while regressive cystic changes in thyroid nodules are very common (**Fig. 5.14**).

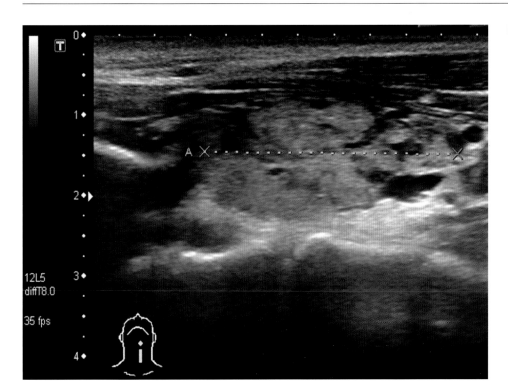

Fig. 5.10 Subacute de Quervain thyroiditis.

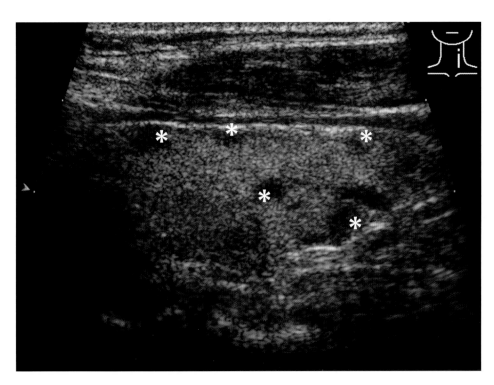

Fig. 5.11 Early-stage lymphocytic Hashimoto thyroiditis: small hypoechoic areas (asterisks).

In the differential diagnosis, secondary regressive cystic changes in a nodule can be distinguished from a true cyst (which has no wall and is avascular) by the presence of a residual solid tissue margin with vascularity seen on color Doppler imaging (**Fig. 5.15**). Most cysts do not cause any symptoms. Acute pain may be a symptom of a recent hemorrhage into a cyst. The cyst no longer appears anechoic but rather shows patchy or striped internal echogenicity due to the hematoma (**Fig. 5.16**).

When symptoms are severe, the treatment of choice is ultrasound-guided fine-needle aspiration and drainage of the cyst under local anesthesia. Thyroid scintigraphy for cysts, which would appear on scans as nonfunctional "cold" nodules, is now obsolete.

Thyroid Nodules

Thyroid nodules are very common in Germany. The prevalence increases with age (the prevalence of nodules is 50% beyond the age of

60 years) and more women are affected than men. In a gland normal on palpation, sonography of the thyroid gland can demonstrate thyroid nodules in up to 50% of patients. The vast majority of these nodules are asymptomatic and are found by chance as so-called incidentalomas. The abundance of cysts and regressive thyroid nodules contrasts with less common findings such as adenomas and very rare malignant tumors.

The assessment of a thyroid nodule must address the following two issues:

- 1. Exclusion of thyroid malignancy
- 2. Assessment of the functional properties of a thyroid nodule (hyper-, hypo-, or normal function).

In addition to the history and clinical examination, laboratory tests (bTSH, free T_3, free T_4, and calcitonin), imaging procedures (ultrasound, scintigraphy), and fine-needle aspiration cytology form part of the diagnostic work-up.

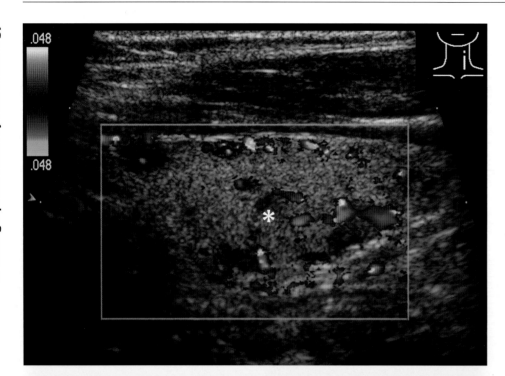

Fig. 5.12 Early-stage lymphocytic Hashimoto thyroiditis: small hypoechoic areas (asterisks) with slightly increased vascularization (color Doppler imaging).

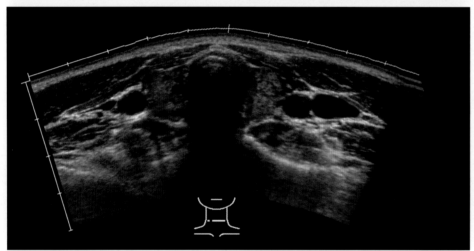

Fig. 5.13 Lymphocytic Hashimoto thyroiditis, small hypoechoic thyroid gland with inhomogeneous echotexture (hypothyroid stage).

Table 5.6 Ultrasound features of a thyroid cyst

- Anechoic
- Smooth, clearly defined margins
- Distal acoustic shadowing
- Avascular
- Compressible

The morphological appearance of thyroid nodules on B-mode scans is very variable. In comparison with the surrounding parenchymal tissue, nodules may be hypoechoic, hyperechoic, or isoechoic, with homogeneous or inhomogeneous echotexture. Many nodules are surrounded by a hypoechoic rim or halo that, unlike in other organs such as the liver, tends to be a sign of a benign lesion in the thyroid gland (**Fig. 5.17**).

In addition, calcification (either central microcalcification [**Fig. 5.18**] or coarse calcifications) or regressive cystic areas (**Fig. 5.19**) may be present.

Color Doppler sonography usually demonstrates a peripheral vascular margin (perinodular flow) in regressive nodules (**Fig. 5.20**). Demonstration of intrinsic hypervascularity suggests an autonomous adenoma, particularly when the patient is known to have clinical hyperthyroidism (**Fig. 5.21**).

However, rare thyroid cancers may also have visible central vessels and it cannot be reliably determined whether a tumor is malignant or benign on the basis of vascularity alone.

Thyroid nodules have to be described in the same way as other focal changes in parenchymatous organs with regard to size, localization (right or left lobe; upper, middle, or lower position), and echogenicity (in comparison with the surrounding thyroid tissue, as described previously); see **Table 5.7**. The dimensions of a solitary nodule or a few nodules (two to five) should be given with the maximum measurements (in millimeters) in the longitudinal and transverse planes (**Figs. 5.22, 5.23**) or by stating the volume of the nodule (length × width × depth × 0.5). With multiple nodules (more than five), details of the largest nodule should be given—echogenicity, maximum diameter, and position (at the upper or lower pole or in the middle of the lobe).

Describing the precise localization of the nodule, as well as providing information on regressive cystic areas, is particularly important should scintigraphy subsequently reveal a focus that needs to be assigned to the corresponding nodule seen on ultrasound. The best solution is to compare the scintiscan results directly with the ultrasound images (**Fig. 5.24a, b**).

Most thyroid nodules (>90%) are benign (**Table 5.8**), but benign regressive nodules have to be distinguished from benign autonomous adenomas (bTSH suppressed) and the rare malignant thyroid nodules (thyroid cancer, metastases).

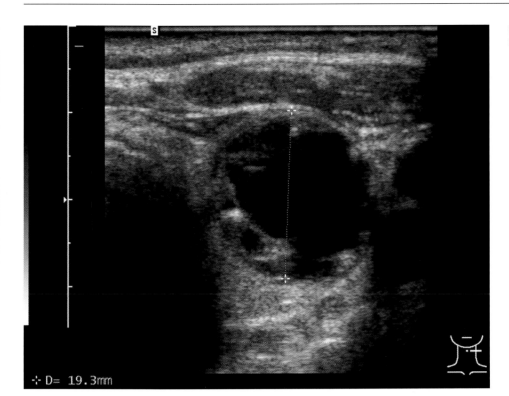

Fig. 5.14 Regressive cystic changes in thyroid nodules.

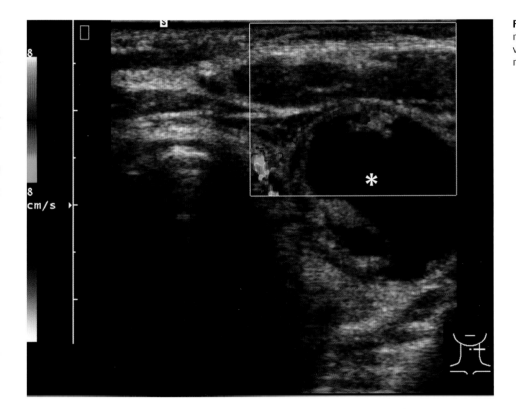

Fig. 5.15 Regressive cystic changes in thyroid nodules (color Doppler imaging): only a little vascularization in the periphery of the nodule; mostly avascular cystic nodule (asterisk).

Thyroid Adenoma

A clinical picture of hyperthyroidism (lowered bTSH and/or raised T_3/T_4) is often the starting point. Thyroid adenomas are epithelial neoplasms, in contrast to the reactive adenomatous nodules in goiter. Thyroid adenomas have a homogeneous, usually slightly hypoechogenic pattern (**Fig. 5.25**). As well as perinodular vascularity, color Doppler images show central vascularity in the case of active endocrine adenomas (**Fig. 5.24**), while regressive thyroid nodules usually display only perinodular flow. Scintigraphy serves to confirm an autonomous adenoma, although nodules of diameter <1 cm cannot always be identified owing to the poor resolution, even in suppression scintigraphy.

Thyroid Cancer

Determining whether a thyroid nodule is malignant or benign is problematic because the prevalence of nodules is very high, being between 10% and 50% depending on age, and cancer is rare. According to data from the German cancer register, the prevalence of thyroid cancer is low, at 0.1%–1%. The annual incidence is 2–5 cases per 100 000. Statistically, therefore, just one cancer occurs in 10 000–30 000 nodules.

The most frequently occurring types of such rare malignancies are differentiated papillary and follicular thyroid cancers. They grow very slowly and, like medullary cancers, have a favorable to very good prognosis with a 5-year survival rate of 70%–90%. Anaplastic cancers with

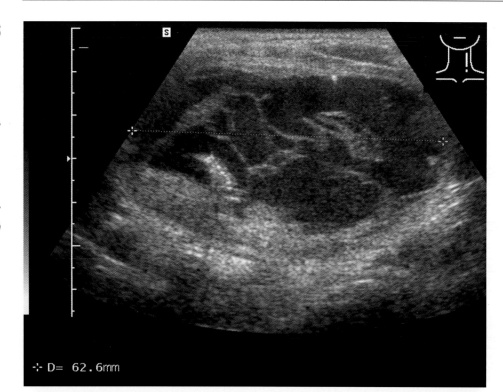

Fig. 5.16 Hemorrhage into a cyst.

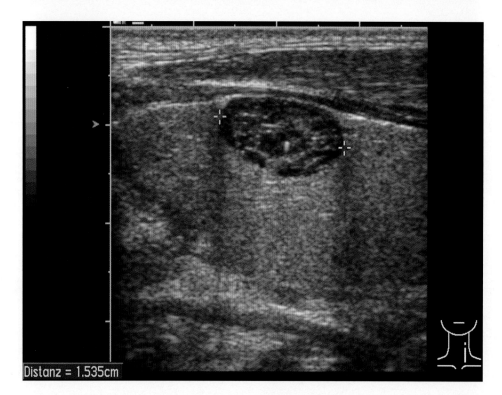

Fig. 5.17 Thyroid nodule. Hypoechoic rim or halo suggestive of a benign lesion.

an extremely poor prognosis are very rare, grow rapidly, and are usually seen in elderly patients. Metastases in the thyroid gland are also rare. Papillary thyroid cancer is often an incidental finding on histology when examining a resected goiter. Papillary thyroid cancer develops more frequently after irradiation (e.g., the incidents at Chernobyl and Fukoshima) and tends to metastasize early to the cervical lymph nodes. Follicular thyroid cancer usually causes very few symptoms and is often not diagnosed until metastases are found (in the bones, lungs, or brain). Medullary thyroid cancer (C-cell cancer) occurs sporadically in 80% of cases and in a familial type, the so-called multiple endocrine neoplasia (MEN2). Chronic diarrhea is a cardinal symptom. Laboratory tests show elevated calcitonin and carcinoembryonic antigen (CEA) levels.

Table 5.9 lists potential clinical signs associated with thyroid cancer.

Thyroid cancers appear hypoechoic on ultrasonography, but have to be distinguished from benign hypoechoic thyroid nodules, which are very much more common.

Local infiltration and frank invasion of adjacent structures (**Fig. 5.26**), with or without pathologically enlarged regional lymph nodes (**Fig. 5.27**), are definite signs of malignancy. Current American Association of Clinical Endocrinologists (AACE) guidelines include a risk assessment based on sonographic criteria (**Table 5.10**).

Should the lesion give rise to any suspicion of malignancy, its nature must be clarified by fine-needle aspiration cytology, irrespective of the size of the nodule. If a nodule is unremarkable on sonography (**Table 5.10**), repeat scanning is performed 6–12 months later to monitor progression. If it remains the same size, follow-up (ultrasound plus bTSH) is required at 1- to 2-yearly intervals.

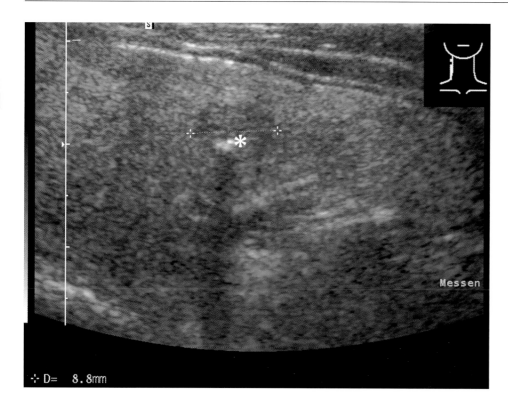

Fig. 5.18 Hypoechoic thyroid nodule with central microcalcification (asterisk).

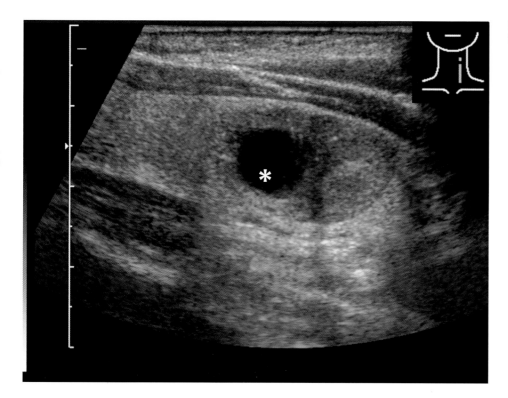

Fig. 5.19 Thyroid nodule: anechoic lesion, indicating regressive cystic area.

Diagnostic Value of Scintigraphy in Thyroid Nodules

Scintigraphy no longer has a key role in the current guidelines for the diagnostic work-up of thyroid malignancies (only ~1% of all hypofunctional nodules found on scintigraphy are malignant; nodules measuring <1 cm are not detected by this method). Nevertheless, scintigraphy is important for the detection of so-called "hot" nodules (showing increased autonomous metabolic activity in the multinodular thyroid gland; autonomous adenoma). Scintigraphy should be performed in the case of reduced bTSH with solid thyroid nodules >1 cm, and also with multinodular goiter in areas of iodine deficiency to determine autonomous activity.

Figure 5.28 shows an algorithm for diagnostic work-up of a solid thyroid nodule found on ultrasound in a euthyroid patient (normal TSH).

Fine-needle Aspiration Biopsy

The quality of the results of a fine-needle biopsy depends greatly on the experience of the person who performs the biopsy and of the pathologist. Malignancy in fine-needle aspiration cytology (FNAC) aspirate was found in the literature with a sensitivity of 83% and a specificity of 92%, with 5% false (combined) results. Sources of inconclusive results include an insufficient aspirate and the presence of autoimmune thyroiditis. Aspiration should be performed under ultrasound guidance, which

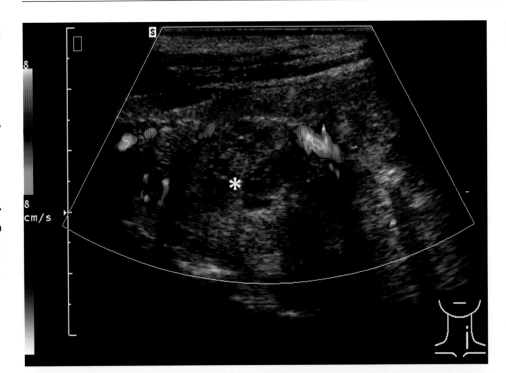

Fig. 5.20 Regressive nodules (color Doppler imaging).

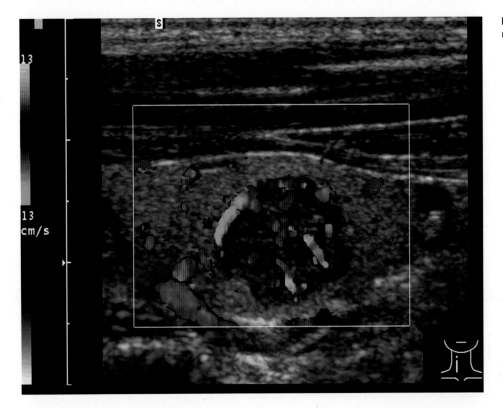

Fig. 5.21 Hypervascularity suggestive of an autonomous adenoma (color Doppler imaging).

Table 5.7 Documentation of thyroid nodules

- Localization (site in right/left lobe of the thyroid; upper pole; lower pole; middle)
- Echogenic texture (anechoic; hypoechoic; isoechoic; hyperechoic)
- Size/volume
- Uniformity (homogeneous; inhomogeneous)
- Margins (clearly defined/distinct; ill-defined)
- Hypoechoic halo (present; not present)
- Vascularity (perinodular flow or also intrinsic vascularity; extent)
- Microcalcification (yes/no)
- Compressibility (elastography may be helpful here)
- Regional lymph nodes

reduces the rate of inconclusive cytology. Surgery (thyroidectomy) is indicated if the FNAC shows malignant cells. Findings are inconclusive if only necrotic or altered cells are visible, and further elucidation is necessary (re-biopsy or definitive surgical resection). Follicular neoplasia is an intermediate finding on cytology. With this cytological finding, no distinction can be made between follicular adenoma and follicular cancer; a core biopsy can overcome this problem. As only ~20% of these follicular neoplasms undergo malignant change, surgery is not always the first-line treatment. The American Thyroid Association (ATA) guidelines recommend scintigraphy if the cytology shows follicular neoplasia. If the scintiscan reveals a "cold" nodule, surgery is indicated on the grounds that there is a considerably increased risk of malignancy. On the other hand, if scintigraphy shows a functionally active or indifferent nodule associated with the follicular neoplasia, a watch-and-wait policy can be followed with repeat ultrasound scanning after 3–6 months.

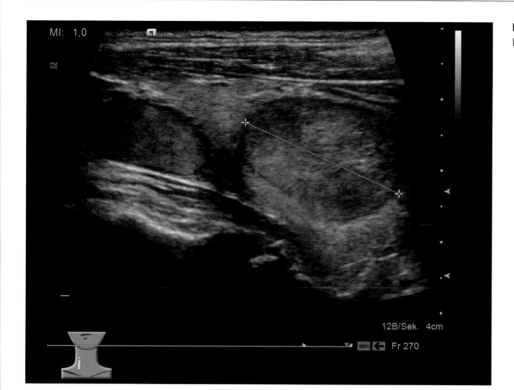

Fig. 5.22 Measurement of nodules (longitudinal plane): maximum longitudinal dimension.

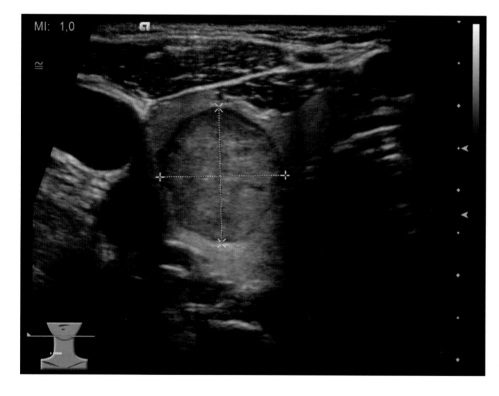

Fig. 5.23 Measurement of nodules (transverse plane): maximum width and depth dimensions.

Table 5.11 lists the limitations of ultrasonography in the diagnosis of thyroid cancer.

Upcoming New Ultrasound Methods (Elastography, Contrast-enhanced Ultrasound) in Thyroid Nodules

Elastography

Hard thyroid nodules are associated with an increased risk of malignancy. New methods such as ultrasound elastography can determine tissue elasticity directly in real time during the ultrasound examination. Calculation of the elasticity coefficient between nodular and normal thyroid tissue allows the differentiation of benign and malignant lesions. A meta-analysis of eight studies with a total of 639 histologically confirmed thyroid nodules showed that malignant nodules were diagnosed with a sensitivity of 92% and a specificity of 90% (95% confidence interval 85–95%), although the specificity in the eight studies concerned showed wide variation. Limitations of elastography include the determination of follicular cancers (false-negative findings) and the evaluation of regressive, fibrosed, and calcified benign nodules (false-positive findings). Cysts, nodules with calcified capsules, and nodules in a multinodular goiter are not suitable for elastography. Large-scale prospective studies are needed to clarify the value of elastography.

Contrast-enhanced Ultrasound

Echo signal enhancers (ultrasound contrast media) are clearly superior to the conventional color or power Doppler techniques in demonstrating microvascularity. Evidence of microperfusion is not clinically relevant in the differentiation of malignant and benign thyroid nodules. However, the use of contrast medium is extremely helpful for assessing the therapeutic success of ablative procedures (percutaneous ethanol injection therapy, thermal ablation), as the extent of necrosis and any possibly vital residual tissue can be determined precisely.

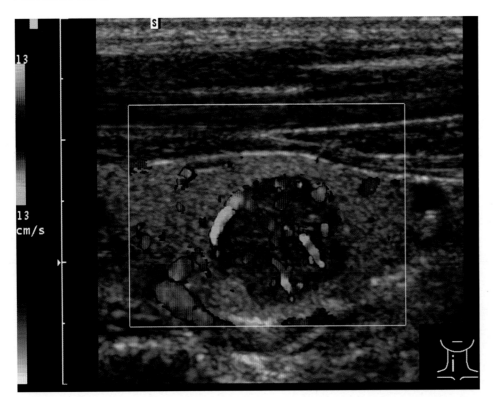

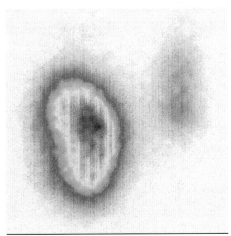

Fig. 5.24 Thyroid adenoma.
a Ultrasound image: 1.5 cm round hypoechoic hypervascular lesion (color Doppler).
b Scintiscan image: in correlation to the ultrasound image, autonomous adenoma of the thyroid gland (right lobe).

Table 5.8 Sonographic criteria of benign nodules

• Multiple nodules, tending to be round or oval in shape
• Homogeneous echotexture
• Clear, well-demarcated margins
• Completely hypoechoic/anechoic rim (halo) around the nodule
• Hyperechoic, isoechoic, or anechoic echotexture
• Perinodular vascularity on color Doppler imaging
• No regional lymph nodes
• Coarse calcifications

Elastography and contrast-enhanced ultrasonography are not routinely used in the diagnostic work-up of the thyroid gland at present.

Summary: Thyroid Gland

Ultrasonography is the primary imaging tool in patients with suspicion of a diseased thyroid gland. It offers the highest resolution of all imaging procedures in real time. As an inexpensive, noninvasive, and widely available procedure, thyroid ultrasonography belongs in the basic diagnostic work-up whenever there is a clinical suspicion of thyroid disease. Taken together with the history, clinical examination, and bTSH as the screening marker for thyroid dysfunction, ultrasound imaging provides valuable diagnostic information. In the clinical situation of hyperthyroidism, additional scintigraphy supplies evidence of autonomous areas.

All thyroid nodules must be stratified for risk on the basis of the clinical picture and the ultrasonographic findings (B-scans, color Doppler imaging). If these findings are suspicious, FNAC should be performed irrespective of the size of the nodule. Surgery is indicated if malignant or suspicious cells are found in the aspirate. Whenever there is a high cancer risk clinically, but the findings according to sonographic criteria

are benign or FNAC has failed to show malignant cells, follow-up with repeat ultrasound scanning after 6–12 months is recommended.

Parathyroid Glands

Normal-sized parathyroid glands cannot be displayed on ultrasonography, even using high-resolution transducers. The four parathyroid glands lie directly at the upper and lower poles of the lobes of the thyroid. In rare cases, there may be more than four parathyroid glands or they may be found at ectopic sites. In the case of primary or secondary hyperparathyroidism, the region is explored in the longitudinal and transverse planes, looking closely at the upper and lower poles of the thyroid for hypoechoic space-occupying lesions lying outside the thyroid gland. It is essential that the polar regions of the thyroid can be seen clearly and that they are well demarcated (beware of a retrosternal goiter!). Parathyroid glands measuring 5 mm or more can be seen on ultrasound images. Parathyroid adenomas usually appear as hypoechoic, homogeneous, smooth, clearly demarcated oval structures lying in the immediate vicinity of the thyroid gland. It is important to discern the thyroid capsule in both planes, so as not to mistake a finding within the thyroid gland for a parathyroid gland finding. If the thyroid capsule is not clearly visible on the ultrasound images, it is impossible to differentiate a parathyroid from a hypoechoic nodule within the thyroid gland itself. Signs of malignancy with respect to a parathyroid cancer are an inhomogeneous echotexture, irregular ill-defined margins, and invasive growth. Every hypoechoic focal lesion at the poles of the thyroid has to be suspected of being an enlarged parathyroid gland.

If there is a clinical picture with hypercalcemia in primary hyperparathyroidism or long-standing hypocalcemia in secondary hyperparathyroidism (with chronic renal insufficiency), enlargement of the parathyroid can be demonstrated with the characteristic ultrasound appearance (**Fig. 5.29**). Ultrasonography is also more suitable than CT or MRI in preoperative diagnostic localization of the parathyroid glands and is surpassed only by surgical exploration.

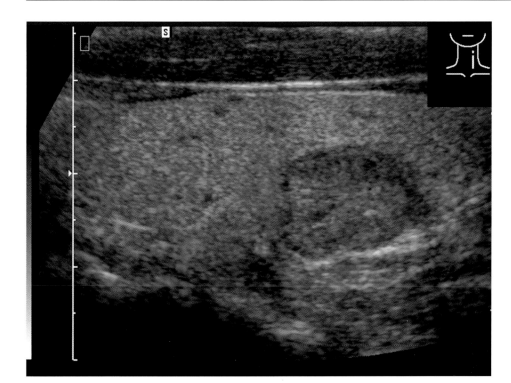

Fig. 5.25 Thyroid adenoma: well-demarcated 1.4 cm nodule with a homogeneous hypoechoic echotexture.

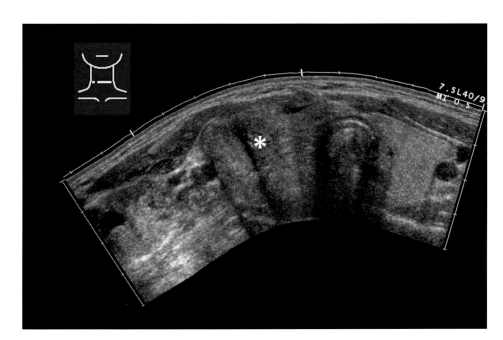

Fig. 5.26 Thyroid cancer: Local infiltration or frank invasion of adjacent structures.

Table 5.9 Potential clinical signs associated with thyroid cancer

History	Family history of thyroid cancer
	Local irradiation of the neck
	General exposure to ionizing radiation
	Aged < 14 or > 70 years
Clinical findings	Hard, immobile nodules on palpation
	Rapid increase in size
	Vocal cord paralysis
	Dyspnea/dysphagia
Laboratory tests	Elevated calcitonin and CEA levels (medullary thyroid cancer)

CEA, carcinoembryonic antigen.

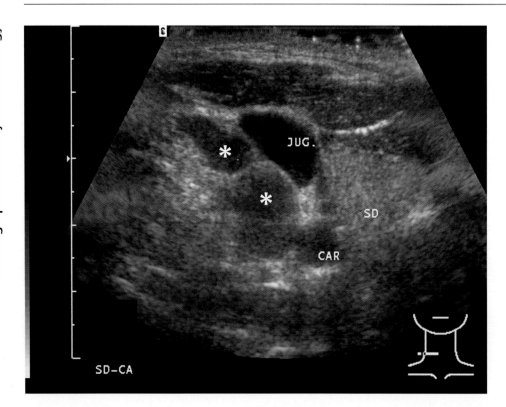

Fig. 5.27 Local infiltration or frank invasion of adjacent structures with pathologically enlarged regional lymph nodes.

Table 5.10 Potential ultrasound signs associated with thyroid cancer

- Solitary nodules
- Ill-defined margins
- Incomplete or absent halo
- Inhomogeneous, anechoic echotexture
- Microcalcification
- Intrinsic vascularity in the case of "cold" nodules seen on scintigraphy
- Local infiltration/frank invasion of adjacent structures
- Pathologically enlarged regional lymph nodes

Table 5.11 Limitations of ultrasonography in the diagnosis of thyroid cancer

- Benign thyroid nodules are common (prevalence up to 50%)
- Thyroid cancers are rare
- Criteria for malignancy may not be met
- False-negative fine-needle aspirates (10–20%)
- 25% of thyroid cancers are <1 cm in size and are incidental findings after partial thyroidectomy

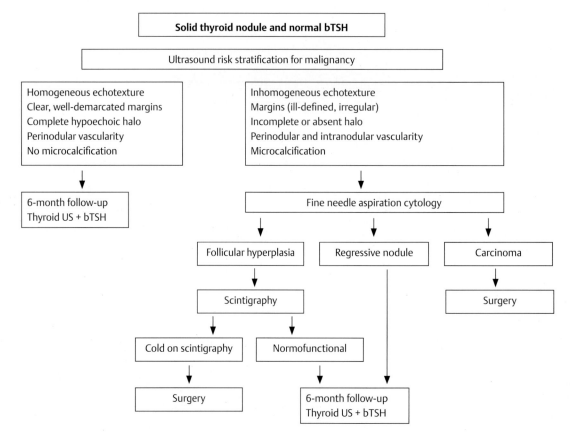

Fig. 5.28 Diagnostic algorithm.

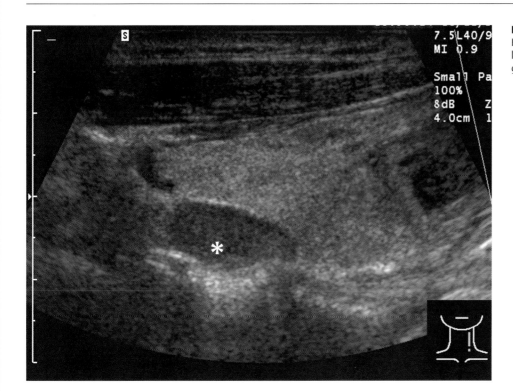

Fig. 5.29 Adenoma of the parathyroid gland. Hypoechoic well-demarcated 1.3 cm lesion located dorsal to the upper pole of the thyroid gland.

Bibliography

Bojunga J, Herrmann E, Meyer G, Weber S, Zeuzem S, Friedrich-Rust M. Real-time elastography for the differentiation of benign and malignant thyroid nodules: a meta-analysis. Thyroid 2010;20(10):1145–1150

Cooper DS, Doherty GM, Haugen BR, et al; American Thyroid Association (ATA) Guidelines Taskforce on Thyroid Nodules and Differentiated Thyroid Cancer. Revised American Thyroid Association management guidelines for patients with thyroid nodules and differentiated thyroid cancer. Thyroid 2009;19(11):1167–1214 Erratum in: Thyroid 2010;20(6):674–675 and Thyroid 2010;20(8):942

Delange F, Benker G, Caron P, et al. Thyroid volume and urinary iodine in European schoolchildren: standardization of values for assessment of iodine deficiency. Eur J Endocrinol 1997;136(2):180–187

Gharib H, Papini E, Valcavi R, et al; AACE/AME Task Force on Thyroid Nodules. American Association of Clinical Endocrinologists and Associazione Medici Endocrinologi medical guidelines for clinical practice for the diagnosis and management of thyroid nodules. Endocr Pract 2006;12(1):63–102 Erratum in: Endocr Pract 2008 Sep;14(6):802–803

Papini E, Guglielmi R, Bianchini A, et al. Risk of malignancy in nonpalpable thyroid nodules: predictive value of ultrasound and color-Doppler features. J Clin Endocrinol Metab 2002;87(5):1941–1946

Paschke R, Reiners C, Führer D, Schmid KW, Dralle H, Brabant G. Recommendations and unanswered questions in the diagnosis and treatment of thyroid nodules. Opinion of the Thyroid Section of the German Society for Endocrinology. [Article in German]. Dtsch Med Wochenschr 2005;130(31–32):1831–1836

Rago T, Scutari M, Santini F, et al. Real-time elastosonography: useful tool for refining the presurgical diagnosis in thyroid nodules with indeterminate or nondiagnostic cytology. J Clin Endocrinol Metab 2010;95(12):5274–5280

Reiners C, Wegscheider K, Schicha H, et al. Prevalence of thyroid disorders in the working population of Germany: ultrasonography screening in 96,278 unselected employees. Thyroid 2004;14(11):926–932

Schilddrüsenstudie Papillon 2003 and 2006. Available at: http://www.schilddruese.de/content/download/download-studie.pdf

6   Neck Lymph Nodes

Anatomy

The use of ultrasound has been validated in examination of the superficial structures of the head and neck as considerably more sensitive than clinical assessment through palpation in the identification and interpretation of the 200–300 lymph nodes of the neck and soft tissues changes in this region. Given the optimal exposure of the cervical soft tissues and the high spatial resolution, diagnostic ultrasonography is the first choice of method, as lymph nodes exceeding 3 mm are easy to identify. The patient is usually examined with the neck hyperextended (see Chapters 3 and 4).

Figure 6.1 shows the histological appearance of a typical cervical lymph node. The sonographic appearance of cervical lymph nodes on high-resolution ultrasound reflects their structure and has some distinctive characteristics.

Lymph nodes in the neck are oval or ellipsoid in shape. Within the node, there is generally a hypoechoic marginal zone, which can be distinguished from the central hyperechoic hilar region (the medullary sinuses with blood vessels and efferent lymph vessels).

Classification of the Cervical Lymph Nodes

Size and Three-dimensional Proportions

Although the size of a lymph node in the neck may be used as a classification criterion, this is not without problems. Owing to the typical physiological configuration of cervical lymph nodes (oval/ellipsoid), the node should always be measured in all three orthogonal planes: the diameter is measured in one long axis and two short axes (**Figs. 6.2a,b**).

> **Pearls and Pitfalls**
>
> There is a danger of confusing lymph nodes in level II, which are commonly found at the posterior border of the submandibular gland, with the posterior belly of the digastric muscle sliced obliquely or in cross-section. The pinnate structure of the muscle can mimic a lymph node hilus. Rotating the probe by 90° "over the finding" allows an identification to be quickly made.

Most work assessing lymph nodes on the basis of their size refers to the short-axis diameter. The existing limits of short-axis size, above which a lymph node is suspected of being malignant, vary with the level of the node (levels IB and II: ~8 mm; levels IA, III, IV, V: ~5 mm). As routine practice shows, these limits cannot be used unreservedly. Small nodes with malignant changes often have measurements below the cut-off value and, conversely, enlarged reactive lymph nodes (e.g., in infectious mononucleosis) can be considerably larger.

The overall clinical constellation is decisive for the assessment.

There is currently no imaging technique that allows the certain classification of micrometastases or small metastases with a maximum diameter of less than 3 mm.

Echogenic Hilum ("Hilar Sign") and Perfusion Pattern

A pinecone-shaped echogenic structure protruding from the center of the node can be seen in grayscale images (**Figs. 6.3, 6.4, 6.5**). It is sometimes referred to as the "hilar sign" or "hilus sign" and is a normal part of the lymph node morphology. Absence of this hyperechoic central structure in the hilar region may be considered a criterion for malignancy.

Malignant transformation causes changes in or loss of the lymph node structure, with reduction or erosion of the central hilar complex.

The "hilar sign" is confirmed by the use of color-coded duplex sonography (CCDS), which shows color-coded hilar perfusion in the echogenic central area. Blood vessels leading to and from the node can be seen in the hilum, corresponding to the histological structure (**Fig. 6.6**; ▶ Video 6.1).

The perfusion pattern can be used to determine the angioarchitecture of the node, so that any pathological changes can be identified. Tschammler and co-workers described distinct patterns for enlarged lymph nodes in CCDS, indicating malignant or nonmalignant origin. Enlarged reactive lymph nodes show a vascular pattern originating in the hilum and branching radially or like the spokes of a wheel (**Figs. 6.5, 6.7, 6.8**; ▶ Video 6.2).

Changes from the normal structure that may be considered suspicious of malignancy include decentralized vascularity, peripheral perfusion or an avascular focus (**Fig. 6.9**). In the characteristic appearance of a metastasis, the vessels are distributed peripherally around the capsule of the node (subcapsular; **Fig. 6.10**; ▶ Video 6.3).

Lymph Node Shape

The rationale for including lymph node shape as a criterion of malignancy is that an oval/kidney-shaped lymph node increases in volume during an inflammatory process. The oval or spindle shape is maintained when changes are reactive (**Figs. 6.3, 6.11, 6.12, 6.13**), but malignant transformation causes the node to become more rounded.

The Solbiati Index (cutoff value 1.5 or 2.0), which represents the lymph node morphology in terms of the ratio of the long- to short-axis ratio (L/S ratio), is frequently used. A node with an index <2.0 is suspected of being malignant.

> **Pearls and Pitfalls**
>
> Lymph nodes in levels IA and IB, the nuchal and the parotid regions, normally have a rounded shape. Beware of suspecting malignancy too quickly when assessing nodes in these areas.

Lymph Node Borders

Cervical lymph nodes are usually well demarcated from surrounding tissues and freely mobile on sonographic palpation. In addition to demonstrating the layers of impedance, the zoom function of the ultrasound system allows a precise determination of the node's movement during arterial pulsation from the surroundings (**Figs. 6.14, 6.15**; ▶ Videos 6.4, 6.5). If a cervical lymph node is not clearly defined, it should first be considered whether the scanning conditions might be unfavorable.

If there are signs of extensive infiltration, the differentiation between strong inflammatory changes and neoplastic enlargement can usually be made on the basis of the clinical situation.

During inflammatory processes, poor demarcation of the lymph node on ultrasound indicates a process extending beyond the capsule, such as an abscess or a phlegmon.

With malignant transformation (metastasis, lymphoma), ill-defined margins or club-shaped thickenings are considered indicative of neoplastic enlargement/infiltration of the lymph node capsule and therefore, with high sensitivity and specificity, as clear criteria of malignancy (**Figs. 6.16, 6.17**). Mobility of the nodes within their sheaths is reduced or absent.

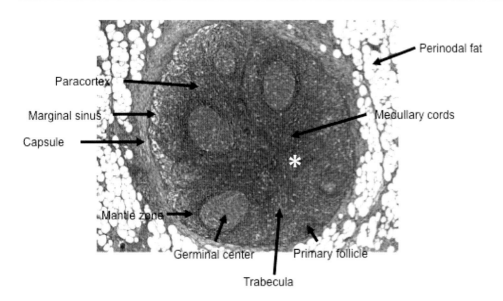

Fig. 6.1 Histology of a typical cervical lymph node. The trabeculae extending centrally from the periphery represent the lymph node hilum and contain, among other things, the blood vessels (asterisk). (Reproduced with kind permission of A. Agaimy MD, Institute of Pathology, Erlangen University Hospital, Germany.)

Perinodal fat
Paracortex
Marginal sinus
Medullary cords
Capsule
Mantle zone
Germinal center
Primary follicle
Trabecula

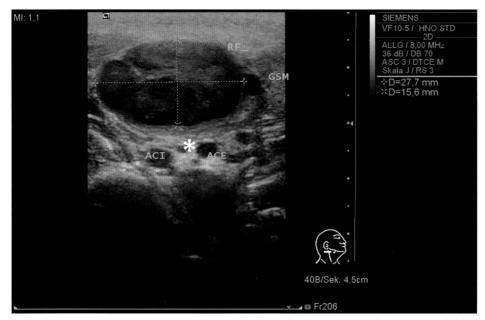

Fig. 6.2a Right side of the neck, transverse, level II. An oval lymph node in **acute lymphadenitis colli** (RF); the node has a delicate internal echo pattern with well-defined margins and measures 30 mm × 15 mm in both short-axis diameters. A clearly visible incidental finding is the nerve bundle of the vagus nerve seen in cross-section between the internal (ACI) and external (ACE) carotid arteries (asterisk). GSM, submandibular gland.

Homogeneity of the Intranodal Echotexture

According to classical teaching, the lymph node cortex (hypoechoic) and hilum (echogenic) show a homogeneous structure on ultrasound (**Fig. 6.18**). The presence of a markedly inhomogeneous echotexture is a relevant criterion of malignancy (**Figs. 6.19, 6.20, 6.21**).

Pearls and Pitfalls

It is becoming problematic that the latest ultrasound scanners with higher resolution and improved displays hardly ever show completely homogeneous lymph nodes; rather they nearly always demonstrate some inhomogeneous—but not actually malignant— textural elements.

If the lymph node structure is altered as the result of a malignant transformation, the distinction between cortex and hilum is lost (**Fig. 6.22**). The echotexture is inhomogeneous with anechoic areas indicating necrosis and reduced perfusion of the center of the tumor (**Figs. 6.23, 6.24**).

On the other hand, a central anechoic area in a reactive cervical lymph node is typical of abscess formation. Liquefaction with a central anechoic area is seen particularly in mycobacteria infections and actinomycosis (see below). In contrast, echogenic reflections or calcification are characteristically seen in tuberculosis and in the case of metastases of papillary carcinoma of the thyroid.

Lymph Node Distribution

Level in the Neck

If there is an inflammatory process, the lymph nodes in the drainage channels of the affected organs show reactive changes. Hugely enlarged cervical lymph nodes in the lower neck are relatively less often affected by inflammation and are therefore detectable more often in the presence of malignancy. The overall clinical situation must also be taken into account to be able to make an appropriate assessment (**Fig. 6.25**).

Noting the distribution of lymphadenopathy helps in narrowing down the differential diagnosis (**Figs. 6.26, 6.27**). Lymph node metastases from solid tumors are usually found initially in groups sited in the relevant lymphatic drainage channels. Particularly in cervical cases, the manifestation of many types of malignant lymphoma tends to appear in a conglomerate pattern.

Pearls and Pitfalls

The ultrasound criteria for assessing whether or not a cervical lymph node is malignant are:

1. Size and three-dimensional proportions
2. Detectability of a lymph node hilus, perfusion pattern
3. Lymph node shape
4. Border of the lymph node
5. Homogeneity of the intranodal structure
6. Distribution of the lymph nodes

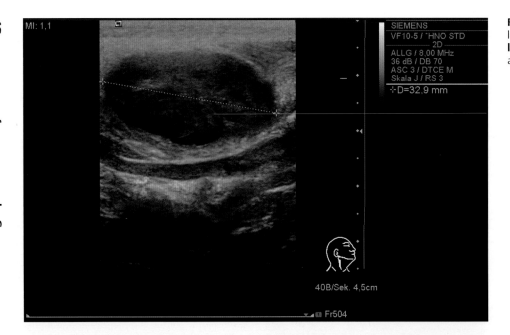

Fig. 6.2b Right side of the neck, longitudinal, level II. The oval lymph node seen in **acute lymphadenitis** colli measures 32 mm on its long axis.

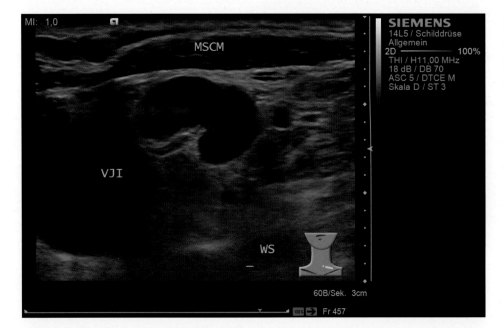

Fig. 6.3 Left side of the neck, transverse, level V. This lymph node shows a characteristic pattern of inflammation (kidney shape, hilar sign, homogeneous texture). MSCM, sternocleidomastoid muscle, VJI, internal jugular vein, WS, vertebral spine.

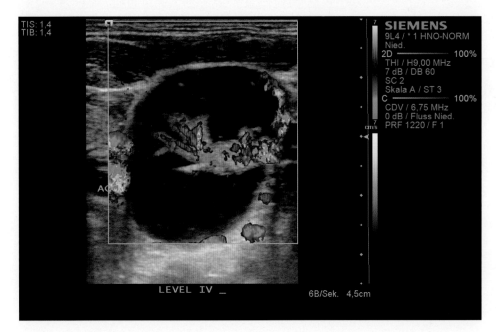

Fig. 6.4 Left side of the neck, transverse, CCDS. A round, clearly defined lymph node lateral to the common carotid artery (ACC), with a classical "hilar sign" and hilar perfusion seen on CCDS. The afferent and efferent hilar vessels can also be identified at the right border of the node. In this case, the massive enlargement of the node with maintenance of the normal vascular and hilar structures was due to **non-Hodgkin lymphoma**. A cystic mass in the lower neck area may also be found with metastases of papillary thyroid carcinomas.

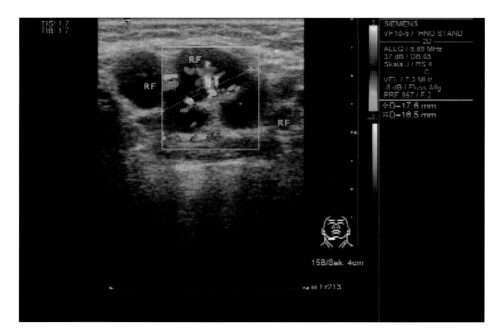

Fig. 6.5 Submandibular, right, transverse, CCDS. An oval lymph node with the classical configuration of an **inflammatory lymph node**: clear "hilar sign," strong hilar perfusion visible with subvessels branching in the periphery.

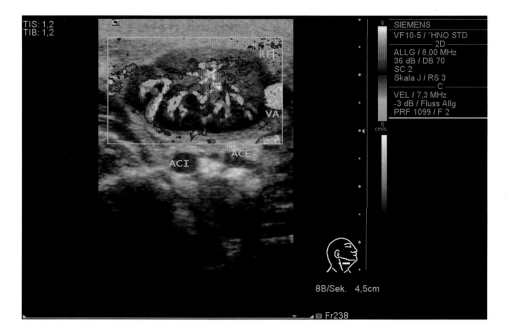

Fig. 6.6 Transverse view of the right side of the neck at level II in a 6-year-old child, CCDS. An oval lymph node in **acute lymphadenitis** colli (RF). The node measures approximately 25 mm (to visually estimate the size the scale at the right-hand side of the image above the pictogram can be used). The central vascular structures can be seen branching out from the left upper side of the echogenic "hilar sign." The perfusion is particularly intensive because the acuteness of the infective process and is consistent with the stage of disease. The facial artery (VA) appears at the right side of the image, the internal carotid artery (ACI) and external carotid artery (ACE) are to be found in level II below the lymph node.

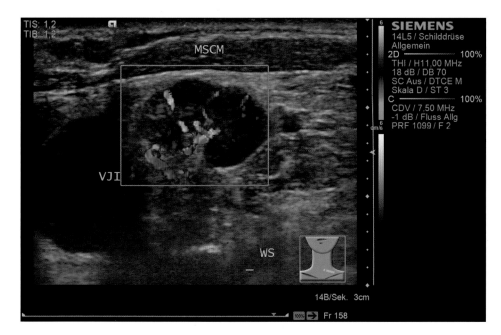

Fig. 6.7 Left side of the neck, transverse, level V, CCDS. A lymph node (see also **Fig. 6.3**) with strong hilar sign and hilar perfusion pattern. VJI, internal jugular; WS, vertebral spine; MSCM, sternocleidomastoid muscle. Diagnosis: **Sarcoidosis**.

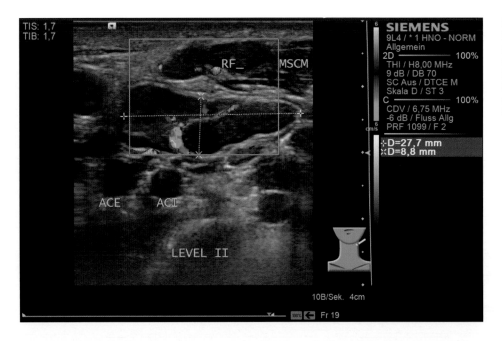

Fig. 6.8 Left side of the neck, transverse, level II, CCDS. Two lymph nodes (RF and caliper marked) can be seen in level II: they are oval and well demarcated. A strong "hilar sign," clearly defined margins and hilar perfusion, together with an L/S ratio > 2.0, indicate a **reactive enlargement**. ACI, internal carotid artery; ACE, external carotid artery; MSCM, sternocleidomastoid muscle.

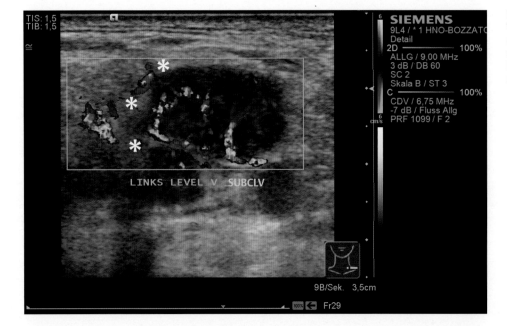

Fig. 6.9 Left side of the neck, transverse, level V, CCDS. A round lymph node with ill-defined contours (asterisks) shows irregular vessel parts and pathways, totally unlike the normal central hilar perfusion pattern. Diagnosis: **Lymph node metastasis**.

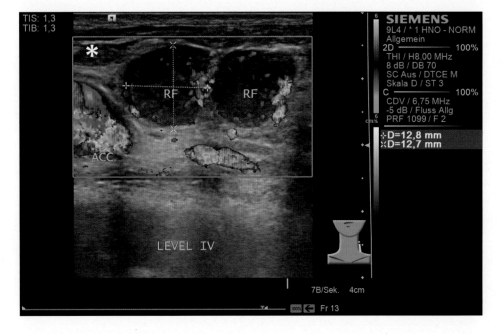

Fig. 6.10 Left side of the neck, longitudinal, level IV, CCDS. Two round metastases without a "hilar sign" (RF) and with **subcapsular perfusion**. Besides the inhomogeneous internal echoes, there is also a more hypoechoic central area. Cranially, the belly of the omohyoid muscle (asterisk) can be seen in cross-section, and the carotid bulb is visible at the left edge of the image, clearly placing the nodes in level IV.

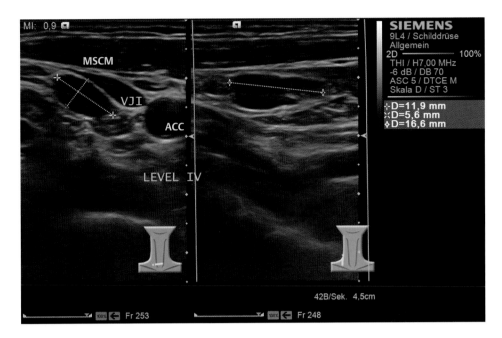

Fig. 6.11 Right side of the neck, level IV, split screen. Lying laterally to the internal jugular vein (VJI) is an enlarged oval, reactive lymph node; it has an L/S ratio of 2.0, is well demarcated, and shows the "hilar sign." On the left of the image, another smaller lymph node with the same configuration can be seen medial to the vein. ACC, common carotid artery; MSCM, sternocleidomastoid muscle. Diagnosis: **Acute lymphadenitis**.

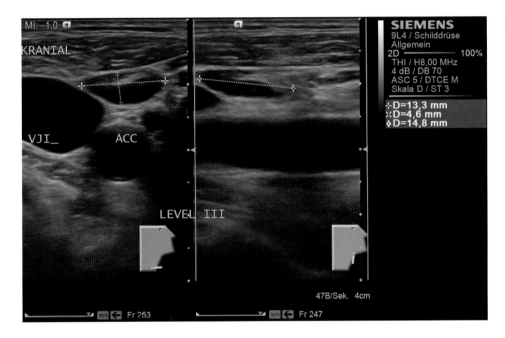

Fig. 6.12 Split screen, right side of the neck, level III. Lying between the internal jugular vein (VJI) and the common carotid artery (ACC) is an enlarged oval **reactive lymph node**; it has an L/S ratio of 2.0, is well demarcated, and shows the "hilar sign."

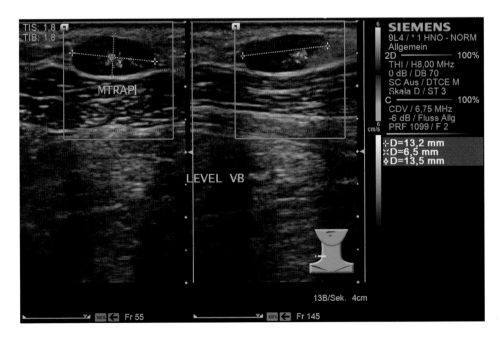

Fig. 6.13 Split screen, left side of the neck, level V, CCDS. An enlarged oval reactive lymph node; it has an L/S ratio of 2.0, is well demarcated, and shows both the "hilar sign" and hilar perfusion. MTRAP, trapezius muscle. Diagnosis: **Toxoplasmosis**.

II Sonographic Anatomy and Pathology

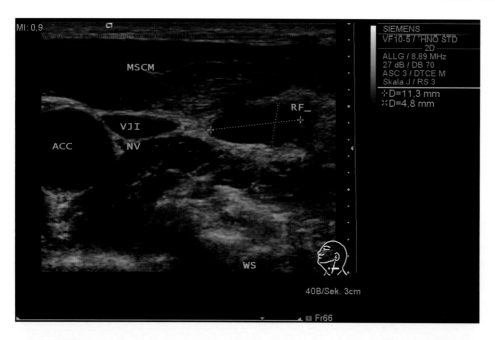

Fig. 6.14 Left side of the neck, transverse, level IV. A lymph node in level IV which, at first glance, appears oval and well demarcated. A polycyclic extension can be seen at the lateral end. This could be considered significant in a patient in whom malignancy is suspected, but the patient concerned had an **acute respiratory tract infection**. ACC, common carotid artery; MSCM, stemocleidomastod muscle; NV, vagus nerve; RF, lymph node; VJI, internal jugular vein; WS, vertebral spine.

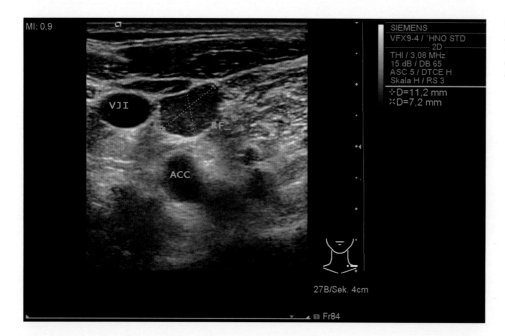

Fig. 6.15 Left side of the neck, transverse, level IV. A **lymph node metastasis** (RF) with an irregular rounded shape and clearly defined margins. The echogenicity is homogeneous. ACC, common carotid artery; VJI, internal jugular vein.

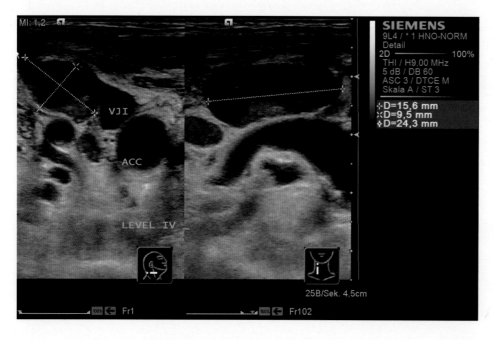

Fig. 6.16 Split screen, right side of the neck, level IV. The lymph node is polycyclic in cross-section and lies directly on the internal jugular vein (VJI). To the right of the image is an oval, well-demarcated lymph node seen in longitudinal section, with a second, more rounded, lymph node lying cranially. No hilum can be distinguished in either the longitudinal or transverse section. ACC, common carotid artery. Diagnosis: **Lymph node metastasis**.

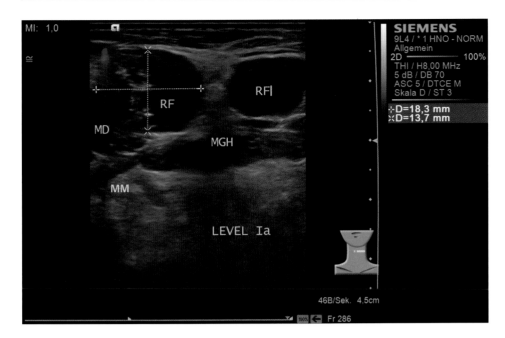

Fig. 6.17 Floor of the mouth, transverse, level IA. Two round, space-occupying lesions (RF) with malignancy of the floor of the mouth. Besides the criterion of malignancy met in the ill-defined borders with the right digastric muscle (MD), both lymph nodes are round or polycyclic in shape. A further suspicious feature is the obvious inhomogeneity of the lymph node at the left edge of the image. MGH, geniohyoid muscle; MM, mylohyoid muscle. Diagnosis: **Lymph node metastasis.**

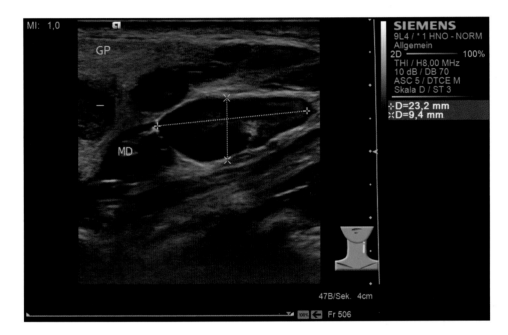

Fig. 6.18 Left side of the neck, longitudinal. An oval, well-demarcated lymph node in level II, bordering the bed of the parotid gland (GP). The echogenic structure corresponds to a "hilar sign." Cranial to the oval, lymph node is what appears to be a further rounded space-occupying lesion with central echogenic septa. This, however, is the digastric muscle (MD) seen in cross-section, which may be confused morphologically with a lymph node. More cranially, three lymph nodes can be identified in the apex of the echogenic lower pole of the parotid. Lymph nodes at the inferior border of the parotid gland that are simultaneously neighbouring the latero-posterior aspect of the submandibular gland are also called "**Küttner's lymph nodes.**" Diagnosis: **Acute lymphadenitis of the neck and the parotid gland in viral infection.**

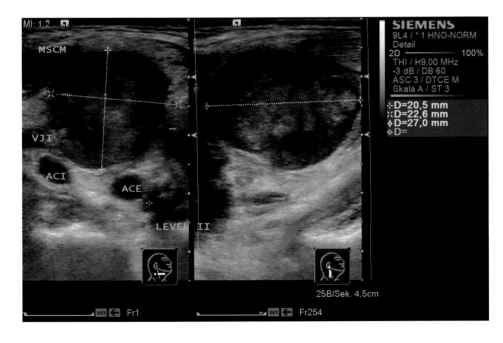

Fig. 6.19 Right side of the neck, level II/III. The space-occupying lesion with an inhomogeneous echo pattern lies on the external carotid artery (ACE) and internal carotid artery (ACI), medial to the internal jugular vein (VJI). Morphologically, a branchial cyst may appear similar, but would not show any intrinsic perfusion. MSCM, sternocleidomastoid muscle. Diagnosis: **Lymph node metastasis.**

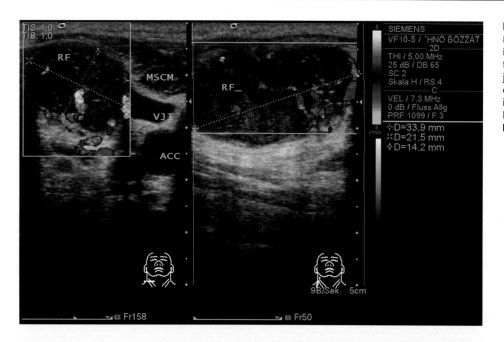

Fig. 6.20 Split screen, right side of the neck, level IV, CCDS. The space-occupying lesion (RF) with an inhomogeneous echo pattern is sited laterally to the common carotid artery (ACC) and the internal jugular vein (VJI). The perfusion is peripheral and decentralized; in addition, irregular echogenic internal echoes are consistent with metastasis. MSCM, sternocleidomastoid muscle. Diagnosis: **Lymph node metastasis**.

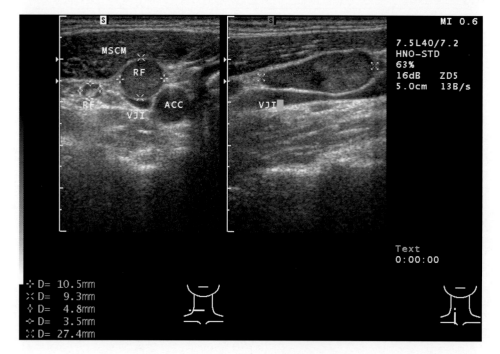

Fig. 6.21 Split screen, right side of the neck, level III. A lymph node (RF) in a patient being followed up for malignant disease; the caudal margins show marked extension. Compared with the normal architecture, there is marked inhomogeneity. ACC, common carotid artery; VJI, internal jugular vein; MSCM, sternocleidomastoid muscle. Diagnosis: **Lymph node metastasis recurrence**, 6 months after initial multimodal treatment.

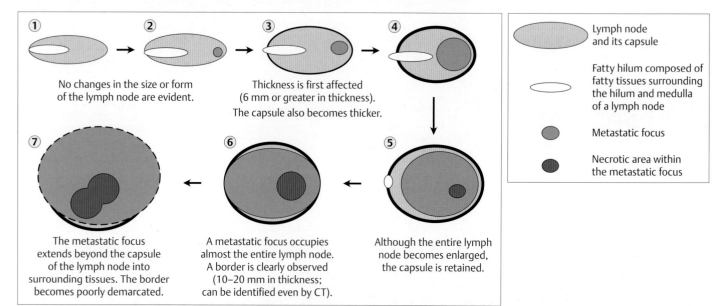

① No changes in the size or form of the lymph node are evident.

② Thickness is first affected (6 mm or greater in thickness). The capsule also becomes thicker.

⑦ The metastatic focus extends beyond the capsule of the lymph node into surrounding tissues. The border becomes poorly demarcated.

⑥ A metastatic focus occupies almost the entire lymph node. A border is clearly observed (10–20 mm in thickness; can be identified even by CT).

⑤ Although the entire lymph node becomes enlarged, the capsule is retained.

Lymph node and its capsule

Fatty hilum composed of fatty tissues surrounding the hilum and medulla of a lymph node

Metastatic focus

Necrotic area within the metastatic focus

Fig. 6.22 A schematic representation of **morphological changes in metastases**. These morphological transformations within a lymph node illustrate sonographic findings of malignancy.

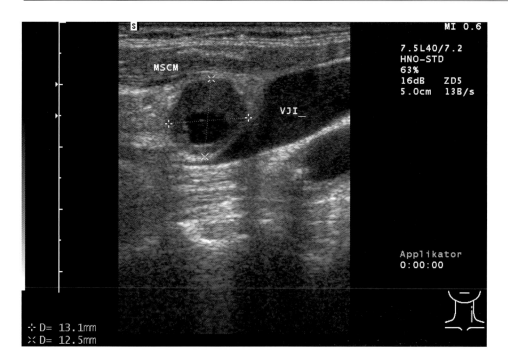

Fig. 6.23 Left side of the neck, longitudinal, level III. A round **lymph node metastasis** with irregular borders has an anechoic center, which is indicative of necrosis caused by the metastatic transformation. VJI, internal jugular vein; MSCM, sternocleidomastoid muscle.

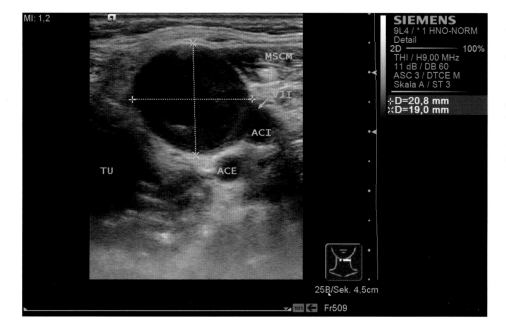

Fig. 6.24 Left side of the neck, level II. Medial to the internal and external carotid arteries, the round metastasis has an anechoic center consistent with **central necrosis**; this is considered to be a sign of malignancy. To the left, medial in the image, is an ill-defined hypoechoic primary tumor (TU) of the left side of the oropharynx. The internal jugular vein (VJI) is compromised and can be seen between the anterior border of the sternocleidomastoid muscle (MSCM) and the internal carotid artery (ACI). The vein can be demonstrated better with a Valsalva maneuver. ACE, external carotid artery.

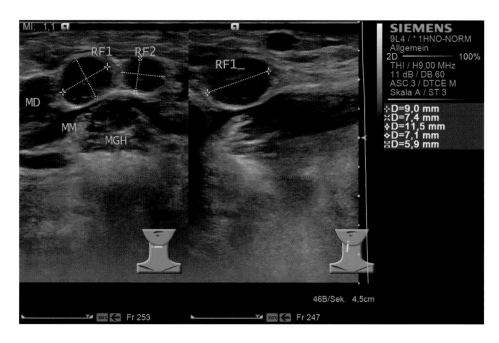

Fig. 6.25 Split screen, right side of the floor of the mouth. The two round paramedian lymph nodes with inhomogeneous internal echoes lie on the right in level IA. If there were an acute dental infection, these two lymph nodes (RF1 and RF2), both showing a weak "hilar sign" and clearly defined margins, would be consistent with reactive enlargement; however, both lymph nodes can definitely be considered possible metastases when there is clinical suspicion of cancer of the floor of the mouth, tongue, or sinonasal area. MD, digastric muscle; MGH, geniohyoid muscle; MM, mylohyoid muscle. Histological diagnosis: **Lymph node metastasis**.

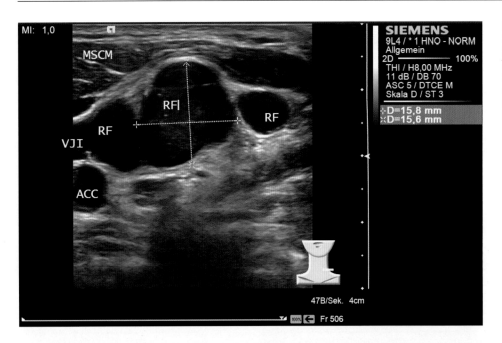

Fig. 6.26 Left side of the neck, transverse, level V. Multiple round supraclavicular and infraclavicular lymph nodes (RF) with a hypoechoic echotexture. The lymph nodes have ill-defined margins in part and no visible echogenic hilar structures. ACC, common carotid artery; MSCM, stermocleidomastoid muscle; VJI, internal jugular vein. Diagnosis: **Metastases of small cell bronchial carcinoma.**

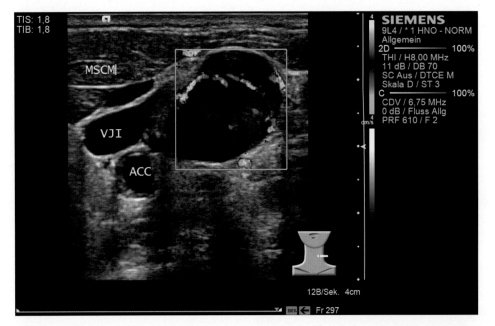

Fig. 6.27 Left side of the neck, transverse, level V, CCDS. The multiple round lymph nodes show strong irregular decentralized perfusion, with no obvious hilum visible even on CCDS. Metastases from a small-cell bronchial carcinoma were confirmed on subsequent lymph node biopsy (see also **Fig. 6.26**). Lymph nodes in the left supraclavicular fossa are also referred to as "**Virchow's nodes**". As they are supplied from abdominal lymph vessels, they may also indicate abdominal cancer. ACC, common carotid artery; MSCM, stermocleidomastoid muscle; VJI, internal jugular vein. Diagnosis: **Metastases of small cell bronchial carcinoma.**

Inflammatory Changes

Acute and Chronic Lymphadenitis

Changes in the perfusion and/or lymph drainage corresponding to the activity as part of the normal immune system can be demonstrated clearly with ultrasound.

A reactive inflammatory stimulus leads to an enlargement of the draining lymph nodes and hyperperfusion can be seen on CCDS.

If the inflammatory process abates, the size of the node and the degree of hyperperfusion regress. Not infrequently, however, the lymph nodes remain in a state of chronic lymphadenitis (see **Figs. 6.2a, 6.2b, 6.3, 6.5, 6.6, 6.8, 6.11, 6.12, 6.14, 6.18**).

Pearls and Pitfalls

Smoking on a regular basis irritates the epithelium of the aerodigestive tract and may cause a marked increase in the number of enlarged lymph nodes, with the clinical picture of chronic lymphadenitis. Another frequent cause of lymph node enlargement is a pathological condition of the dental apparatus.

Epstein–Barr Virus/Mononucleosis

The clinically enlarged lymph nodes of mononucleosis seen in children and young adults may form conglomerates. These—sometimes very large—lymph nodes illustrate, among other things, the fact that lymphatic tissue in children, adolescents, and young adults is much more reactive to immunological stimuli than that of adults (**Fig. 6.28**).

The cervical masses usually have a soft consistency and are tender to palpation. Depending on the site of the underlying organ infection, the (usually multiple) lymph nodes are localized on one or both sides of the neck (**Figs. 6.29, 6.30, 6.31**). Distribution and size may also mimic the clinical picture of lymphoma in adolescents.

Abscess Formation in Lymph Nodes

With progression of the inflammatory process, bacterial infections may give rise to liquefaction, seen on ultrasound imaging as anechoic areas with irregular borders. Distal acoustic enhancement is characteristic, as is the visible movement of fluid secretions on applying pressure with the probe (**Fig. 6.32**).

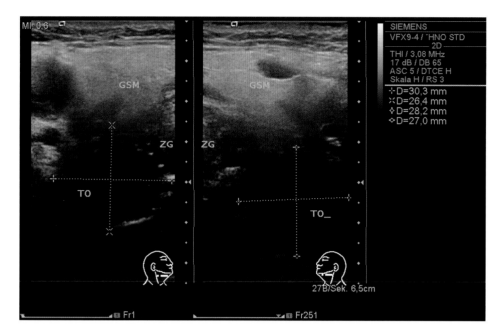

Fig. 6.28 Split screen, submandibular areas on both sides. Both tonsils (TO) are considerably enlarged in a 21-year-old patient with acute **mononucleosis**. GSM, submandibular gland; ZG, base of the tongue.

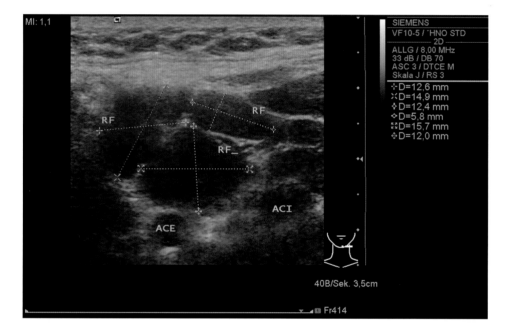

Fig. 6.29 Left side of the neck, transverse, same patient as in **Fig. 6.28**. Acute **mononucleosis** and typical lymph node enlargement. The multiple lymph nodes (RF) in this case form a conglomerate lying superficially to the bifurcation in level II (ACI/ACE).

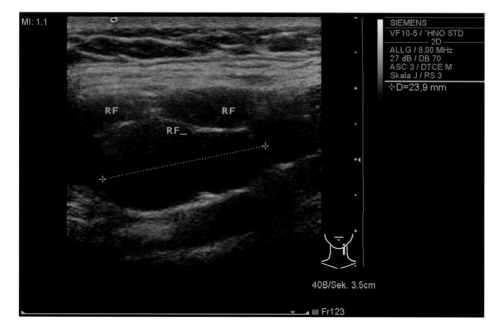

Fig. 6.30 Left side of the neck, longitudinal. Same patient as in **Fig. 6.28** and **6.29**, with **mononucleosis**. In the longitudinal view, the individual nodes are separated from each other by thin connective-tissue septa that are ill defined in parts. The loss of clear demarcation is due to periadenitis. In this clinical setting, the loss of demcarcation can be falsely interpreted as a sign of malignancy. RF, lymph nodes.

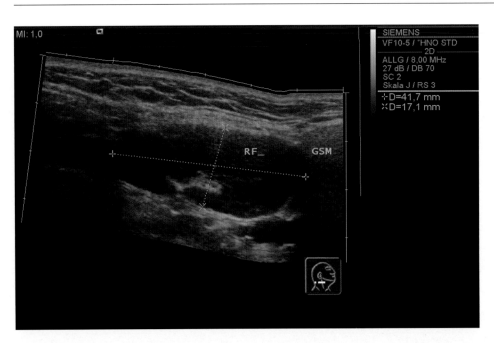

Fig. 6.31 Panoramic view, right side of the neck, longitudinal, level II, same patient as in **Figs. 6.28–6.30**. On the contralateral side, a lymph node in level II reaches maximum dimensions of 42 mm × 17 mm. Cranially the node extends to the submandibular gland (GSM).

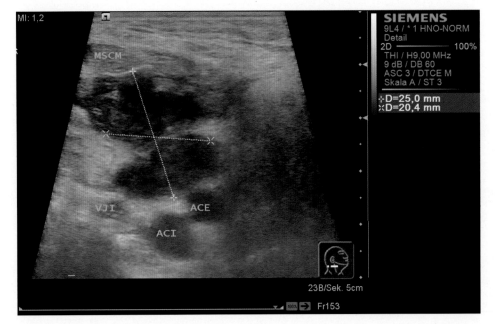

Fig. 6.32 Right side of the neck, transverse. Abscess formation in a level II lymph node. Lying anterior to the internal (ACI) and external (ACE) carotid arteries and beneath the sternocleidomastoid muscle (MSCM) are two polycyclic space-occupying lesions with inhomogeneous, hypoechoic echo patterns. A central anechoic area can be identified, although it is not well demarcated from the surrounding tissues. Distal acoustic enhancement is only weakly demonstrated on the compound imaging setting with high gain. VJI, internal jugular vein.

CCDS reveals no vascularity of the abscess cavity, although there is hyperperfusion of the adjacent tissues (**Fig. 6.33**; ▶ Videos 6.6, 6.7). Tissue affected by periadenitis is hypoechoic and the associated reaction may cause thickening or loosening of its structure.

Cervical Abscess

The main causes of cervical abscesses are lymphadenitis with abscess formation (see also Chapter 8, p. 98); tonsillar or dental infections; peritonsillar abscesses; mastoiditis; mucosal lesions of the mouth or pharynx; and foreign bodies. Ultrasound images of cervical abscesses are, of course, similar to images of an abscess in a lymph node, with progressive extension along the fascial plane of the neck (**Figs. 6.34, 6.35, 6.36**; ▶ Video 6.8).

Mycobacteria other than Tuberculosis (MOTT)

Infection with nontuberculous mycobacteria (NTM)—scrofula—is common in children under the age of 6 years. Cervical lymphadenitis

(submandibular, preauricular, and submental) leads to intranodal abscess formation and fistulas draining to the skin. The affected lymph nodes often have a lobulated shape with central or decentralized anechoic areas (**Figs. 6.37, 6.38, 6.39**). The fistulas extend as hypoechoic channels from the skin into the suppurating lymph nodes. Affected nodes may also be found in the submandibular bed and within the parotid gland (**Figs. 6.40, 6.41**).

Tuberculosis

The multiple enlarged lymph nodes seen as cervical manifestations of tuberculosis (TB) are firm on palpation with an inhomogeneous internal structure with irregular anechoic areas consistent with cystic lesions on ultrasound (**Fig. 6.42**). The anechoic zones correspond to areas of caseating necrosis. Because of the strong echogenicity, intranodal calcification can be observed with distal acoustic shadowing (**Fig. 6.43**). The irregular lymph node contours are a result of periadenitis.

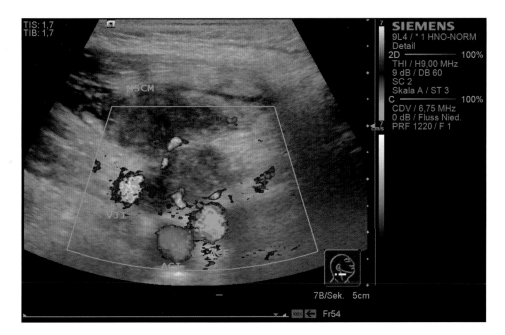

Fig. 6.33 Right side of the neck, transverse, same patient as in **Fig. 6.32**. **Abscess** formation in a level II lymph node. It lies anterior to the internal and external carotid arteries as well as to the internal jugular vein (VJI), and beneath the sternocleidomastoid muscle (MSCM). No hilar perfusion is detectable, but an irregular peripheral vascularity can be seen on CCDS.

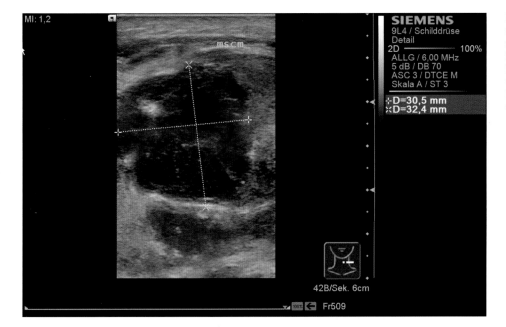

Fig. 6.34 Left side of the neck, transverse. An **abscess** beneath the anterior border of the sternocleidomastoid muscle (MSCM) shows an inhomogeneous hypoechoic internal structure indicating the different liquid and viscous components of the purulent secretions. The polycyclic border of the abscess is not clearly demarcated lateral to the muscle belly.

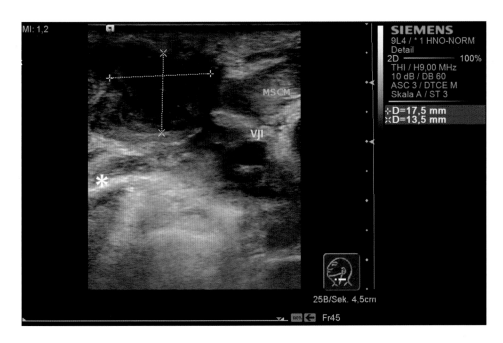

Fig. 6.35 Left side of the neck, transverse. The cervical **abscess** seen here is sited superficially between the thyroid cartilage (echogenic oblique band in the lower left of the image, asterisk) and the sternocleidomastoid muscle (MSCM). Lateral to this, the tissue is hypoechoic and ill defined with a loosened structure lying more deeply. The inflammatory process extends beneath the anterior border of the MSCM into the deeper soft tissues of the neck. VJI, internal jugular vein.

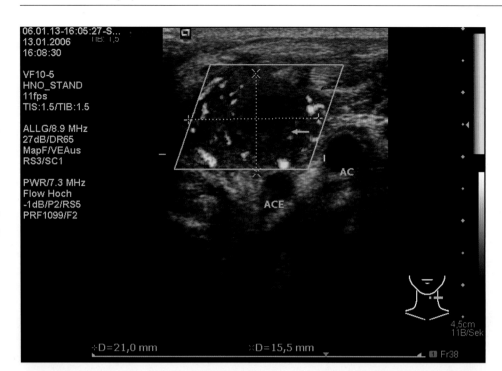

Fig. 6.36 Right side of the neck, transverse, CCDS. A circumscribed cervical **abscess** from a suppurating lymph node. The area of the abscess lateral to the branches of the carotid artery (ACE, ACI) is ill defined and hypoechoic, showing an anechoic area in the center. CCDS shows that the inflamed tissues are hyperperfused, but no color coding can be seen in the liquefied central zone.

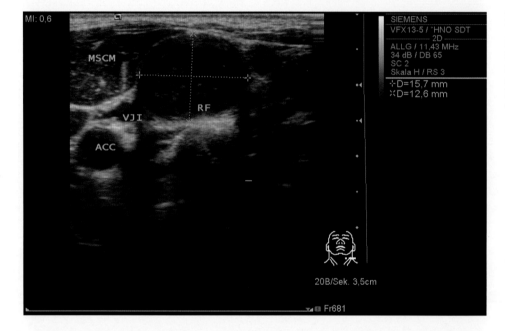

Fig. 6.37 Left side of the neck, transverse, level V. This round, inhomogeneous, painful hypoechoic lymph node (RF) in an 8-year-old child lies lateral to the vascular sheath (ACC; VJI) and the sternocleidomastoid muscle (MSCM). The "hilar sign" is absent. ACC, common carotid artery; VJI, internal jugular vein. Diagnosis: **Mycobacteriosis other than tuberculosis (MOTT)**.

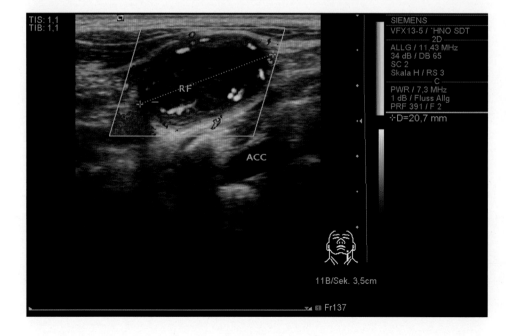

Fig. 6.38 Left side of the neck, longitudinal, level V, CCDS. The well-demarcated oval node (RF) shows peripheral vascularity and becomes increasingly hypoechoic toward the center. ACC, common carotid artery. Diagnosis: **Mycobacteriosis other than tuberculosis (MOTT)**.

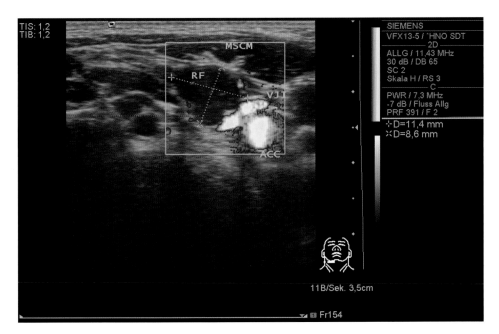

Fig. 6.39 Right side of the neck, transverse, level II. Small polycyclic lymph nodes (RF) can be seen on the contralateral side. These nodes do not have any visible "hilar sign"; the perfusion is decentralized and more pronounced at the periphery. ACC, common carotid artery; MSCM, sternocleidomastoid muscle; VJI, internal jugular vein. Diagnosis: **Mycobacteriosis other than tuberculosis (MOTT)**.

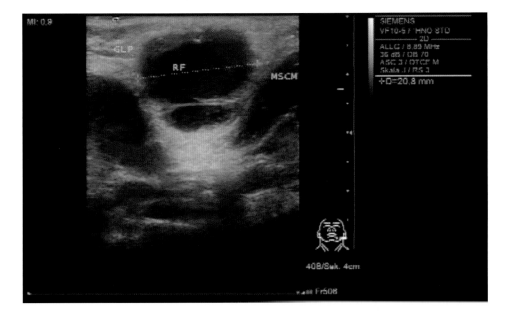

Fig. 6.40 Left side of the neck, transverse, level II. Manifestation of NTM infection at the transition to the parotid bed (GLP) in level II. The hypoechoic polycyclic lymph nodes (RF) are forming a conglomerate. MSCM, sternocleidomastoid muscle. Diagnosis: **Mycobacteriosis other than tuberculosis (MOTT)**.

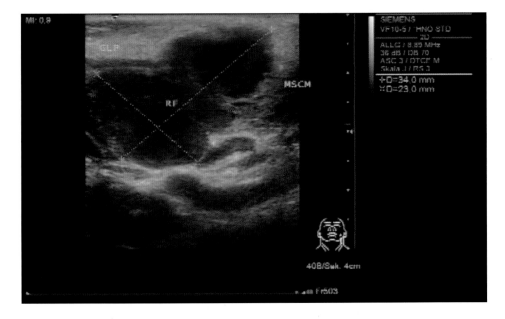

Fig. 6.41 Left side of the neck, longitudinal, level II. Manifestation of NTM infection at the transition to the parotid bed (GLP) in level II. The hypoechoic polycyclic lymph nodes (RF) also extend into the parotid gland (GLP). MSCM, sternocleidomastoid muscle. Diagnosis: **Mycobacteriosis other than tuberculosis (MOTT)**.

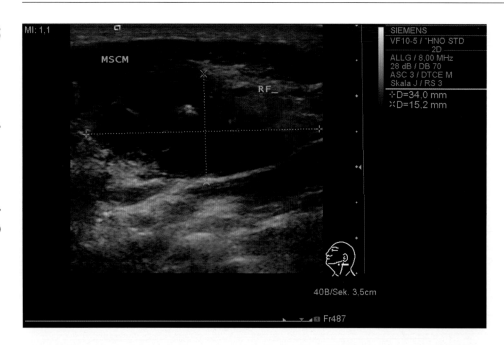

Fig. 6.42 Left side of the neck, transverse, level II. Lymph node enlargement in TB. A spindle-shaped lymph node (RF) with an inhomogeneous, partly anechoic echotexture shows a central echogenic reflection that should not be confused with a "hilar sign." MSCM, sternocleidomastoid muscle. Diagnosis: **Tuberculosis**.

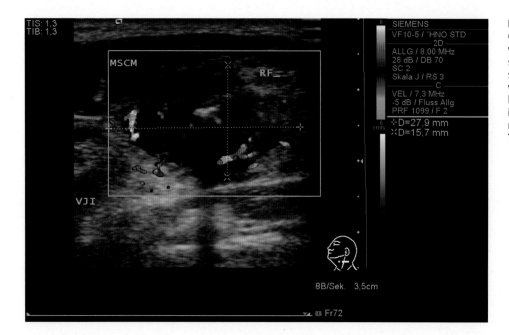

Fig. 6.43 Left side of the neck, transverse, level II, CCDS. On the CCDS setting, the central reflection within the lymph node (RF) shows distal acoustic shadowing, similar to the appearance seen with salivary stones. There is peripheral perfusion without any central hilar vascularity, as the central lymph node architecture has been altered by the infective process. MSCM, sternocleidomastoid muscle; VJI, internal jugular vein. Diagnosis: **Tuberculosis**.

Actinomycosis

Actinomycosis is caused by infection with the Gram-positive anaerobic bacterium *Actinomyces israelii*, which affects the face and neck in many (>50%) cases. It shows a boardlike infiltration of the subcutaneous tissues with indurated nodes, fistulas, and ulceration. Ultrasound imaging shows precisely how far the abscesses and fistulas extend into the tissues (**Figs. 6.44, 6.45**). Circumscribed abscesses can be aspirated and drained under ultrasound guidance.

Differential Diagnosis in Lymphadenopathy

There are numerous additional infective or inflammatory conditions responsible for neck lymph node enlargement. It is, however, not possible to assign characteristic sonomorphological characteristics to these heterogeneous entities (**Table 6.1**). Depending on the clinical presentation, further laboratory testing or bio-optical confirmation may be required.

Table 6.1 Differential diagnosis of lymphadenopathy of the neck

Non-infectious causes	Sarcoidosis (**Figs. 6.3, 6.7**)
	Kikuchi–Fujimoto disease (histiocytic necrotizing lymphadenitis)
	Rosai–Dorfman syndrome (sinus hitiocytosis)
	Castleman's disease (angiofollicular lymph node hyperplasia)
Infectious causes	Viral agents such as Epstein–Barr virus infection (**Fig. 6.28–6.31**), cytomegalovirus, Rubella, human immunodeficiency virus
	Fungal infection
	Toxoplasmosis (**Fig 6.13**)
	Tuberculosis (**Fig. 6.42, 6.43**), MOTT (**Fig. 6.37–6.41**), Bartonellosis, cat scratch disease, Yersiniosis, Listeriosis, Lues, Tularemia, Brucellosis, Actinomycosis (**Fig. 6.44, 6.45**)

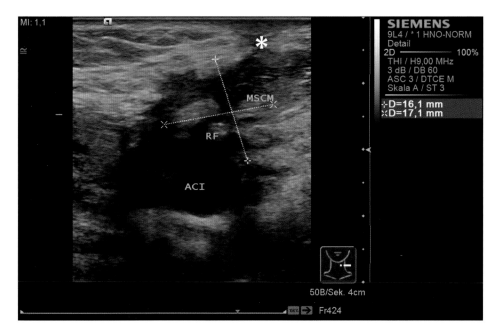

Fig. 6.44 Left side of the neck, transverse, level II. In a case of **actinomycosis**, the infected lymph nodes liquefy and form abscesses, leading to periadenitis with an ill-defined hypoechoic reaction in the surrounding tissue. The lymph node next to the carotid artery can no longer be distinguished clearly. The inflammatory process has already extended to the subcutaneous tissue; quite often a fistula is formed to the outside (asterisk). ACI, internal carotid artery; MSCM, sternocleidomastoid muscle.

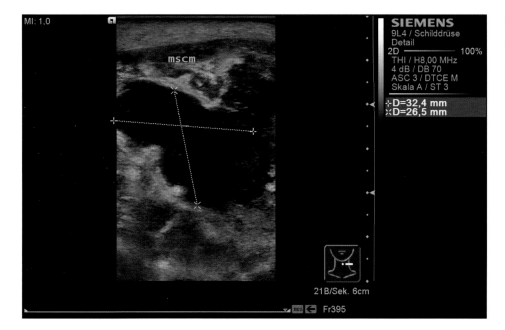

Fig. 6.45 Left side of the neck, transverse. The inflammatory process is anechoic with a polycyclic configuration, but no connection to the skin. In some cases, the picture is one of a cervical **abscess**, seen here beneath the anterior border of the sternocleidomastoid muscle (MSCM).

Benign Tumors

Although several conditions affecting the neck soft tissues are mentioned elsewhere (Chapter 10, p. 152, and Chapter 12, p. 173) two entities should be described here because of their positions and frequent occurrence in the soft tissues of the neck.

Lipomas

Lipomas are usually superficial, spindle shaped, well demarcated, and hypoechoic, showing a characteristic echogenic striped pattern or "pinnate" structure (**Figs. 6.46, 6.47**). The capsule is often clearly visible in superficial lesions, while the more infiltrative growth of deeper lipomas can also be identified on ultrasound by their ill-defined margins. In the generalized types (Madelung disease/Launois–Bensaude syndrome/horse collar), multiple lipomas of varying size and extent are present.

Lymphangioma/Cystic Hygroma

Lymphangiomas arise from aberrant sequestration of portions of the primitive lymphatic systems after the sixth week of embryonic development; they have no connection to the venous system and degenerate to form cystic cavities. They are characterized by extensive, infiltrative growth. Lymphangiomas are typically sited laterally in the neck. They have a soft cushionlike consistency on both manual and sonographic palpation.

Ultrasonography allows the true extent of the lesions to be demonstrated, something that is often underestimated by palpation on clinical examination (**Figs. 6.48, 6.49, 6.50, 6.51, 6.52, 6.53**).

Pearls and Pitfalls

Sclerosants can be applied precisely to macrocystic lesions under ultrasound guidance.

Similar topics covered elsewhere include the following:
- Neck abscess and neck phlegmon (Chapter 8, p. 98)
- Paragangliomas (Chapter 7, p. 91)
- Branchial cyst (Chapter 8, p. 98)
- Ranula (Chapter 8, p. 99)
- Epidermoid cysts (Chapter 10, p. 152)

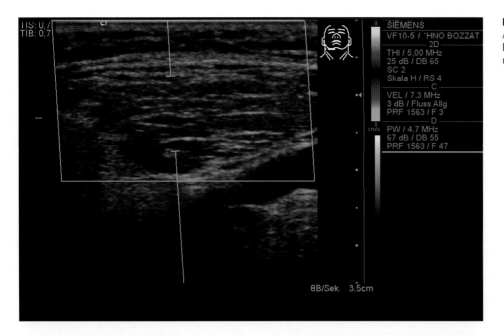

Fig. 6.46 Right submandibular region, transverse. A subcutaneous **lipoma** is spindle shaped and hypoechoic, with no signs of perfusion on Doppler ultrasound.

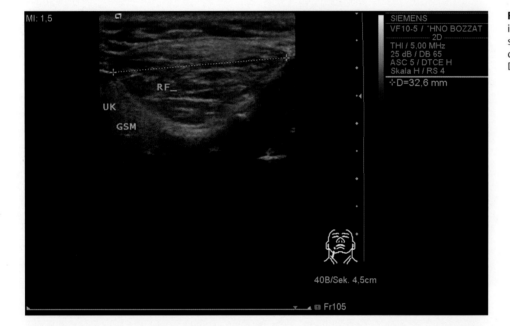

Fig. 6.47 Right submandibular region, longitudinal. The **lipoma** (RF) lies superficially to the submandibular gland (GSM) and can easily be distinguished from the gland. UK, mandible. Diagnosis: **Lipoma**.

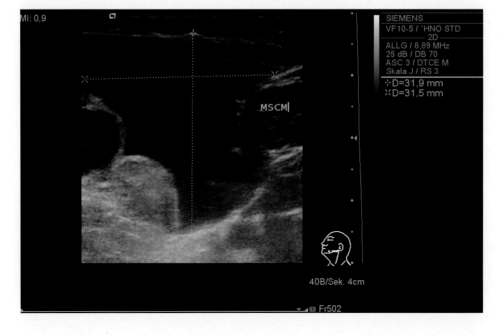

Fig. 6.48 Left submandibular region, transverse. A **macrocystic lymphangioma** with an anechoic internal space and fine echogenic septa. In this case, the anterior border of the sternocleidomastoid muscle (MSCM) forms the lateral border of the lymphangioma.

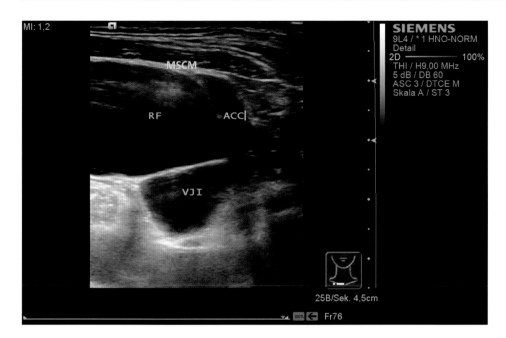

Fig. 6.49 Right side of the neck, transverse, level V. A well-demarcated, anechoic lesion (RF) lies laterally to the internal jugular vein (VJI) and common carotid artery (ACC). MSCM, sternocleidomastoid muscle. Diagnosis: **Lymphangioma**.

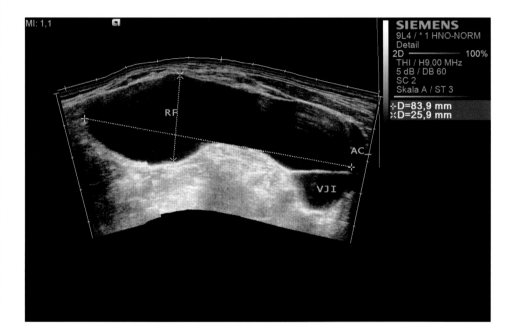

Fig. 6.50 Panoramic view: right side of the neck, transverse, level V. The **lymphangioma** extends laterally for almost 100 mm. The lesion (RF) is soft to sonographic palpation and does not pulsate. AC, common carotid artery; VJI, internal jugular vein.

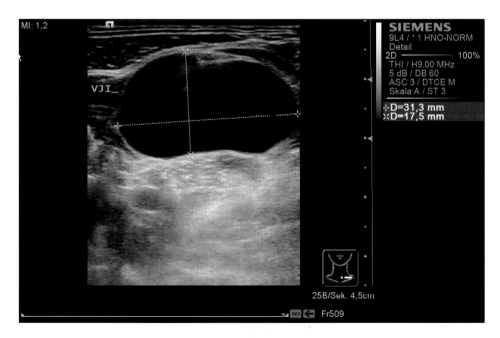

Fig. 6.51 Left side of the neck, transverse. An anechoic lesion can be seen on the left side of the neck; there is no evidence of intrinsic perfusion on CCDS and the consistency is soft to palpation. Lymphangiomas may be bilateral. A branchial cyst has to be considered in the differential diagnosis of a solitary lesion. VJI, internal jugular vein.

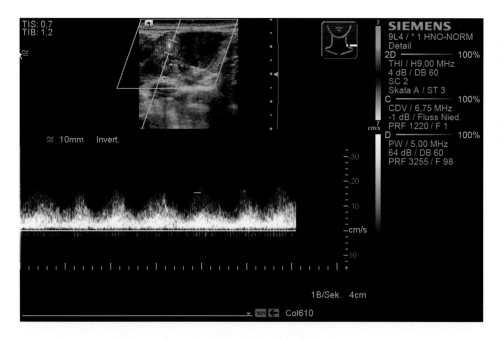

Fig. 6.52 Left side of the neck, transverse, CCDS. CCDS is used to differentiate a lymphangioma in the left supraclavicular region. The internal jugular vein, here coded red, lies medially, adjacent to the malformation, which does not show any intrinsic perfusion. The sensitive CCDS setting also reveals small vessels, but gives rise to color-coded pixel artifacts. The Doppler spectrum also shows some arterial flow signals, which are coming from the common carotid artery and are picked up by the Doppler scanner.

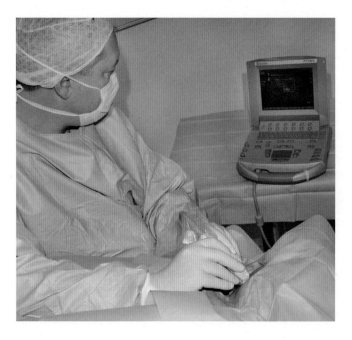

Fig. 6.53 Imaging during aspiration/injection of a **lymphangioma** on the right side of the neck/parotid. A sclerosing agent is instilled under aseptic conditions, after drainage of the lymphangioma.

Malignant Tumors and Metastases

Malignant Lymphomas

Malignancies arising from the lymphatic system, such as Hodgkin and non-Hodgkin lymphomas, have to be distinguished from metastases of other histological primary tumor origin. Certain subtypes of malignant lymphoma present particularly in the head and neck. Malignant lymphomas may be localized (e.g., early stages of Hodgkin disease), but are usually systemic, affecting several groups of lymph nodes. Sites of extranodal disease are not rare: for example, the spleen, liver, lungs, skeleton, mucosa (mucosa-associated lymphatic tissue, MALT), elements of the pharyngeal (Waldeyer) lymphatic ring (especially with

B-cell lymphomas), and the skin (especially with T-cell lymphomas). Ultrasound examination of the neck shows that the lymphomas are typically arranged in groups as lymph node conglomerates near the blood vessels. The submandibular, cranial, and posterolateral cervical lymph nodes are predominantly affected (**Fig. 6.4**).

The "bunch of grapes" or "string of pearls" appearance is pathognomonic for the presence of a lymphoma (**Fig. 6.54**). The echo pattern is usually hypoechoic or even anechoic. The shape is often round or oval, with clearly defined margins. Distal acoustic enhancement and intranodal reticulation have been described for non-Hodgkin lymphomas (**Figs. 6.55, 6.56**). Perfusion seen on CCDS often shows marked central vascularity (**Fig. 6.57**). Peripheral vascular patterns can also be present, and no angioarchitecture typical of lymphoma has yet been identified (**Fig. 6.58**).

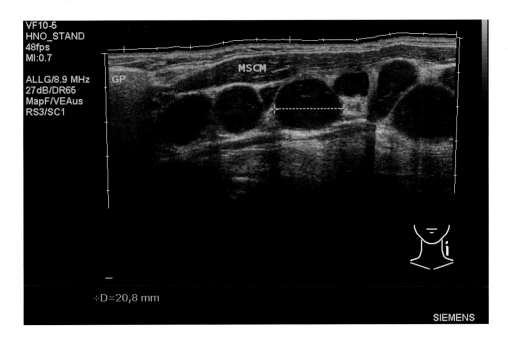

Fig. 6.54 Panoramic view, left side of the neck, longitudinal. Cervical **lymphoma** manifestation with the typical string of pearls appearance of a lymph node conglomerate. MSCM, sternocleidomastoid muscle.

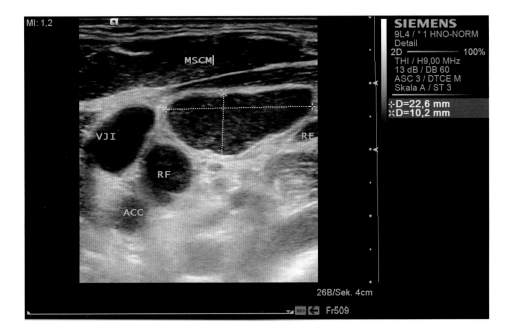

Fig. 6.55 Left side of the neck, transverse. Cervical non-Hodgkin **lymphoma** showing an oval node (RF) with the frequently observed fine reticular echotexture. ACC, common carotid artery; VJI, internal jugular vein; MSCM, sternocleidomastoid muscle.

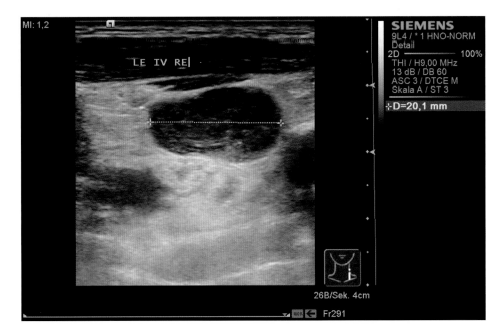

Fig. 6.56 Left side of the neck, longitudinal. Cervical non-Hodgkin **lymphoma** with an oval node seen in the longitudinal view. The intranodal reticulation is clearly visible in this image.

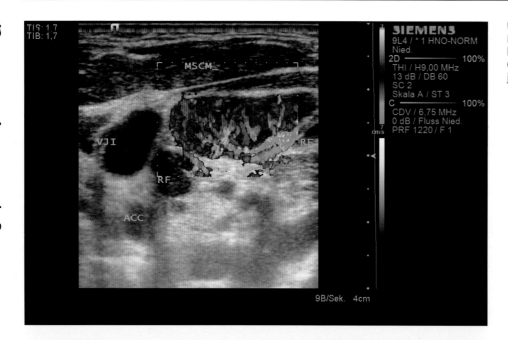

Fig. 6.57 Left side of the neck, transverse, CDDS. Malignant **lymphoma** manifestation with an oval lymph node (RF) showing strong perfusion on CCDS. ACC, common carotid artery; VJI, internal jugular vein; MSCM, sternocleidomastoid muscle.

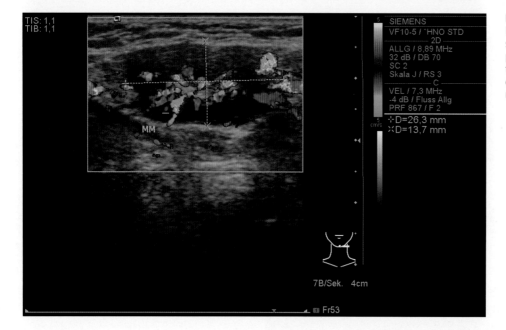

Fig. 6.58 Left side of the neck, transverse level IB, CDDS. Cervical **lymphoma** with an oval submandibular lymph node showing strong perfusion on CCDS. The vessels extend from the visible central echogenic hilum and branch centrifugally in the periphery. MM, mylohyoid muscle.

Sarcoma

Sarcomas are rare mesenchymal tumors (e.g. rhabdomyosarcoma and angiosarcoma), mainly situated in the parotid region and neck soft tissues. Rapid progression and agressive infiltration of neighbouring structures characterize these tumors clinically. On ultrasound examination they often show classic signs of malignancy: Poor demarcated borders, inhomogenous echotexture, irregular pattern of perfusion, and necrotic/hypoechoic areas (see **Fig. 9.78**).

Metastases

Cervical lymph node metastases in the regional spread of squamous cell carcinomas are of both therapeutic and prognostic relevance in the management of this patient group. The precise staging examination is extremely important. Ultrasonography plays an essential role in primary staging and cancer aftercare.

After the clinical and endoscopic assessment of the primary tumor, the lymph nodes in the soft tissues of the neck have to be evaluated according to a set protocol. The lymph nodes thereby observed are classified according to the criteria mentioned previously (**Figs. 6.9, 6.10, 6.15, 6.16, 6.17, 6.19, 6.20, 6.21 6.23, 6.24, 6.25, 6.26, 6.27**). In classifying enlarged lymph nodes, it must be mentioned once again that

attention should be paid to the size and biology of the primary tumor as well as to its typical drainage channels. The assessment of the blood vessels (infiltration of the internal jugular vein, flow area of the carotid artery; **Figs. 6.59, 6.60**), nerve plexuses, and muscles is also essential before any surgery, to determine how radical a procedure is required.

Infiltration of the extracranial segments of the carotid artery is of particular importance (**Figs. 6.61, 6.62, 6.63, 6.64**; ▶ Videos 6.9, 6.10, 6.11). Sheathing of the common or internal carotid artery by more than two-thirds of its circumference means that infiltration of the wall is likely. With the aid of the zoom function and high-resolution B-mode scanning, it is possible to demonstrate infiltration in these cases.

Melanoma Metastases

Depending on the site of the primary tumor, ultrasound assessment of cervical lymph nodes and melanomas of the face and neck may reveal lymph node metastases in the draining lymphatics and the salivary glands. Metastases show a characteristic malignant configuration with ill-defined margins, inhomogeneous echo pattern, infiltration into the adjacent tissues, absence of a "hilar sign," and irregular decentralized perfusion on CCDS (**Fig. 6.65**).

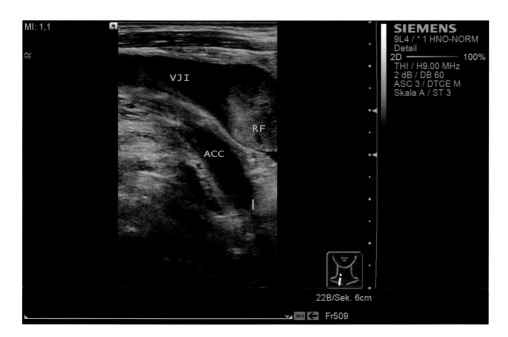

Fig. 6.59 Right side of the neck, longitudinal, level V. **Metastasis** compressing the jugular vein (VJI) may cause thrombosis. The thrombus (RF) in the vein lumen is hyperechoic and prevents the vein being occluded by manual compression. ACC, common carotid artery.

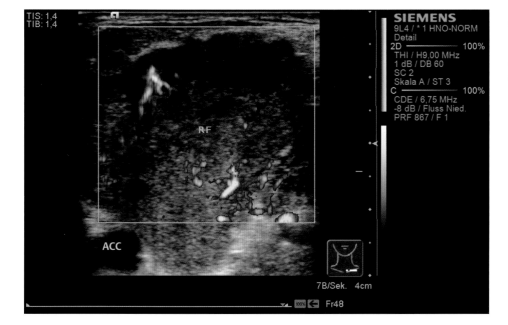

Fig. 6.60 Left side of the neck, transverse, level V, CCDS. A supraclavicular cN3 **metastasis** (RF) allows the carotid artery to be defined only at the left edge of the image. Infiltration of the jugular vein and branches of the brachial plexus is to be expected here. ACC, common carotid artery.

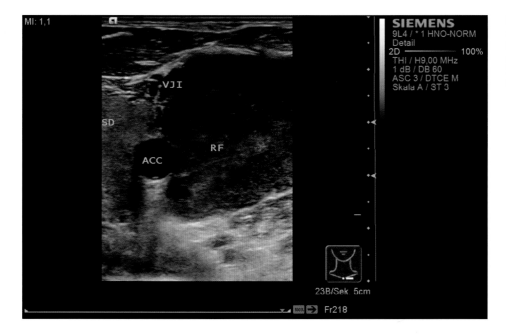

Fig. 6.61 Left side of the neck, transverse, level IV. An ill-defined hypoechoic metastasis (RF) surrounds about one-third of the common carotid artery (ACC) and the jugular vein (VJI). Infiltration is difficult to assess in cross-section and freeze-frame. SD, thyroid gland.

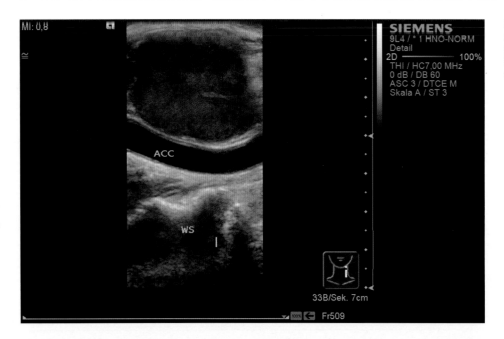

Fig. 6.62 Left side of the neck, longitudinal. A metastasis lies on the common carotid artery (ACC). There is no evidence of vessel wall infiltration, as can be seen clearly in the longitudinal view. WS, spine.

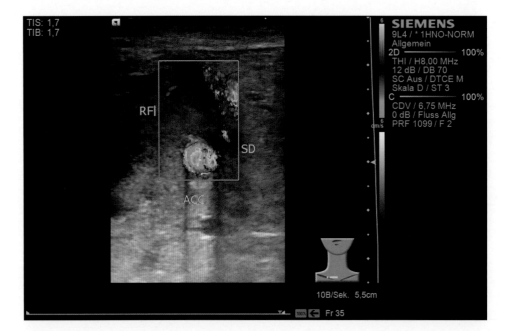

Fig. 6.63 Right side of the neck, transverse, CCDS. A metastasis (RF) completely surrounds the common carotid artery (ACC). The ill-defined margins are also consistent with infiltration of the thyroid gland (SD).

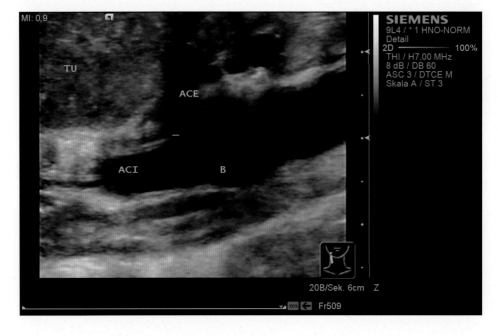

Fig. 6.64 Right side of the neck, longitudinal, level II. Infiltration of the internal and external carotid arteries (ACI, ACE). The metastasis (TU) lies on the carotid bulb and continuity of the surface is lost. Infiltration of the vessel wall was therefore to be expected and resection of the common, external and internal carotid arteries was required during the operation. After these findings on ultrasound, a balloon occlusion test was conducted. During surgery the infiltration of both arterial segments was confirmed. B, bifurcation.

Cancer of Unknown Primary (CUP) Syndrome

This entity, consisting of lymph node metastasis from an unknown primary tumor, is often detected as a clinically or sonographically suspicious solitary space-occupying lesion in the neck (**Fig. 6.66**). It is not possible to localize the primary tumor from the ultrasound morphology of the metastasis. Detailed ultrasound examination of the tonsillar region, the base of the tongue, the remaining soft tissues of the neck, and the salivary glands may, however, reveal a mass that was not discovered previously on inspection, palpation, or endoscopy.

In this context, another rare malignant mass must also be mentioned: **Cystic malignoma**. Whether or not these cystic tumors are a "primary" malignant entity remains controversial. On intial examination these cystic formations at the mid-neck level may be mistaken for lateral cervical cysts. In the majority of cases they are specially configred metastases of squamous cell carcinomas or lymphoepithelial carcinomas orginating from the oropharynx or nasopharynx. At the lower neck level, cystic tumors or lymph nodes should bring the focus on the thyroid gland as they may be metastases of a papillary carcinoma (**Fig. 6.4**).

Ultrasound in Oncological Follow-up

Clinical follow-up of head and neck cancer at regular intervals allows the early recognition of local or regional recurrence.

In our experience, the frequency of ultrasound examinations of the neck as part of routine cancer aftercare depends on several factors: initial TNM stage, site of the primary tumor, and the treatment given. Thus, there is no hard and fast rule for follow-up intervals. Diseases with a low risk of recurrence (e.g., cT1 glottis carcinoma) are not as closely monitored with ultrasound as those with a high risk (e.g., cT4, R1, G4, uvula).

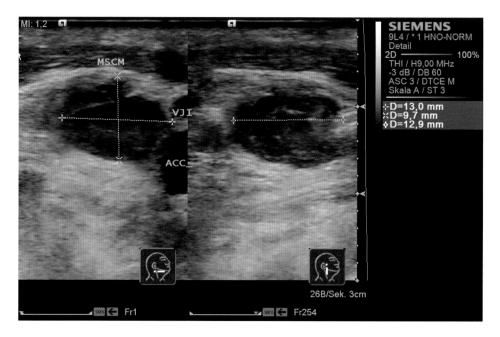

Fig. 6.65 Split screen, right side of neck. A **melanoma metastasis** is round in shape with an inhomogeneous echo pattern, which appears "cuboidal." The node also has ill-defined margins. It lies beneath the sternocleidomastoid muscle (MSCM), lateral to the internal jugular vein (VJI) and the common carotid artery (ACC).

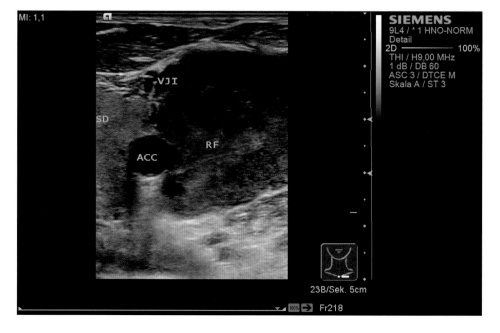

Fig. 6.66 Left side of the neck, transverse, level IV. A solitary enlarged node (RF) lying on the left side of the lower neck was classed as CUP in the subsequent diagnostic work-up. Lateral to the vascular sheath (VJI, ACC) is an ill-defined hypoechoic, inhomogeneous tumor, which lies directly on the carotid artery (ACC) laterally and compresses the internal jugular vein (VJI) medially. SD, thyroid gland. Diagnosis: **Squamous cell carcinoma in CUP syndrome**.

Regional Follow-up

One of the following situations usually applies to follow-up of cervical lymph nodes.

Primary Tumor Resection without Neck Dissection

With an initial cN0 situation, the neck has to be monitored closely once the postoperative swelling has subsided (in 2–4 weeks), to detect any abnormal lymph nodes promptly.

Primary Tumor Resection and Neck Dissection with/without Subsequent Radiotherapy

Once postoperative changes have subsided, the first follow-up examination is performed 4 weeks after surgery when only neck dissection has been performed. If radiotherapy has also been given, marked lymphedema often prevents an adequate assessment for 4–6 weeks after its completion. Attention must be paid to residual lymph nodes and any progression in their size (**Figs. 6.67, 6.68**). Assessment through the beginnings of scar tissue formation is much easier once the lymphedema has subsided.

Primary Radiochemotherapy with/without Subsequent Neck Dissection

If neck dissection is not performed after primary radiochemotherapy, the findings after completion of therapy and subsidence of inflammatory swelling count as baseline.

Lymphedema has an echogenic, dense, cloudlike subcutaneous appearance and, if pronounced, may make the identification of deeper structures much more difficult.

Therapeutic irradiation can alter the visibility of structures to varying degrees. In a large number of patients treated with radiotherapy, the altered tissues are more difficult to see with ultrasound, but in other patients, organ structures are seen with greater contrast. Patients often have enlarged residual lymph nodes in the neck after treatment. Typically, the number of identifiable nodes is greatly reduced. In this situation, the same criteria are used to determine the benign or malignant nature of each node. We find that the nodes described previously have now clearly regressed in size. The specification of a limit for the percentage reduction in lymph node volume found on ultrasound examination as a criterion of success, when comparing values obtained before and after radiotherapy or chemotherapy, has to be viewed critically. (Several ways of calculating the volume have been proposed, such as $1/6 \times \pi \times diameter1 \times diameter2 \times diameter3$).

The internal echotextures seen on ultrasound are more compact and inhomogeneous, and tend to be more echogenic (**Figs. 6.69, 6.70, 6.71, 6.72, 6.73, 6.74, 6.75, 6.76**). The internal echo pattern is often coarse. Perfusion previously seen within the lymph nodes on CCDS is no longer visible or is considerably weaker. If signs of intrinsic perfusion are still to be found on CCDS, it generally means that the node still contains viable cells. However, there are no reliable studies on the correlation between perfusion and tumor viability, so that we determine the indication for surgical treatment (neck dissection) on an individual basis, using PET-CT if necessary.

An increase in size or changes in the echo pattern during the course of disease, especially in the draining lymphatic channels, indicates activity/viability of the node, which is highly suspicious for a new metastasis (**Figs. 6.77, 6.78**).

As a noninvasive procedure, ultrasonography can be repeated as often as necessary in the follow-up of malignant disease; it is inexpensive, does not take up much time, and is freely available. One advantage of ultrasound is that it can be performed by the treating physician, who knows about the progression of the disease and endoscopic findings. This overall picture allows the changes in the findings with time—by imaging before and after treatment—to be interpreted correctly and the right decisions to be made.

Finally, it should be mentioned that the use of ultrasound in the search for tumors and in their follow-up is an indispensable part of the treatment protocol.

Pearls and Pitfalls in Sonographic Oncological Follow-up

1. Consider presurgical neck lymph node status and changes over time (number, shape and size, region)
2. Consider the tumor site, biology and probable metastatic pattern
3. Consider that, immediately after a surgical intervention, lymph nodes may be reactively enlarged
4. Keep a strict and standardized oncological follow-up schedule
5. In cases where a lymph node has undergone a change not correlating to the whole clinical situation, additional check-ups may be helpful
6. Implement standardized regimes and vocabulary for documentation and reports
7. Assessment after neck dissection is difficult because of scarring or altered anatomical relations.

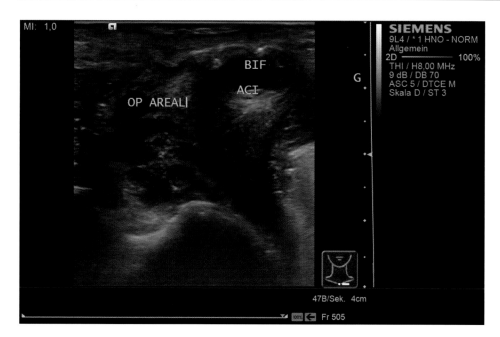

Fig. 6.67 Right side of the neck, transverse, level III, same patient as in **Fig. 6.66**. Following neck dissection and radiotherapy, the bifurcation (BIF) has been displaced anteriorly. The surgical bed of the cervical lymph node metastasis (OP AREAL) lies laterally and appears hypoechoic, ill defined and inhomogeneous. ACI, internal carotid artery.

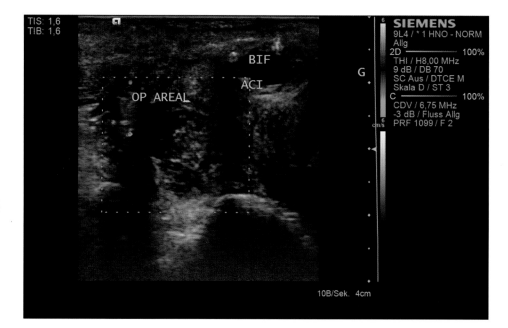

Fig. 6.68 Right side of the neck, transverse, level III, CCDS. Following neck dissection and radiotherapy, the bifurcation (BIF) has been displaced anteriorly. The surgical bed of the cervical lymph node metastasis (OP AREAL) lies laterally and appears hypoechoic, ill defined and inhomogeneous. Perfusion without any significant vascularity indicates scarring rather than recurrence. ACI, internal carotid artery.

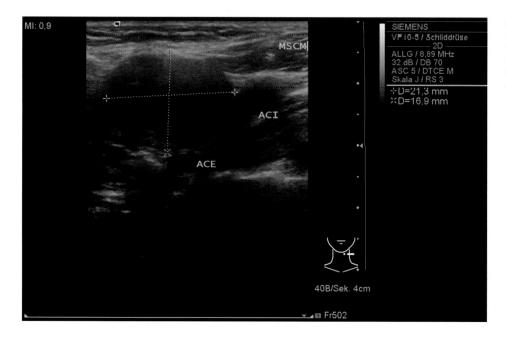

Fig. 6.69 Transverse view of the left side of a cN2c neck, lateral to the carotid arteries (ACE/ACI), prior to concomitant radiochemotherapy. The depicted lymph node metastases show an irregular hypoechoic picture with an inhomogeneous echotexture. MSCM, sternocleidomastoid muscle.

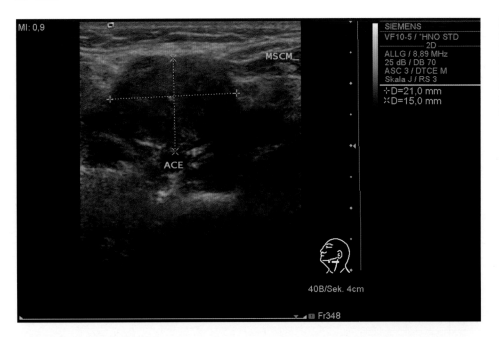

Fig. 6.70 Transverse view of the left side of the neck after radiochemotherapy. The internal echotexture of the metastases is more echogenic and inhomogeneous in appearance. No conclusions about the residual viability of the tumor cells can be made from the B-mode scan. ACE, external carotid artery; MSCM, sternocleidomastoid muscle.

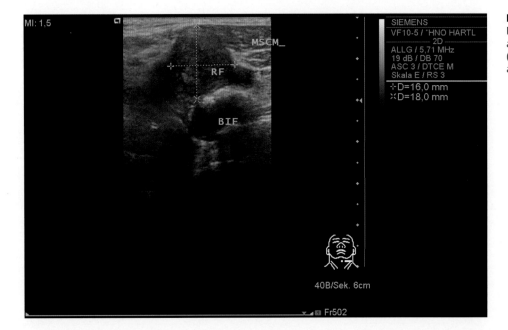

Fig. 6.71 Left side of the neck, transverse. Metastasis (RF) on the bifurcation (BIF) at the anterior border of the sternocleidomastoid muscle (MSCM). The inhomogeneous metastasis is round and measures 16 mm × 18 mm.

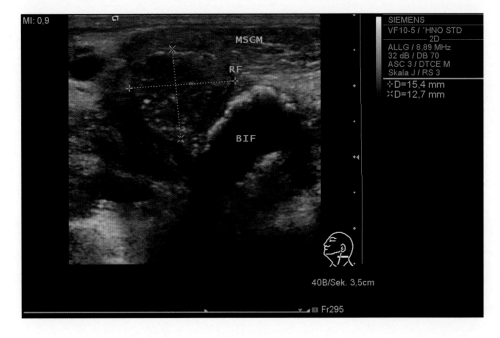

Fig. 6.72 The metastasis is smaller (12 mm × 13 mm) following radiochemotherapy. The inhomogeneity of the echo has increased with a highly echogenic parenchymal pattern. As an incidental finding, the vascular walls are thickened and exhibit echogenic changes as an expression of the sclerotic changes caused by radiotherapy. BIF, bifurcation; MSCM, sternocleidomastoid muscle. Histological diagnosis: **No vital tumor cells of squamous cell carcinoma**.

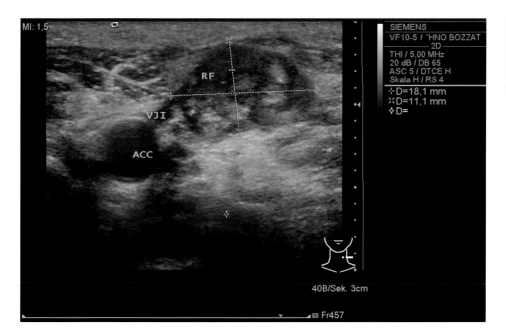

Fig. 6.73 Left side of the neck, transverse, level III. cN1 metastasis (RF) (18 mm × 11 mm) lateral to the internal jugular vein (VJI) and common carotid artery (ACC). Histological diagnosis: **Several nests of vital tumor cells of squamous cell carcinoma.**

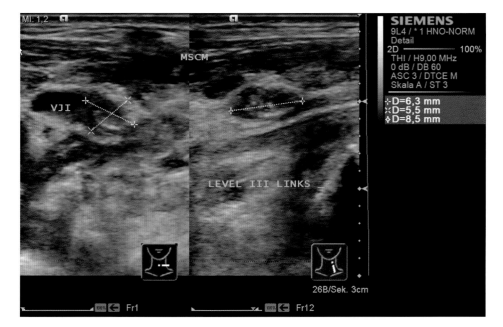

Fig. 6.74 Split screen, left side of the neck, transverse, level III. Clear reduction in the size of the metastasis (5 mm × 6 mm) lateral to the internal jugular vein (VJI), following radiochemotherapy. MSCM, sternocleidomastoid muscle. Histological diagnosis: **No vital tumor cells of squamous cell carcinoma.**

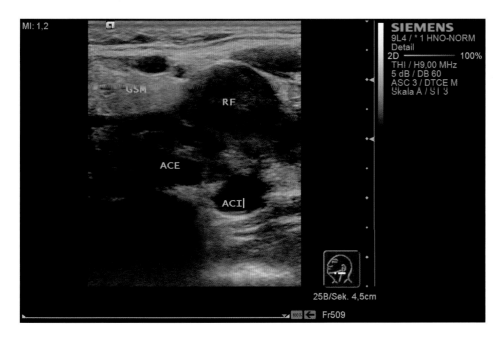

Fig. 6.75 Left side of the neck, level II. Metastasis (RF) lying above the bifurcation (ACE, ACI) at the posterior border of the submandibular gland (GSM).

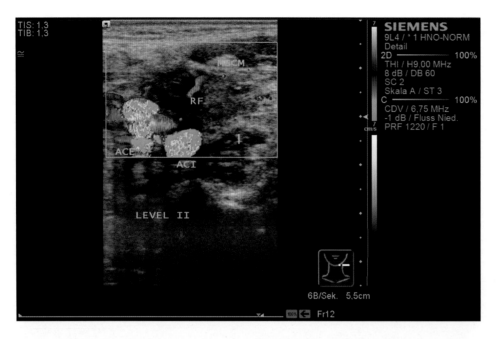

Fig. 6.76 Left side of the neck, level II, CCDS. Following radiochemotherapy, there is a hypoechoic area with ill-defined margins, at the site where the cervical lymph node metastasis (RF) used to be. A solid change can no longer be distinguished. As well as the clear color duplex signal of the branches of the carotid artery (ACE, ACI), isolated punctate vascular signals can be seen in the area of the metastasis. MSCM, sternocleidomastoid muscle. Diagnosis: **Tissue changes after multimodal therapy.**

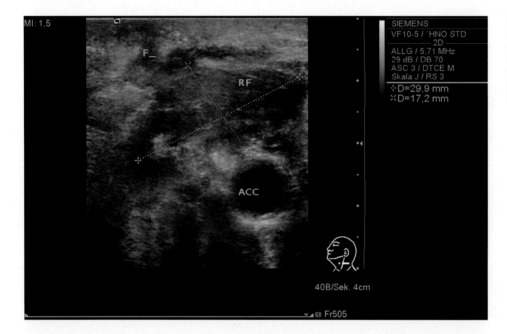

Fig. 6.77 Left side of the neck, transverse, level III. Two years after neck dissection and radiochemotherapy, this patient presented with a weeping wound. Ultrasound showed an echogenic, ill-defined structure medial to the carotid artery (ACC), with a fistula (F) reaching the skin surface. Diagnosis: **Fistula after multimodal therapy.**

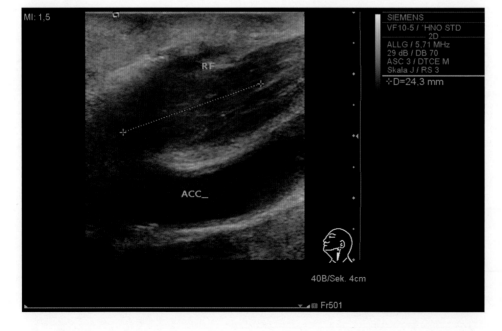

Fig. 6.78 Left side of the neck, longitudinal, level III (see also **Fig. 6.77**). In the longitudinal view, there is clear demarcation from the artery, but an ill-defined border with the sternocleidomastoid muscle (MSCM). Biopsy confirmed recurrence of the earlier oropharyngeal carcinoma. ACC, common carotid artery.

Ultrasound-guided Needle Biopsies

As a rule, needle biopsies are performed for diagnostic purposes. The results provide information on the cytopathology, histopathology, and/or microbiology of the lesion (**Fig. 6.79**; ▶ Videos 6.12, 6.13, 6.14).

Such investigations in the head and neck involve the salivary glands (parotid gland, submandibular gland) and the cervical lymph nodes. Fine-needle aspiration is also appropriate for draining cysts and abscesses and for the insertion of catheters into the blood vessels. With diagnostic needle biopsies, a distinction hats to be made between fine-needle aspiration (aspiration biopsy, fine-needle aspiration biopsy [FNAB]), fine-needle aspiration cytology (FNAC), and core-needle biopsy (**Fig. 6.80**) (specimen for histology). Whereas fine-needle biopsies are defined as using needles with an outer diameter of less than 1 mm (usually 0.7–0.8 mm), core-needle biopsy systems use needles with a diameter of 1 mm and above (**Fig. 6.81**).

Needle biopsies, and in particular fine-needle aspiration biopsies, are considered problematic to distinguish between malignant lymphomas, as an assessment of the histological architecture of an entire lymph node forms the basis of the differential diagnosis. Suspected mesenchymal tumors and cystic/necrotic lesions provide difficult starting conditions. Diagnostic accuracy is determined by the experience of the physician and the pathologist in harvesting, processing, and interpreting the specimens.

If the general problem is restricted to differentiating between benign and malignant, then both methods are often sufficient to give an adequate response; this may help to avoid surgical biopsy in patients with multiple morbidity.

In summary, needle biopsy is a comparatively simple, minimally invasive diagnostic procedure that can be performed on an outpatient basis. Plausible positive results rule out the need for more major diagnostic investigations, but the informational value of the method is limited when findings are negative. These basic reservations persist even though performing the biopsy under ultrasound guidance can increase the sensitivity and the negative predictive value. There are no absolute contraindications to needle biopsy; the procedure is particularly suitable as the primary diagnostic method when there is a high anesthetic risk or when anesthesia is not possible. Caution should be exercised if the patient has a severe coagulation disorder.

Ultrasound-guided Injection

Needle guidance by ultrasound as a precise targeting tool is increasingly being described by anesthesiologists for regional nerve anesthesia, sclerotherapy of cysts and lymphangiomas (see **Fig. 6.53**) as for injection of Botulinum toxin (**Fig. 6.82**, ▶ Video 6.15).

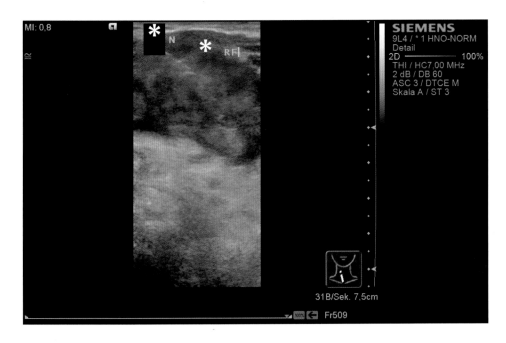

Fig. 6.79 Right side of the neck, transverse oblique. Needle biopsy of a lesion (RF) with a hypoechoic, inhomogeneous structure, suspected of being malignant. Biopsy using the BARD Magnum Core High Speed Biopsy System. The hyperechoic needle (N, asterisk) can be seen as an oblique line; it is advanced carefully into the biopsy area. Diagnosis: **Sarcoma**.

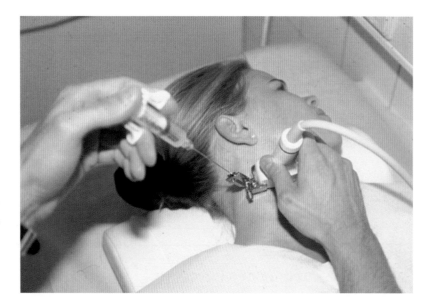

Fig 6.80 Ultrasound-guided fine-needle biopsy performed using a needle guidance attached to the transducer.

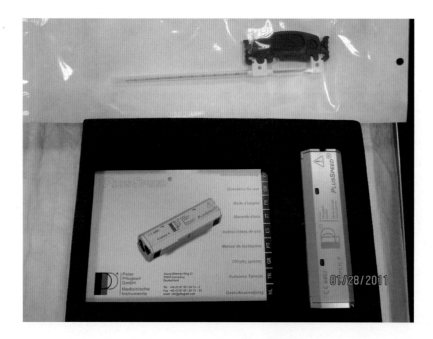

Fig. 6.81 High-speed core-needle biopsy system, "Plus Speed" by Peter Pflugbeil. In the upper part of the image a white coded 14 gauge (2.11 mm) needle can be seen.

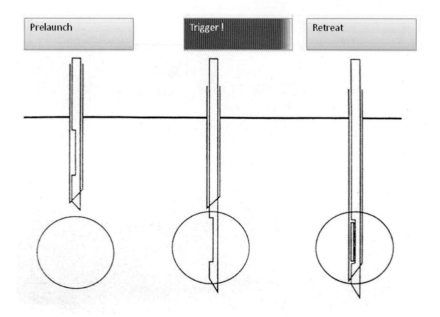

Fig. 6.82 Scheme of a modern core-needle biopsy system. First, the needle is placed in front of the lesion. After triggering the needle, the biopsy stylet is brought into the lesion and harvests the specimen cylinder followed by the outer blade. Finally, both components are extracted.

7   Extracranial Nerves

Anatomy

The extracranial nerves are only partly accessible to ultrasonography. The only cranial nerve regularly displayed on ultrasound imaging is the vagal nerve, the cervical part of which can be easily identified between the carotid artery and the internal jugular vein (**Figs. 7.1, 7.2**). It descends from the skull base along the lateral wall of the internal carotid artery; after the division of the common carotid artery it runs in the caudal cervical part between the internal jugular and the common carotid artery.

As a general rule, the components of the brachial plexus can be seen in level V. They are located laterally to the anterior scalene muscle and appear as hypoechoic oval structures as they are displayed obliquely cut (**Fig. 7.3**). Therefore, they should not be confused with lymph nodes lying in groups.

Ultrasound visualization of the brachial plexus is increasingly used in plexus anesthesia. There are no definite landmarks to facilitate the positive identification of the other cranial nerves, such as the hypoglossal, facial, and accessory nerves. It is therefore not possible to classify them in relation to a pathological process in the vicinity. In thin people or in patients whose anatomy has been altered by surgery, it is possible to see the spinal cord within the spinal canal in the transverse and longitudinal views of the spine (▶ Video 7.1).

Inflammatory Changes

The clinical picture of **carotidynia**, a painful syndrome in the neck with tenderness over the carotid bifurcation, is rare. Despite controversy over the existence of this syndrome, changes are often seen on ultrasound examination when the relevant clinical symptoms and signs are present. At the carotid bulb, the maximum site of local tenderness, patients exhibit a hypoechoic thickening of the carotid artery wall, sometimes in two layers of the wall. This causes a slight narrowing of the lumen and leads to a pronounced outward enlargement of the vessel (**Fig. 7.4**).

Benign Tumors

Paragangliomas

Paragangliomas are neuroendocrine tumors that arise from extra-adrenal paraganglionic cells of the autonomic nervous system. In the neck, they can be found in the region of the infra- and supralaryngeal ganglia, along the path of the vagus and carotids, as well as beyond ultrasound access in the jugulotympanic area.

In B-mode, carotid paragangliomas found in the bifurcation appear as an oval tumor, oval structures with smooth outlines (**Fig. 7.5**). The echotexture is inhomogeneously hypoechoic with internal reflections of greater echogenicity (**Fig. 7.6**). The main ultrasound feature of cervical paragangliomas is the marked hyperperfusion regularly seen in color-coded duplex sonography (CCDS) (**Fig. 7.7**; ▶ Videos 7.2, 7.3). This extreme vascularity goes by the graphic description of color/power Doppler "inferno."

Afferent arteries (feeders) branch off from the internal and external carotid arteries into the lesion (▶ Video 7.4). On sonographic palpation, the forceful pulsations are often perceptibly transmitted to the transducer.

> **Pearls and Pitfalls**
>
> If a lesion consistent with a paraganglioma is seen on ultrasound examination, the carotid bifurcation on the other side must be looked at very carefully. Bilateral and multilocular tumors have been reported in 3%–26% of cases. Further imaging by PET scanning may be required.

Neuromas

The two main entities in this rare class of tumor are neurofibromas and schwannomas. Both of these neurogenic tumors regularly show distal acoustic enhancement, helping to distinguish them from lymph nodes in the individual case.

Neurofibromas are nonencapsulated, hypoechoic, inhomogeneous masses in the immediate vicinity of the nerves from which they arise and they may have irregular outlines (**Figs 7.8, 7.9, 7.10**; ▶ Videos 7.5, 7.6). Malignant transformation occurs in up to 5%; rapid clinical progression and ill-defined margins between the tumor and the adjacent tissue may indicate malignancy.

In B-mode imaging, **schwannomas** are also seen as hypoechoic, inhomogeneous lesions, which can sometimes be assigned to the nerve of origin (e.g., the vagus nerve, a branch of the plexus). Intrinsic anechoic areas consistent with a cyst are common. If the lesion is assigned to a visible nervous structure, it frequently shows a bulb-shaped (tumorous) enlargement (**Fig. 7.11**).

Although schwannomas tend to be better perfused than neurofibromas on CCDS, it is certainly difficult to tell the difference on this basis alone (**Figs. 7.12, 7.13**).

> **Pearls and Pitfalls**
>
> In distinction from carotid paragangliomas, neuromas tend to lie distally or dorsally to the carotid bifurcation.

Malignant Tumors

The most common malignant entities to affect the cranial nerves are malignant mesenchymal tumors, squamous cell carcinomas, and their cervical lymph node metastases. In level V, stage cN3 metastases not infrequently infiltrate or surround the branches of the brachial plexus, which can be diagnosed on ultrasound. If the metastasis extends into the deeper tissues between the sternocleidomastoid and the trapezius muscles, the nerve damage to be expected during resection can be assessed in the presurgical work-up (**Figs. 7.14, 7.15**).

The extremely rare **Merkel cell carcinoma** is usually seen as a solid, reddish-purple hemispherical or spherical tumor (**Figs. 7.16, 7.17**).

There may be secondary cutaneous ulceration. Most tumors present have a diameter of less than 20 mm. The predominant ultrasound finding is of an inhomogeneous lesion with ill-defined margins (**Fig. 7.18**). Any abnormal cervical lymph nodes around a lesion are an indication for neck dissection.

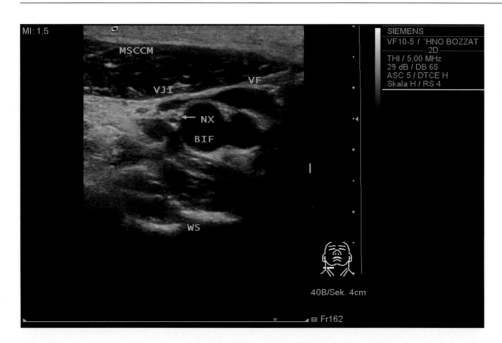

Fig. 7.1 Neck, right, transverse. In level III, the round hypoechoic lumen of the **vagus nerve** (NX, arrow) can be seen at the junction of the facial vein (VF) with the internal jugular vein (VJI), lateral to the bifurcation (BIF). MSCM, sternocleidomastoid muscle; WS, vertebra.

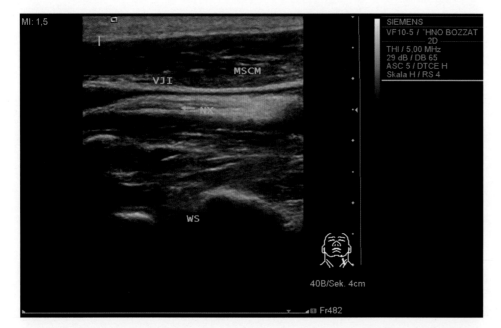

Fig. 7.2 Neck, right longitudinal. In the longitudinal view, the **vagus nerve** (NX, arrow) can be seen as a hypoechoic ribbonlike structure. MSCM, sternocleidomastoid muscle; VJI, internal jugular vein; WS, vertebra.

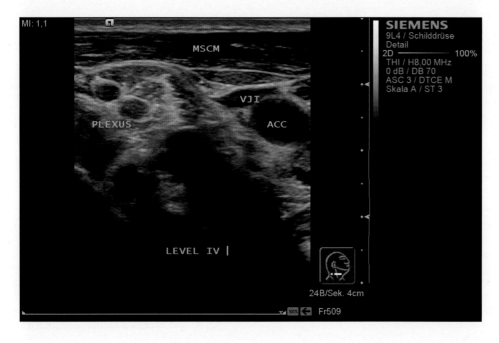

Fig. 7.3 Neck, right, transverse. The **branches of the plexus** are cut obliquely and appear oval; they may be mistaken for lymph nodes. ACC, common carotid artery; MSCM, sternocleidomastoid muscle; VJI, internal jugular vein.

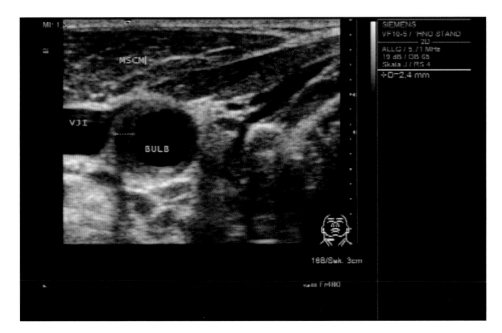

Fig. 7.4 Neck, transverse, right. There is a sickle-shaped thickening of the media of the carotid artery (BULB) wall in the region of the carotid bulb. This corresponds to the site of maximum tenderness reported. MSCM, sternocleidomastoid muscle; VJI, internal jugular vein. Diagnosis: **Carotidynia.**

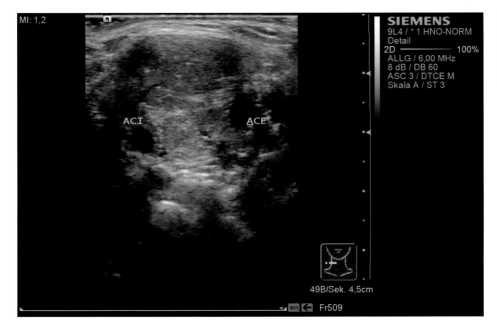

Fig. 7.5 Neck, right, transverse. A hypoechoic, inhomogeneous lesion appears to surround the internal carotid artery (ACI) and external carotid artery (ACE), forcing the two vessels away from each other in the middle of the bifurcation. Diagnosis: **Paraganglioma.**

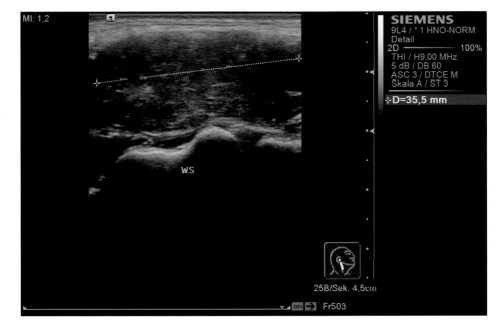

Fig. 7.6 Neck, right, longitudinal. The lesion now appears oval and lies on the spine (WS), although it can be felt to slide easily over the vertebra when pushed with the probe. Diagnosis: **Paraganglioma.**

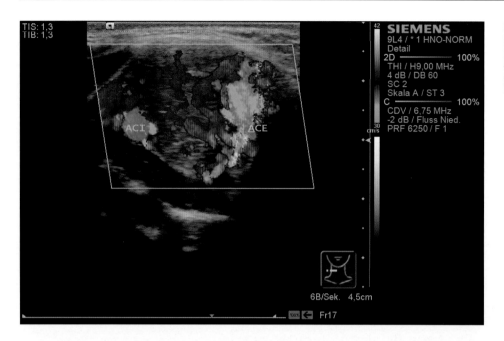

Fig. 7.7 Neck, right, transverse. In CCDS, the **paraganglioma** shows a characteristically strong perfusion (PRF 6250). Although the vessels are arranged irregularly, feeders from the internal (ACI) or external (ACE) carotid arteries can often be demonstrated precisely.

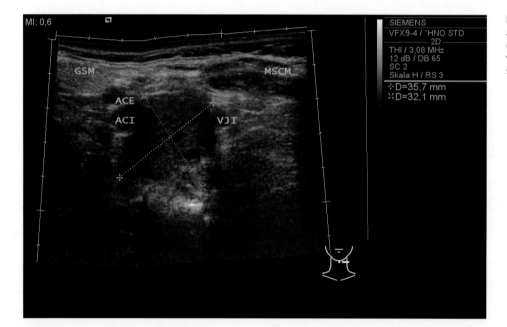

Fig. 7.8 Neck, left, transverse. A **neurofibroma** at a typical site lateral to the carotid bifurcation (ACE/ACI) and medial to the internal jugular vein (VJI). GSM, submandibular gland; MSCM, sternocleidomastoid muscle.

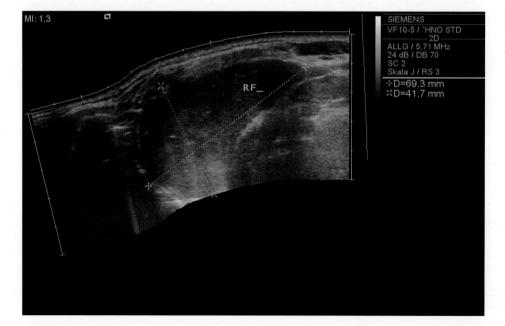

Fig. 7.9 Panoramic view—neck, left, longitudinal, level II. A **plexus neurofibroma** with hypoechoic homogeneous texture. Deeper, the tumor extends fingerlike into the posterior tissues.

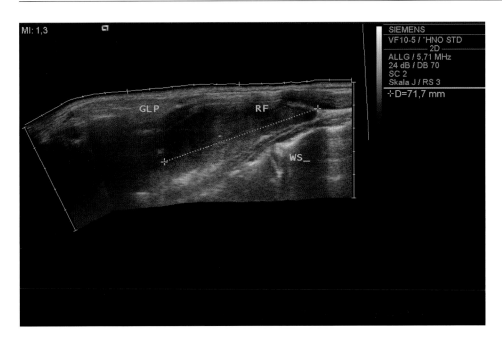

Fig. 7.10 Panoramic view—neck, left, longitudinal, level II. This view shows the **neurofibroma** more clearly in its relation to the parotid gland (GLP) and spine (WS).

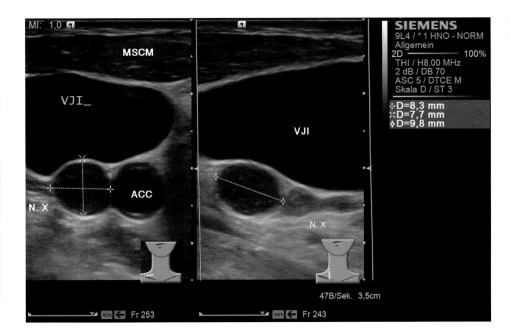

Fig. 7.11 Split-screen, right, level IV. A grape-shaped alteration of the tenth cranial nerve (N.X) in the longitudinal (right) image depicts a tumorous thickening of the nerve. In the transverse (left) view, the diameter of the nerve almost equals that of the common carotid artery (ACC). Apart from the sonomorphological presentation, the diagnosis of a **schwannoma** of the vagus nerve is assumed by the position of the lesion sitting between the carotid and internal jugular vein (VJI). MSCM, sternocleidomastoid muscle.

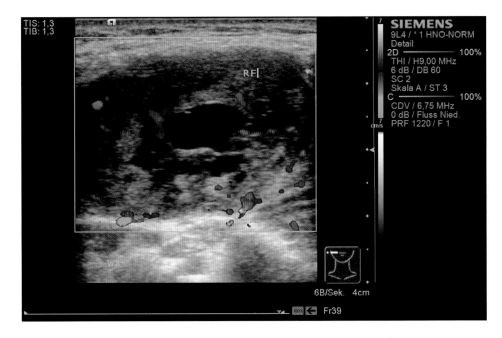

Fig. 7.12 Submandibular, right, transverse, level II. A **schwannoma** (RF) with hypoechoic, partly anechoic echo texture shows diffuse forceful perfusion on CCDS. There is no perfusion to be seen in the central anechoic area, which is probably cystic.

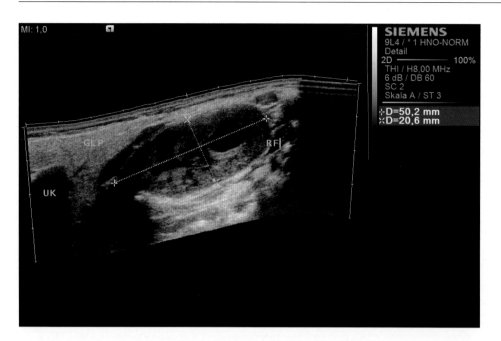

Fig. 7.13 Panoramic view—neck, right, longitudinal, level II. The **schwannoma** (RF) measures up to 50 mm in its craniocaudal extension; it is oval in shape with distinct margins. The inhomogeneous echotexture with anechoic areas caudally is well demonstrated. GLP, parotid gland; UK, mandible.

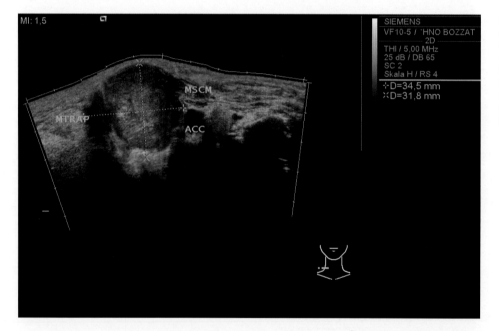

Fig. 7.14 Neck, right, transverse, level V. A cervical lymph node metastasis (35 mm × 32 mm) of a hypopharyngeal carcinoma in level V. A **cN3 cervical lymph node metastasis**, lying between the posterior border of the sternocleidomastoid muscle (MSCM), the trapezius muscle (MTRAP), and the common carotid artery (ACC). In a neck dissection, several branches of the plexus have to be resected to achieve a complete resection.

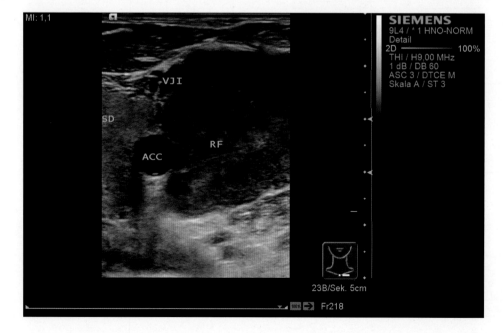

Fig. 7.15 Neck, left, transverse, level V. Another example of **soft-tissue infiltration**. A metastasis (RF) extends to the common carotid artery (ACC), thyroid gland (SD), and internal jugular vein (VJI). In a neck dissection, several branches of the plexus have to be resected to achieve a complete resection.

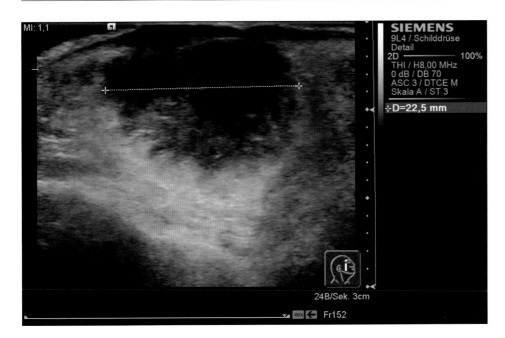

Fig. 7.16 Zygotic arch, right, longitudinal. **Cutaneous Merkel cell carcinoma** is hypoechoic and inhomogeneous, with indistinct margins in the periphery.

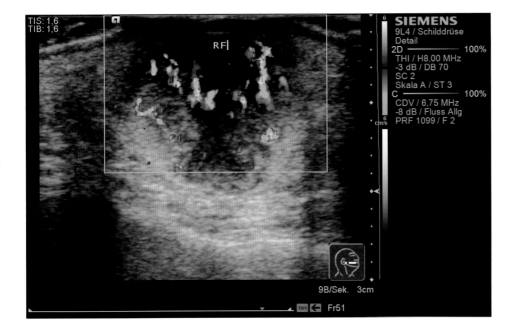

Fig. 7.17 Zygomatic arch, right, transverse. CCDS shows a **Merkel cell carcinoma** with diffuse irregular perfusion.

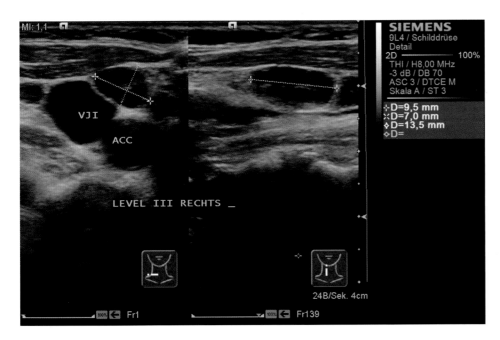

Fig. 7.18 Split screen, cervical, right. Several oval lymph nodes with a hyperechoic central structure (the "hilum sign") can be seen in level III on the affected side. The largest lymph node measures 13.5 mm × 7 mm x 9.5 mm and shows a distinct "hilum sign." The inhomogeneous internal echogenicity seen in the longitudinal view on the right side of the image is suspicious. ACC, common carotid artery; VJI, internal jugular vein. Diagnosis: **Lymph node metastasis in Merkel cell carcinoma**.

8   Floor of the Mouth and Oropharynx

Anatomy

Inspection, bimanual palpation, and laryngoscopy are the classic procedures for examining the tongue, floor of the mouth, and oropharynx.

There are two basic ways of performing an ultrasound examination in this area: transcutaneously, that is, through the soft tissues of the neck, and intraorally, in which the ultrasound probe is covered, for example, with a glove, and inserted into the mouth (**Figs. 8.1, 8.2**). However, special probes exist for application in the oral cavity and deeper areas of the oropharynx and hypopharynx.

Bony structures (the horizontal ramus of the mandible and the hyoid bone), which can be seen as hyperechoic reflections with distal acoustic shadowing, are initially used as landmarks when examining the floor of the mouth, tongue, and oropharynx. Like the other muscles in the head and neck, muscles in the floor of the mouth are hypoechoic, while the intrinsic muscles of the tongue appear homogeneously echogenic. The longitudinal, transverse, and vertical groups of muscle fibers can be seen in both transverse and longitudinal views as more echogenic or punctate hyperechoic reflections. The surface of the tongue is easily recognized from the hyperechoic curved line of the air–tissue interface. The penetration depth for examining the whole tongue should be set at 70 mm, with appropriate adjustments of the frequency, focus, and gain.

A routine demonstration of the palate and posterior wall of the pharynx with the transcutaneous approach is hampered by the reflection of the ultrasound waves due to the air within the oral cavity. Demonstration of the tip of the tongue, which is surrounded by air, is similarly problematic in transcutaneous ultrasonography, but this area can easily be examined clinically by inspection and palpation. In addition, intraoral ultrasound may be of use here.

After the acoustic shadow of the mandible, the first structures to be identified on transcutaneous examination in the transverse plane, starting at the point of the chin, are the rounded anterior bellies of the digastric muscles (**Fig. 8.3**; ▶ Video 8.1).

The geniohyoid muscles, which lie between the mylohyoid muscles spanning the horizontal rami of the mandible and the genioglossus muscles, can be identified from their typical hypoechoic structures and distinguished from the echogenic intrinsic muscles of the tongue.

The entire length of the tongue, including its base, can be assessed by moving the ultrasound probe down to the hyoid. The lingual arteries can be demonstrated at the transition of the middle to posterior third of the tongue as round hypoechoic or anechoic structures (**Figs. 8.4, 8.5**; ▶ Video 8.2).

The tonsillar bed can be examined if the ultrasound probe, held slightly above the hyoid bone in the transverse plane, is tilted laterally in the submandibular region. The tonsil appears as a hypoechoic, relatively well-defined structure with multiple echogenic reflections due to small inclusions of air (**Fig. 8.6**). The sonographic appearance of the paltine tonsils may resemble the shape of a scallop. The size of the tonsils depends on age and shows great interindividual variation.

Below the hypoechoic infrahyoid muscles, the somewhat more echogenic preepiglottic fatty tissue can be demonstrated between the hyoid and upper edge of the thyroid cartilage (**Fig. 8.7**).

After identification of these landmarks, both the transverse and longitudinal views must be checked carefully for any pathological findings.

Inflammatory Changes

In infections and inflammatory conditions of the floor of the mouth, tongue, and oropharynx, a distinction has to be made between a phlegmon and an abscess.

A **phlegmon** in the floor of the mouth can be identified as diffuse hypoechoic areas lying between the different layers of tissue, which often appear blurred and loosely structured (**Figs. 8.8, 8.9**), while an **abscess** in the floor of the mouth can be recognized as a clearly defined hypoechoic space-occupying lesion, containing hypoechoic to anechoic central structures with distal acoustic enhancement (**Figs. 8.10, 8.11**). Perfusion in the inflamed tissue areas is usually increased.

A visible gap in the hyperechoic contour line may be identified at the position where a dental abscess has breached the mandible (**Fig. 8.12**).

Acute inflammatory conditions affecting the palatine tonsils are seen as an enlargement with hypoechoic change and loss of clear demarcation from the surrounding tissues. It is not possible to use ultrasound to unambiguously distinguish an intra-, peri-, or retrotonsillar abscess from an acute tonsillitis, but ultrasound may support the provisional diagnosis (**Figs. 8.13, 8.14, 8.15**; ▶ Videos 8.3, 8.4, 8.5).

A hypoechoic, clearly defined space-occupying lesion touching the tonsillar bed can be identified on the ultrasound image. It shows the typical signs of an abscess: a central anechoic area, possibly with isolated internal echoes indicating cell debris, and distal acoustic enhancement. Ultrasound may sometimes be a very useful diagnostic tool and examination can also be performed when there is trismus related to infection or inflammation.

Progression of the infection may result in a parapharyngeal abscess (**Figs. 8.16, 8.17, 8.18**) or phlegmon (**Figs. 8.19, 8.20**; ▶ Video 8.6) in the neck.

> **Pearls and Pitfalls**
>
> Comparison of the two sides is invaluable in deciding whether there is a tonsillar abscess. A split-screen display is extremely helpful here, as the two sides can be seen simultaneously in the corresponding plane and compared directly with each other.

Benign Tumors

Branchial Cysts

Branchial cysts and **fistulas** lying laterally in the neck are mostly related to the second branchial (pharyngeal) cleft, as this is the largest in size and persists longest during embryonic development. A cyst or fistula developing here has a close positional relationship to the carotid bifurcation; if there is an internal sinus, it opens into the supratonsillar fossa (**Fig. 8.21**). The cyst sac usually lies laterally to the internal jugular vein and caudally to the posterior belly of the digastric muscle. Malformations of the second, third, and fourth branchial clefts are considerably less common. Ultrasound scans show clearly defined cysts that are round or oval, lying in levels II and III. Sonographic palpation allows the fluid contents to be felt. The homogeneous internal echoes range in the classic description from anechoic to hypoechoic and are more echogenic when infected. Likewise, distal acoustic enhancement is characteristic, as is the lack of perfusion seen in the inner space on color-coded duplex sonography (CCDS) (**Figs. 8.22, 8.23, 8.24**; ▶ Videos 8.7, 8.8). Modern high-resolution ultrasound systems even demonstrate the glycoproteins as finely dispersed "floating" echoes.

Under favorable conditions, the path of a branchial fistula or sinus can be followed right into the oropharynx (**Figs. 8.25, 8.26, 8.27**; ▶Videos 8.9, 8.10).

Infected Branchial Cysts

Correlating with the clinical picture, the distinct margins of a branchial cyst can be partially or completely lost and the demarcation from the sternocleidomastoid muscle becomes indistinct when an acute super-infection intervenes. CCDS shows considerable hyperperfusion of the tissue periphery. The internal echotexture is inhomogeneous with echogenic secretory elements (**Fig. 8.28**; ▶ Videos 8.11, 8.12).

Thyroglossal Duct Cysts and Fistulas

The pathogenesis of thyroglossal duct cysts and fistulas, lying in the midline, is closely linked to the embryonic development of the thyroid gland in the neck. The frequently extremely elastic space-occupying lesions found in the midline between the chin and the thyroid gland (very rarely, also suprasternally) are usually noted during or after an infection. Thyroglossal duct fistulas become apparent from the opening found at the level of the superior thyroid notch and the secretions released at this point: infections with corresponding purulent secretions and abscess formation may occur.

As expected, B-mode ultrasonography shows the cysts lying in close anatomical proximity to the hyoid bone (**Figs. 8.29, 8.30**; ▶ Video 8.13). The cyst sac is situated caudal, cranial, anterior, and/or posterior to the hyoid bone. The extent of a sinus or cyst can be determined precisely during the preoperative planning; how far it extends into the base of the tongue can be assessed without difficulty in the transverse and longitudinal ultrasound views. The differential diagnosis includes cysts originating from the base of the tongue and larnygoceles.

Other Benign Tumors

The ultrasound characteristics of **benign tumors** in the floor of the mouth, tongue and oropharynx are no different from the findings for similar tumors elsewhere in the head and neck.

Lipomas, **hemangiomas**, and **lymphangiomas** can be assessed in relation to surrounding structures. The surgical approach (transoral or transcervical) can be selected on the basis of the findings. Benign tumors are described in more detail in Chapters 6 and 10.

> **Pearls and Pitfalls**
>
> Solid tumors of the oral cavity, particularly those suspected of being associated with the small salivary glands, are more frequently malignant than tumors of the parotid or submandibular glands.

Salivary gland retention cysts can, similarly to the **ranula**, be identified on the basis of the typical ultrasound criteria for a **cyst** containing clear secretions: they are clearly defined, are homogeneously anechoic, and exhibit a marked distal acoustic enhancement without perfusion on CCDS (**Figs. 8.31, 8.32**). This usually makes it possible to distinguish a cyst from a solid thyroid tumor.

The hour-glass figure of a "**plunging ranula**" extends outward through the muscles of the floor of the mouth to the submandibular bed. The possibility of an **epidermoid cyst** should be considered if the constellation of features consists of the typical site for a ranula together with an echogenic internal echo pattern (**Figs. 8.33, 8.34**; ▶ Video 8.14).

A hypoechoic, cloud-shaped extension of the base of the tongue with central echogenic reflections corresponds to the endoscopic finding of lymphatic hyperplasia of the **lingual tonsil** (**Fig. 8.35**).

Cystic changes in the base of the tongue must be assessed in relation to the hyoid bone to distinguish a **tongue-base cyst** from a **thyroglossal duct cyst** (**Fig. 8.36**).

If a space-occupying lesion that appears homogeneously hyperechoic is found at the base of the tongue, the possibility of ectopic thyroid tissue has to be considered (**Fig. 8.37**). This may show marked perfusion on CCDS.

> **Pearls and Pitfalls**
>
> Ectopic thyroid tissue of clinical relevance is frequently found in patients following a thyroidectomy. Surgical removal of this tissue may result in a hormonal insufficiency.

Solid benign tumors are rare and can often be falsely identified as cysts (**Figs. 8.38, 8.39**).

Malignant Tumors

Malignant tumors are seen on ultrasound examination as hypoechoic and inhomogeneous lesions. Their margins are frequently ill defined, although this is not an essential sonographic sign of malignant growth seen with ultrasound. As already indicated, the diagnosis must be confirmed on histology.

Ultrasonography helps to determine the approximate size and extension of most primary tumors prior to therapy.

The location of solid nonneoplastic and malignant lesions in relation to the middle of the tongue is of great importance from a surgical point of view (**Figs. 8.40, 8.41, 8.42, 8.43, 8.44**). The relationship of a carcinoma of the tongue or floor of the mouth to the midline can be assessed better by ultrasound, even for tumors growing submucosally, as these are occasionally wrongly assessed on clinical examination. In addition, ultrasonography can be used to demonstrate the relationship of the malignant growth to the lateral pharyngeal wall. It can also be determined whether there is any direct tumor invasion ("per continuitatem") to the soft tissues of the neck (**Figs. 8.45, 8.46, 8.47**).

In malignant disease of the tongue base and/or supraglottic region, ultrasonography can also show whether there is any infiltration of the preepiglottic fat (**Fig. 8.48**; see also **Figs. 8.7, 12.1, 12.19**).

Alterations of bony structures—malignant infiltration in particular—cannot usually be assessed on ultrasonography. Other methods of diagnostic imaging (CT and MRI) have to be used in these cases and whenever the full extent of the primary tumor cannot be demonstrated because of its size.

As well as in examination of the primary tumor, ultrasound scanning of the relevant lymphatic drainage is also very important (see Chapter 3, **Fig. 3.12**).

Ultrasonography allows the early detection of recurrence in tissues that are edematous (lymphedema), scarred, and fibrotic after cancer treatment (**Fig. 8.49**).

Both local and regional recurrences, which very often may not be detected on palpation in the early stages, can be seen as hypoechoic lesions that usually have ill-defined, but occasionally distinct, margins (**Figs. 8.50, 8.51, 8.52**). In the follow-up of patients with cancer, comparison with earlier images to note any possible dynamic changes in the tissues is absolutely essential for ultrasound findings that are difficult to interpret (recurrence versus scarring) and the subsequent application of the therapeutic algorithm (see Chapter 6, p. 83).

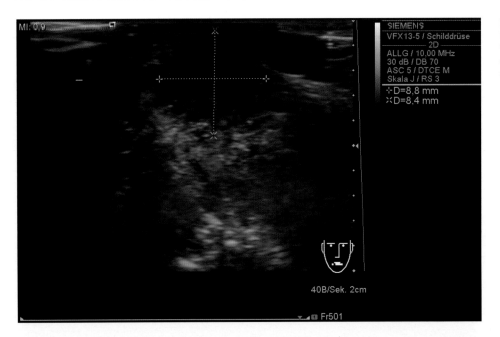

Fig. 8.1 Tongue, intraoral, transverse. There is a hypoechoic space-occupying lesion in the tip of the tongue, at the transition to the back of the tongue. It measures 9 mm × 8 mm and extends with ill-defined margins into the muscle. Diagnosis: **Angioma**.

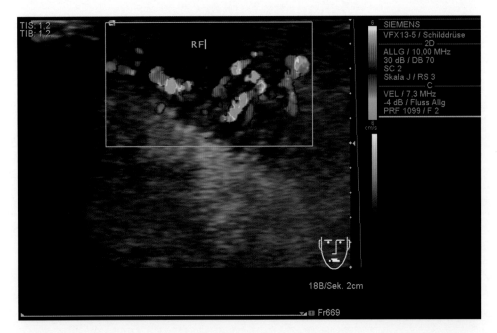

Fig. 8.2 Tongue, intraoral, transverse, CCDS. Color Doppler sonography shows strong perfusion of the mass, which suggests that it is an **angioma**.

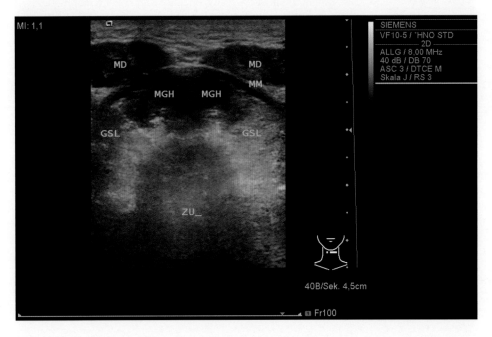

Fig. 8.3 Floor of the mouth, anterior transverse. The anterior belly of the digastric muscle (MD) can be seen on both sides in the transverse view. Below them is the tent-shaped mylohyoid muscle (MM). Deeper still is the hypoechoic geniohyoid muscle (MGH). The sublingual glands (GSL) can be seen laterally in the floor of the mouth, lying medial to the mandible. ZU, body of the tongue. Diagnosis: **Normal findings**.

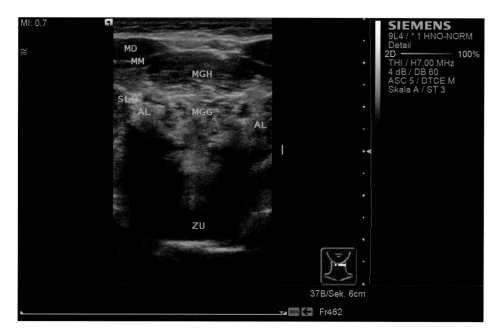

Fig. 8.4 Tongue, midline, transverse. The body of the tongue (ZU), horseshoe shaped in cross-section, can be seen with the landmarks of the floor of the mouth: the digastric muscle (MD), the geniohyoid muscle (MGH), the more echogenic genioglossus muscle (MGG) below and the mylohyoid muscle (MM). Lying laterally at the base of the tongue are the paired sublingual glands (SLG). The lingual arteries (AL), intersected transversely or obliquely in the body of the tongue, can be identified by their pulsation. Diagnosis: **Normal findings**.

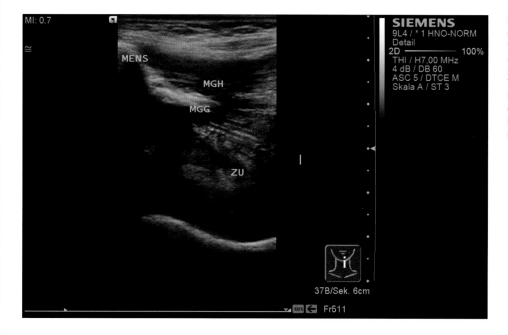

Fig. 8.5 Tongue, midline, longitudinal. The point of the chin (MENS) and the anterior insertions of the muscles of the floor of the mouth can be seen at the left edge of the image, with the geniohyoid muscle (MGH) and genioglossus muscle (MGG). The tongue muscles (ZU) per se are hypoechoic but permeated with a filigree of echogenic stripes (muscle fiber bundles). The surface of the tongue is easily identified by its echogenic contour. Diagnosis: **Normal findings**.

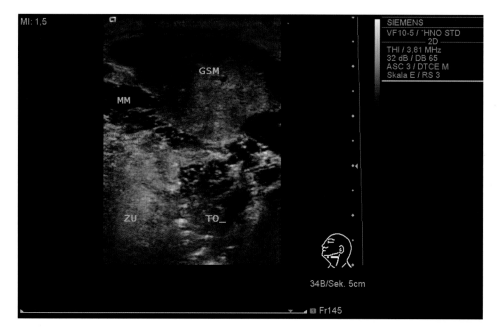

Fig. 8.6 Submandibular region, left, transverse. The tonsillar bed can best be assessed in this classic view. The submandibular gland (GSM) and the border of the tongue (ZU) form a triangle, within which the tonsil (TO) can be identified as a hypoechoic structure. Anteriorly, the muscles of the floor of the mouth, including the mylohyoid muscle (MM), separate the bed of the submandibular gland from the tongue. Diagnosis: **Normal findings**.

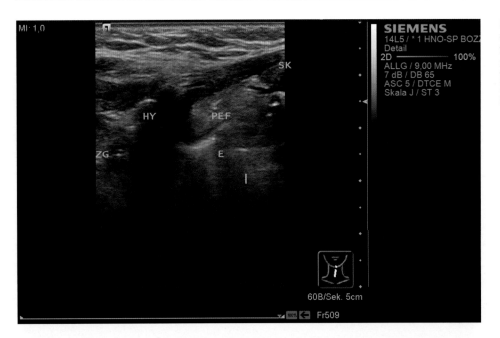

Fig. 8.7 Base of the tonque, lonqitudinal. The pre-epiglottic fat (PEF) is found in the area between the base of the tongue (ZG), the hyoid (HY), the upper edge of the thyroid cartilage (SK) and the epiglottis (E). Above this can be seen the hypoechoic band of the prelaryngeal muscles. Diagnosis: **Normal findings**.

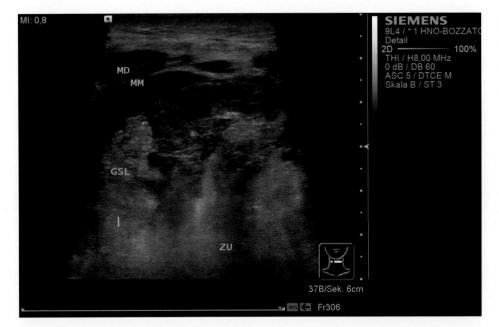

Fig. 8.8 Floor of the mouth, midline, transverse. **Phlegmon**. The muscles (MM, MD) and the adjacent tissues, such as the sublingual gland (GSL), are hypoechoic, loosely structured and clearly enlarged. There is no anechoic formation with distal acoustic enhancement, such as would be seen with an abscess. ZU, tongue. Diagnosis: **Normal findings**.

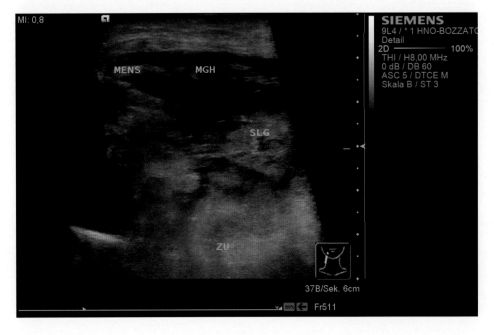

Fig. 8.9 Floor of the mouth, midline, longitudinal. **Phlegmon**. Besides the muscles of the floor of the mouth (MGH) and the sublingual gland (SLG), the muscles of the tongue (ZU) are also hypoechoic and loosely structured due to inflammatory infiltration. MENS, point of the chin.

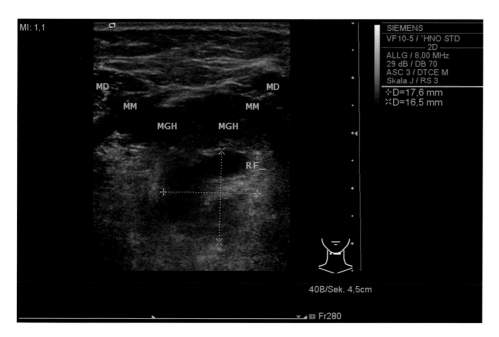

Fig. 8.10 Floor of the mouth, midline, transverse. Left-sided abscess. In contrast to a phlegmon, an **abscess** can be seen as a circumscribed hypoechoic area (RF) with ill-defined inhomogeneous contours. Muscle elements can be clearly distinguished in this view. MD, digastric muscle; MGH, geniohyoid muscle; MM, mylohyoid muscle.

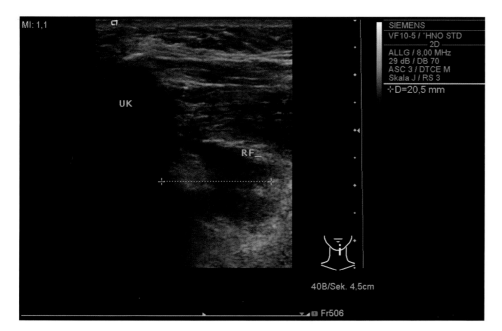

Fig. 8.11 Floor of the mouth, midline, longitudinal. **Left-sided abscess.** The longitudinal view confirms the circumscribed sagittal extent of the inflammatory process (RF) and its relation to the point of the chin (UK).

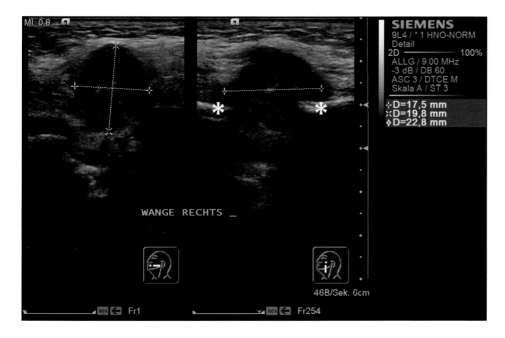

Fig. 8.12 Split screen—mandibular arch, left. The spread of a **dental abscess** has led to the destruction of the horizontal ramus of the mandible.

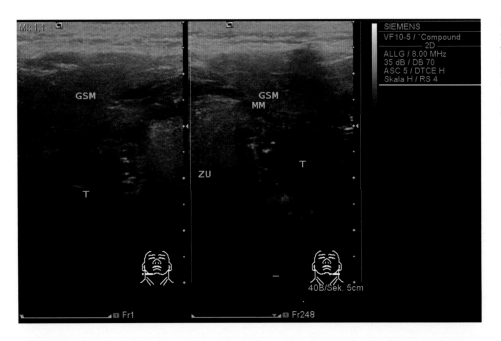

Fig. 8.13 Split screen—submandibular region, transverse. With the clinical picture of **acute tonsillitis**, the two tonsils (T) are enlarged, but show no significant difference in size. However, the acute infection causes the demarcation from the surrounding tissues to become less clear. MM, mylohyoid muscle; GSM, submandibular gland; ZU, tongue.

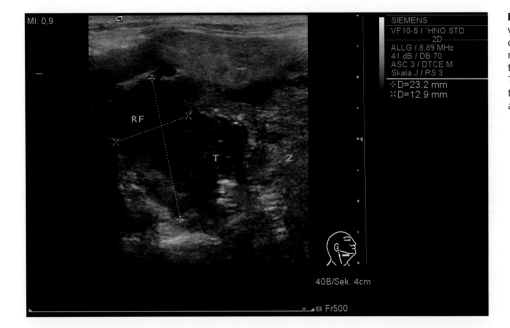

Fig. 8.14 Submandibular region, right, transverse. Even without comparing the two sides, close observation of the right tonsil (T) reveals a mediolateral anechoic **abscess** zone (RF) within the tonsil, showing distal acoustic enhancement. The solid horizontal striped texture of the tonsil that can still be seen medially is elevated by the abscess formation. Z, tongue.

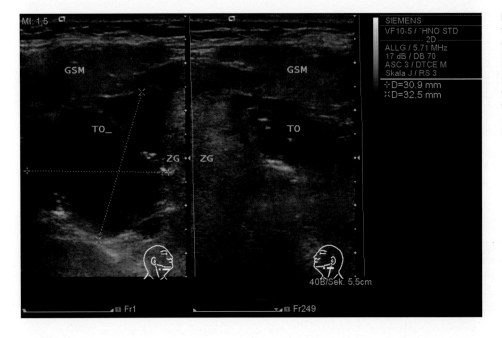

Fig. 8.15 Split screen—submandibular region, transverse. Compared with the small tonsil (TO) on the left side, a lateral anechoic area with an irregular margin is easily discerned in the tonsillar bed on the right. The medial border with the base of the tongue (ZG) can be seen better than the lateral, but it is possible to determine that the lesion measures ~30 mm × 30 mm in the two planes. GSM, submandibular gland. Diagnosis: **Peritonsilar abscess**.

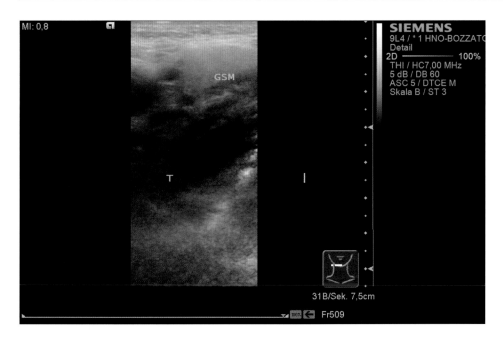

Fig. 8.16 Submandibular bed, right, transverse. A parapharyngeal abscess can be seen on the right, extending from a **peritonsillar abscess** (T); it is demarcated medially from the submandibular gland (GSM).

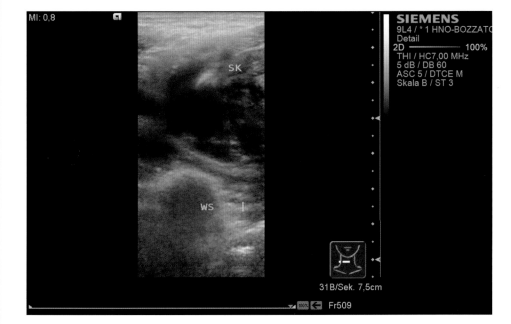

Fig. 8.17 Right side of the neck, paralaryngeal, transverse. The **parapharyngeal abscess** can be demonstrated extending caudally to the level of the right lateral edge of the thyroid cartilage (SK), seen here as a hypoechoic band. The ultrasound morphology of the abscess shows a hypoechoic to anechoic area with distal acoustic enhancement. WS, anterior surface of the vertebral body.

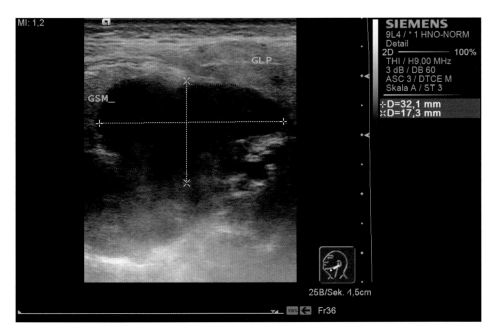

Fig. 8.18 Left side of the neck, paralaryngeal, transverse. A **parapharyngeal dental abscess** on the left at level II, bordering the parotid gland (GLP) and submandibular gland (GSM). The abscess has a cloud-shaped contour and is hypoechoic to anechoic with distal acoustic enhancement. The dynamic assessment reveals fluid within the abscess cavity; moving particles can be seen when pressure is applied with the probe and this effect is related to vascular pulsations.

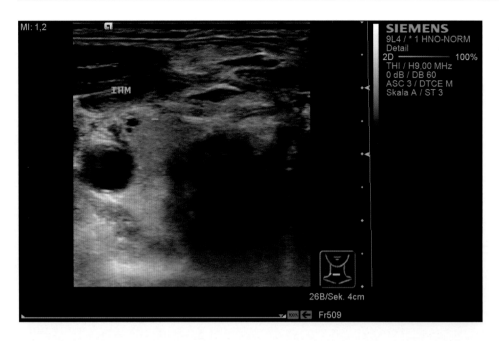

Fig. 8.19 Right side of the neck, transverse, level IV. A **phlegmon** in the parapharyngeal space. An ill-defined mass can be seen lying medial to the thyroid gland and infrahyoid muscles (IHM). The margins of the muscles and thyroid gland appear poorly defined and diffuse. The phlegmon has descended along the fascial spaces and obliterated margins of the muscles and thyroid gland, which appear poorly defined and blurred.

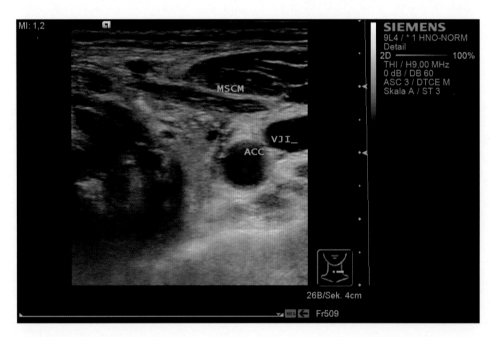

Fig. 8.20 Left side of the neck, transverse, level IV. Demarcation of the muscles and the thyroid gland appears ill defined and diffuse. The **phlegmon** has extended into the neighbouring tissues blurring their boundaries; medial to the thyroid gland, the transition to the parapharyngeal space can only be surmised. ACC, common carotid artery; VJI, internal jugular vein; MSCM, sternocleidomastoid muscle.

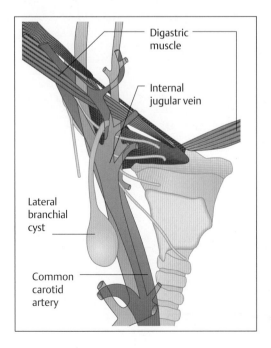

Fig. 8.21 Lateral cervical (branchial) **cyst** (second branchial cleft). The structure demonstrated in the image is found at the most common site for branchial cysts in the neck. Strictly speaking in this case, it is a lateral internal sinus of the neck arising from the second branchial cleft. The internal opening is in the supratonsillar fossa. From: Probst R, Grevers G, Iro H. Basic Otorhinolaryngology. Stuttgart: Thieme; 2006.

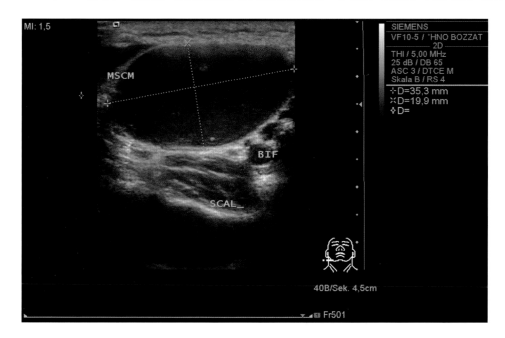

Fig. 8.22 Right side of the neck, transverse. A **branchial cyst** in the neck with an oval, clearly defined morphology and distal acoustic enhancement. The cyst lies laterally to the arteries (BIF); the jugular vein is compressed by the pressure of the ultrasound probe and is not visible. The cyst is bordered laterally by the sternocleidomastoid muscle (MSCM), while the scalene muscle (SCAL) can be seen distinctly in the deeper tissues.

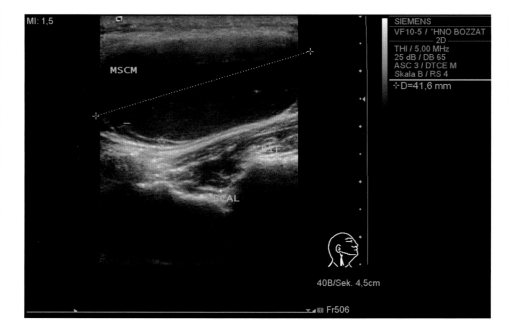

Fig. 8.23 Right side of the neck, longitudinal. The extent of the oval **cyst** with well-defined margins is clearly seen in the longitudinal view (40 mm). The cyst is bordered laterally by the sternocleidomastoid muscle (MSCM), while the scalene muscle (SCAL) can be seen distinctly in the deeper tissues.

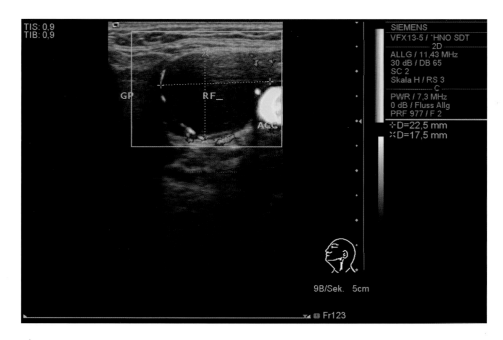

Fig. 8.24 Left side of the neck, longitudinal. **Lateral cysts of the neck** often lie cranially to the parotid gland (GP) and/or are bordered by the submandibular gland. No perfusion into the lumen of the classic, noninfected branchial cyst (RF) is seen on CCDS. ACC, common carotid artery.

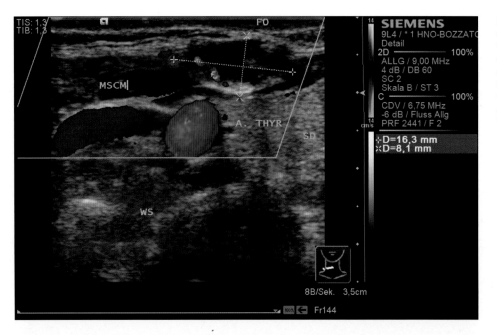

Fig. 8.25 Right side of the neck, transverse, CCDS. From its opening on the skin, a **branchial fistula** can be identified as a hypoechoic, clearly defined oval structure in the subcutaneous tissue, depending on how full it is. CCDS distinguishes it from a subcutaneous vein. A. THYR, superior thyroid artery; FO, fistula opening; MSCM, sternocleidomastoid muscle; SD, thyroid gland; WS, spine.

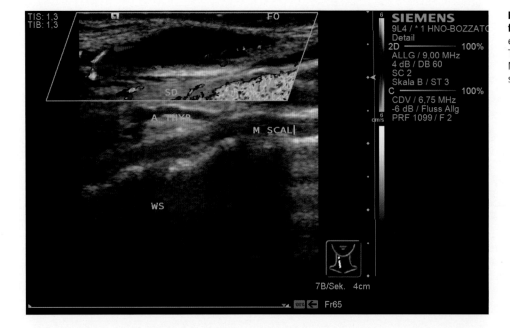

Fig. 8.26 Right side of the neck, longitudinal. The **fistula**, first seen in the cutaneous tissues, can be easily identified as such in the longitudinal view. A. THYR, superior thyroid artery; FO, fistula opening; M. SCAL, scalene muscle; SD, thyroid gland; WS, spine.

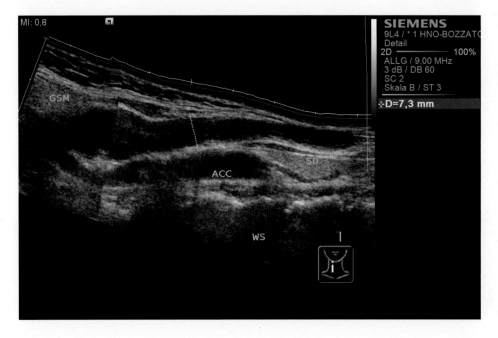

Fig. 8.27 Right side of the neck, longitudinal, panoramic view. The full extent of a **branchial fistula**, running past the submandibular gland (GSM) and as far as the oropharynx, can be seen with the aid of a panoramic procedure; a panoramic view is particularly suitable to demonstrate the entire length of such a lesion. ACC, common carotid artery; WS, spine.

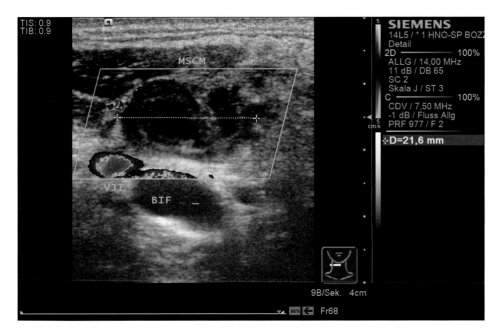

Fig. 8.28 Right side of the neck, transverse. A 39-year-old patient presenting with redness and swelling on the right side of the neck. On ultrasonography, an oval, hypoechoic, inhomogeneous space-occupying lesion can be seen at the anterior border of the sternocleidomastoid muscle (MSCM), medial to the carotid bifurcation and the internal jugular vein (VJI). As in previous examples, CCDS shows no intrinsic perfusion. Toward the midline, the **cyst** cannot be distinguished from the surrounding tissues. BIF, carotid bifurcation.

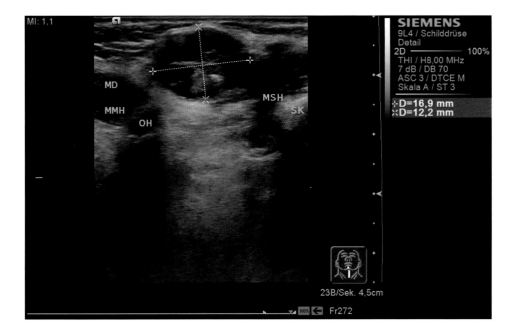

Fig. 8.29 Neck, midline, longitudinal. A midline **thyroglossal duct cyst** has an anechoic lumen with echogenic septa seen inside the cyst. The cyst lies subcutaneously, between the hyoid bone (OH) and the upper edge of the thyroid cartilage (SK). MD, digastric muscle; MMH, mylohyoid muscle; MSH, sternothyroid muscle.

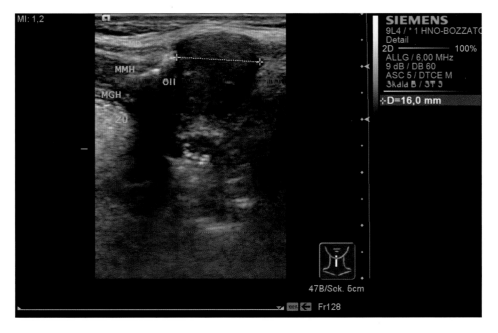

Fig. 8.30 Neck, midline, longitudinal. Depending on its consistency, a **cyst in the neck** may also show echogenic contents, which indicates increased viscosity of the secretions. The cyst lies between the hyoid bone (OH) and the upper edge of the thyroid cartilage. The cyst points behind and under the posterior surface of the hyoid. A subcutaneous opening cannot be ruled out with the ultrasound scan. MD, digastric muscle; MGH, geniohyoid muscle; MMH, mylohyoid muscle; ZU, tongue.

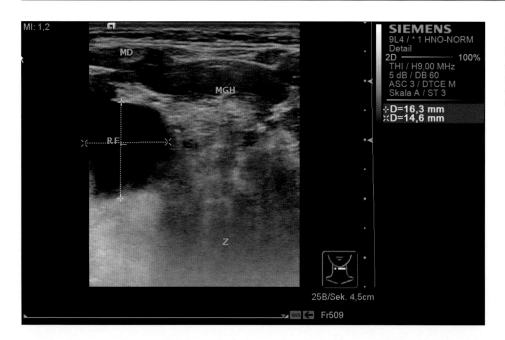

Fig. 8.31 Floor of the mouth, transverse. A right-sided spherical, anechoic space-occupying lesion in the floor of the mouth, seen with the digastric muscle (MD) and the geniohyoid muscle (MGH), shows the clearly defined margins and distal acoustic enhancement characteristic of the **ranula**. Z, tongue.

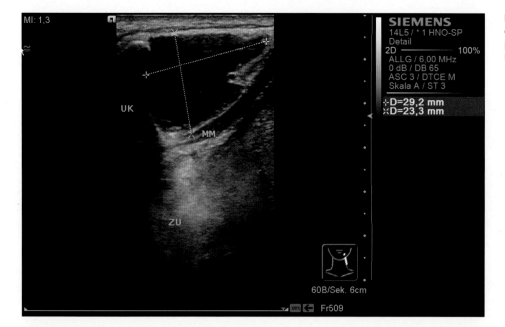

Fig. 8.32 Floor of the mouth, longitudinal oblique. In this view, the **ranula** lies between the point of the chin (UK), the tongue (Z) and the mylohyoid muscle (MM).

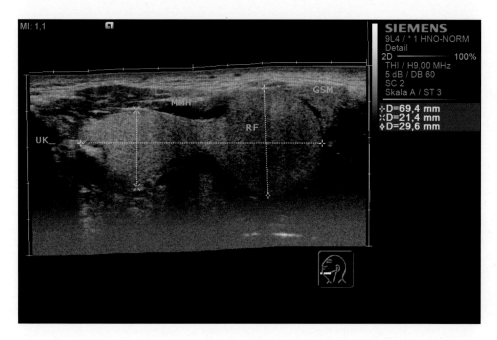

Fig. 8.33 Submandibular region, left, transverse. The hour-glass–shaped space-occupying lesion (RF) lies between the submandibular gland (GSM) and the mandible (UK). It shows an unusually echogenic pattern, although in shape and site it has the typical features of a **plunging ranula**. In fact, in this case, it is an epidermoid cyst, consistent with the firm pastelike consistency found intraoperatively.

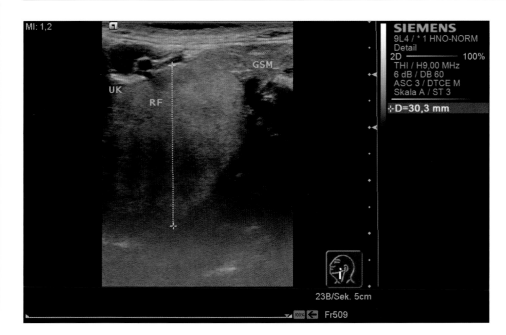

Fig. 8.34 Submandibular region, left, longitudinal oblique. The **epidermoid cyst** has a triangular appearance caudally on the upper pole of the submandibular gland. It demonstrates an anteroposterior extension of 30 mm. UK, mandible.

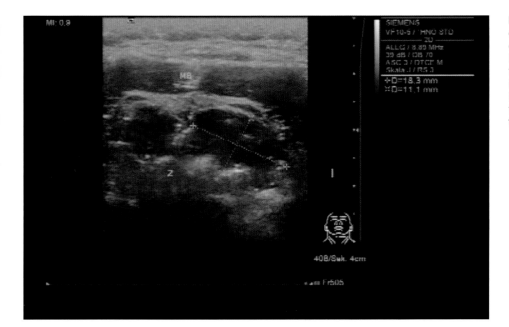

Fig. 8.35 Base of the tongue, transverse. The base of the tongue is hypoechoic and more prominent/curved on the left side than on the right. The irregular echogenic border of the tongue (Z) toward the lumen, seen in the deeper tissues, is due to increased impedance at the air–tissue interface. MB, posterior muscles of the floor of the mouth. Diagnosis: **Hyperplasia of the lingual tonsil**.

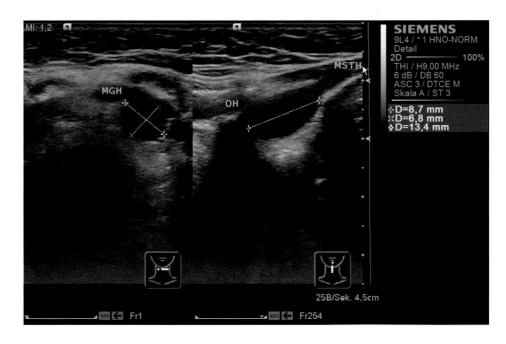

Fig. 8.36 Split screen—base of the tongue. The left-sided paramedian anechoic space-occupying lesion seen in the right half of the picture can be identified as a **cyst** from its clearly defined margins and the distal acoustic enhancement; the longitudinal view on the left indicates its position below the hyoid. MGH, geniohyoid muscle; MSTH, sternothyrohyoid muscle; OH, hyoid bone.

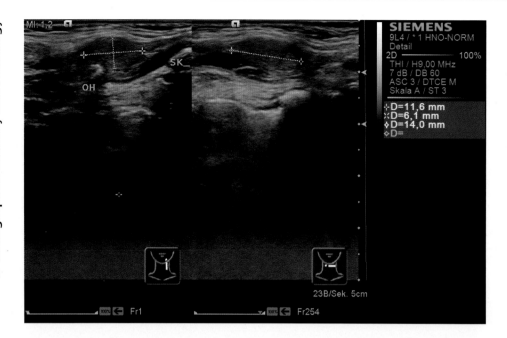

Fig. 8.37 Split screen—base of the tongue. The left longitudinal view shows an oval echogenic lesion with clearly defined margins. It lies anterior and caudal to the hyoid bone (OH) and cranial to the thyroid cartilage (SK). The transverse view confirms the oval shape and good demarcation. Diagnosis: **Ectopic thyroid tissue**.

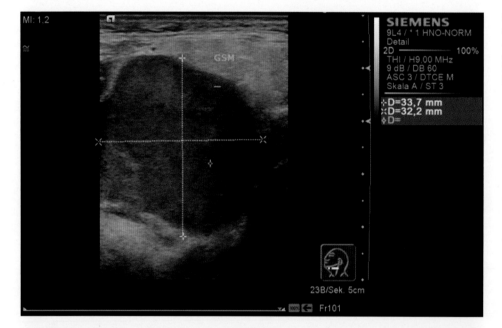

Fig. 8.38 Level IB, left, transverse. In the submandibular space a hypoechoic lesion with a round shape and distinct margins, apparently originating from the floor of the mouth, extends into the neck. A ranula was suspected at first (see **Fig. 8.37**).

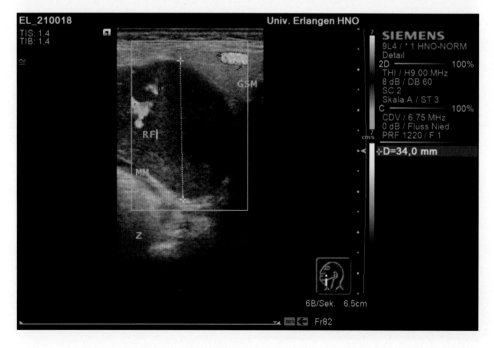

Fig. 8.39 Level IB, left, transverse. Activation of CCDS revealed an irregular perfusion, so a cyst could be excluded. During surgery a solid tumor could be completely extirpated. Histological diagnosis was **rhabdomyoma**.

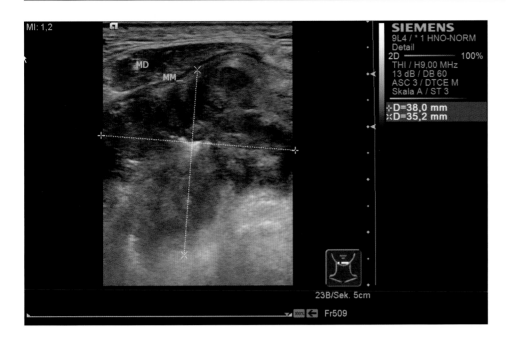

Fig. 8.40 Floor of the mouth, anterior transverse. **Carcinoma, cT3** (caliper). An irregular hypoechoic tumor of the floor of the mouth can be seen crossing the midline and infiltrating the tongue. MD, digastric muscle; MM, mylohyoid muscle.

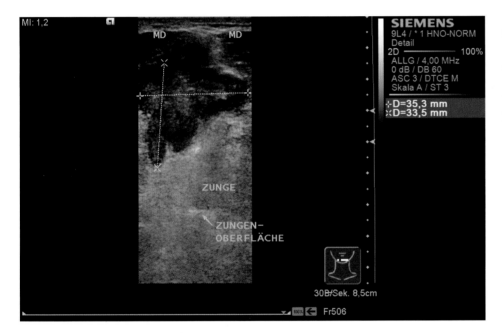

Fig. 8.41 Floor of the mouth, transverse. **Carcinoma, cT3**. The tumor of the floor of the mouth is infiltrating the basal intrinsic muscles of the tongue and is also crossing the midline. The position of the midline can be determined by looking for the line separating the bellies of the two digastric muscles. MD, digastric muscle, ZUNGE, tongue, ZUNGENOBERFLÄCHE, surface of the tongue.

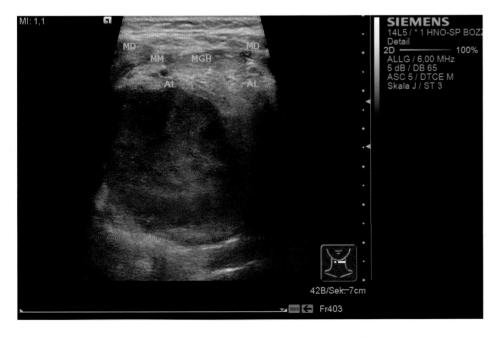

Fig. 8.42 Tongue, transverse. A space-occupying lesion, measuring more than 30 mm, at the right edge of the tongue crosses the midline of the tongue near the surface. The lesion is inhomogeneously hypoechoic and does not have distinct contours. MGH, geniohyoid muscle; MD, digastric muscle; MM, mylohyoid muscle; AL, lingual artery. Diagnosis: **Carcinoma of the tongue, crossing the midline**.

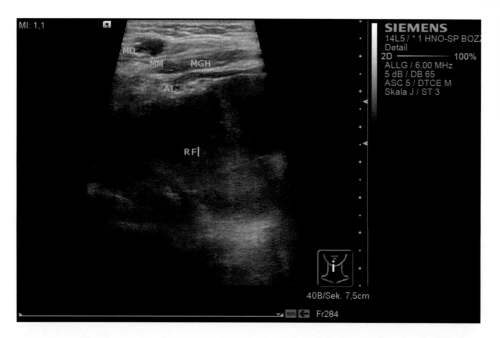

Fig. 8.43 Tongue, longitudinal. The longitudinal view demonstrates the almost 40 mm anteroposterior extension of the tumour (RF) in the base of the tongue. It is even more obvious here that the margins are ill defined. MGH, geniohyoid muscle; MD, digastric muscle; MM, mylohyoid muscle; AL, lingual artery. Diagnosis: **Carcinoma of the tongue**.

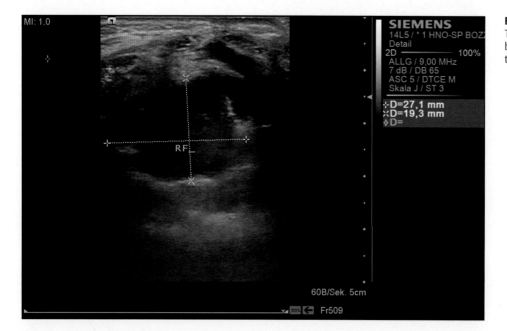

Fig. 8.44 Floor of the mouth, midline transverse. The inhomogeneous hypoechoic lesion seen in the base of the tongue is a **carcinoma**; the primary tumor measures 27 mm × 19 mm.

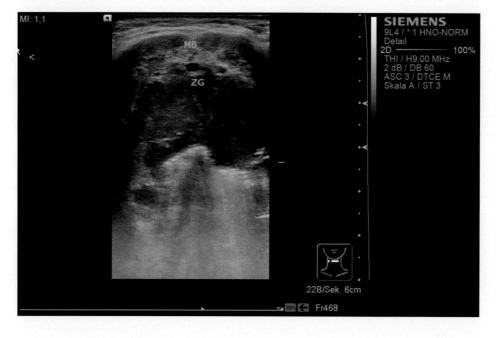

Fig. 8.45 Floor of the mouth, midline, transverse. **cT3 carcinoma of the tongue** extending into the tongue base (ZG). Hypoechoic, inhomogeneous margins. Superficially, the muscles of the floor of the mouth (MB) seem to be separate from the tumor.

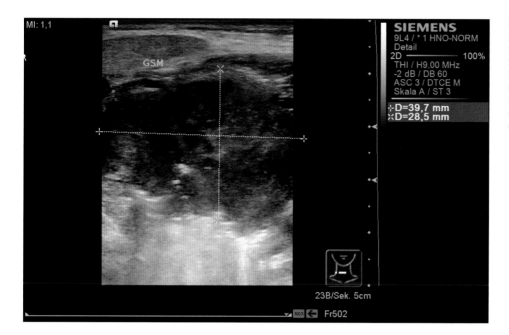

Fig. 8.46 Floor of the mouth, midline, transverse. **cT3 carcinoma of the tongue** extending into the tongue base and floor of the mouth, and invading the soft tissues of the neck. Hypoechoicity and inhomogeneity provide distinction from the submandibular gland (GSM), although this is still separated from the tumor by a muscle margin. The extensive lateral growth raises a strong suspicion of direct spread into the neck.

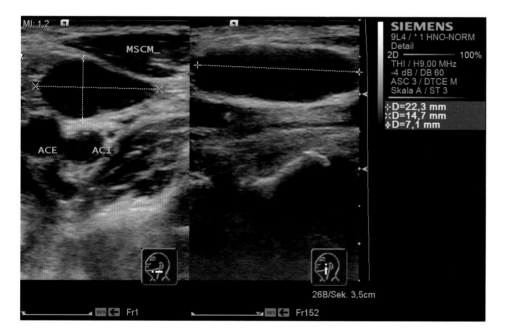

Fig. 8.47 Split screen—left side of neck, level III. Contralateral lymph node seen to be oval in shape but with abnormally turbulent internal echoes. ACI, internal carotid artery; ACE, external carotid artery; MSCM, sternocleidomastoid muscle. Diagnosis: **Carcinoma of the tongue, suspected regional metastasis**.

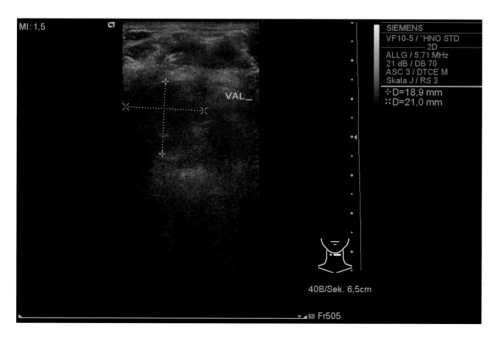

Fig. 8.48 Base of the tongue, midline, transverse. When comparing the two sides at the level of the tongue base (VAL), the ill-defined margins of a T1 **carcinoma of the vallecula**, measuring 19 mm × 21 mm, with inhomogeneous internal echoes can be made out on the right just below the hyoid bone (not actually visible in this transverse view).

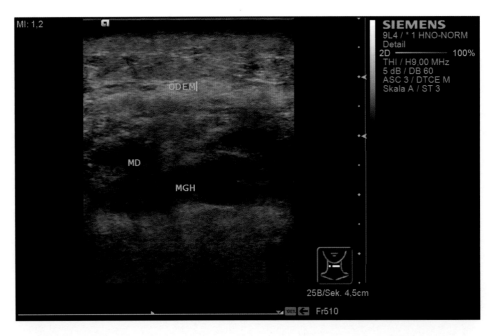

Fig. 8.49 Floor of the mouth, transverse anterior. **Lymphatic edema (ODEM) after radiotherapy.** The subcutaneous tissues are echogenic and thickened following radiation therapy. The blocked lymphatic drainage channels can be seen as hypoechoic cloud-shaped loose tissue structures. Another characteristic feature is the reduction in contrast of individual structures such as the muscles of the floor of the mouth. MD, digastric muscle, MGH, geniohyoid muscle.

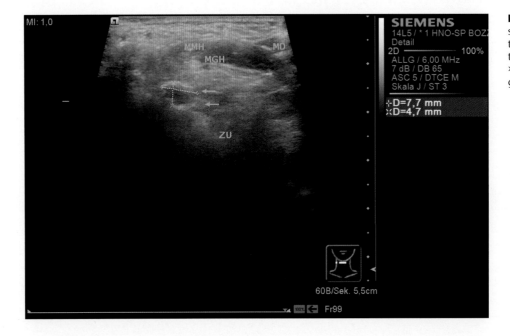

Fig. 8.50 Floor of the mouth, transverse. Right-sided **recurrence of carcinoma** of the floor of the mouth. Within the body of the tongue (ZU), there is a new hypoechoic lesion measuring 7 mm × 5 mm (arrows). MD, digastric muscle; MGH, geniohyoid muscle; MMH, mylohyoid muscle.

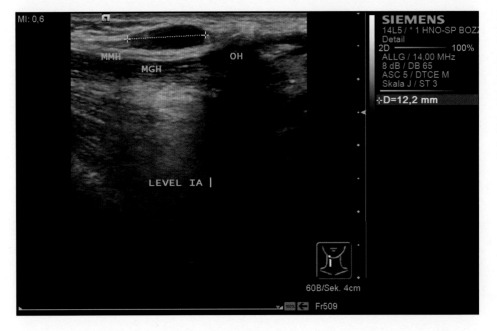

Fig. 8.51 Right side of the floor of the mouth, longitudinal. Right-sided recurrence of carcinoma of the floor of the mouth. In relation to this recurrence, there is highly **suspicious lymph node enlargement**. Although the configuration of the node concerned is oval and the margins are clearly defined, it contains an anechoic area. On the basis of its position in the lymphatic drainage channels of the tongue and the appearance of its internal echoes, this lymph node is to be classified as a metastasis. MGH, geniohyoid muscle; MMH, mylohyoid muscle; OH, hyoid bone.

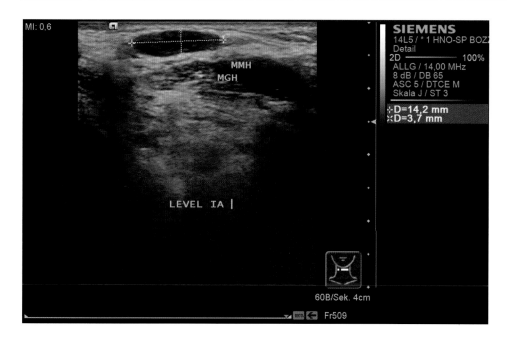

Fig. 8.52 Right side of the floor of the mouth, transverse. MGH, geniohyoid muscle; MMH, mylohyoid muscle.

9   Salivary Glands

Anatomy

Thanks to their superficial location, the three major salivary glands—the parotid, the submandibular, and the sublingual glands—are easily accessible to ultrasound examination. As a basic rule, the glands addressed in this chapter are seen as solid, homogeneous, echogenic structures with clearly defined margins and similar to the thyroid gland in appearance (**Fig. 9.1**).

Parotid Gland

In the transverse plane, the parotid gland is a smoothly contoured, homogeneous, echogenic organ. It can be clearly distinguished from the subcutaneous fatty tissues. The anterior superficial lobe of the gland lies on the masseter muscle. The anterior end of the muscle can be differentiated from the hypoechoic buccal fat pad by getting the patient to contract and relax the muscles of mastication. Bordered anteriorly by the ascending ramus of the mandible and posteriorly by the mastoid and the sternocleidomastoid muscle, the main lobe of the gland lies in the retromandibular fossa. The posterior belly of the digastric muscle, the internal carotid artery, and the internal jugular vein can be identified lying mediocaudally to the lower pole of the parotid (**Figs. 9.2, 9.3**; ▶ Video 9.1). The retromandibular vein lying in the parenchyma of the gland can be seen particularly well in the longitudinal view (▶ Video 9.2). In the transverse view, the styloid process often projects beneath the vein as a hyperechogenic reflection in the parenchyma of the gland.

Pearls and Pitfalls

The hyperechoic signals from the styloid process may be mistaken for a salivary stone.

With the high-resolution transducers currently available (7.5–18 MHz), it is also possible to demonstrate part of the parotid duct (Stensen duct) with ultrasound. However, it is generally not possible to see the duct clearly in the course of routine examinations if it is not obstructed.

Pearls and Pitfalls

The facial nerve itself and lymph nodes within the gland that are not enlarged are not visible on an ultrasound scan.

Submandibular Gland

In the longitudinal view, the submandibular gland has a pinecone-shaped appearance in the submandibular trigone, reaching cranially to the mandible and the mylohyoid muscle; it lies in close proximity to the anterior belly of the digastric muscle, as well as to the tongue and tonsillar bed (**Figs. 9.4, 9.5, 9.6**; ▶ Video 9.3).

The submandibular gland arches over the posterior border of the mylohyoid muscle and often extends as far as the sublingual gland in the ventromedial direction as an "uncinate process."

Pearls and Pitfalls

An echogenic structure with distal acoustic shadowing can occasionally be seen projecting into the hilum of the submandibular gland. This could be either part of the hyoid bone or a salivary stone and these must be differentiated. The hyoid bone can be seen to move on swallowing, which helps to distinguish between the two.

The ultrasound appearance of the submandibular gland is echogenic with a uniform texture, similar to the parenchymal echo pattern of the parotid gland (**Fig. 9.7**). Using a high-resolution ultrasound probe, segments of the submandibular (Wharton) duct can sometimes be seen even when it is not obstructed. Toward the mandible, where it runs close to the surface, the facial vein can be seen where it joins the internal jugular vein and can be compressed with the probe. The facial artery and vein, which can be demonstrated clearly on ultrasound, cross over the posterior part of the gland. The facial artery, originating from the external carotid artery, reaches the posterior margin of the gland or runs through the parenchyma in the shape of a walking stick (**Fig. 9.8**; ▶ Video 9.4).

Sublingual Gland

It can sometimes be difficult to demonstrate the sublingual gland. The gland lies typically beneath the mucosa of the floor of the mouth, close to the frenulum, with the tip of the tongue lying above it. The posterior aspect of this gland, the smallest of the three major salivary glands, often touches the submandibular gland. The anterior and medial borders are formed by the geniohyoid and genioglossus muscles, with the mandible lying caudolaterally (**Fig. 9.9a**; ▶ Video 9.5a).

Gaps in the musculature of the floor of the mouth may lead to a prolapse of the sublingual gland outwards (**Fig. 9.9b** and ▶ Video 9.5b).

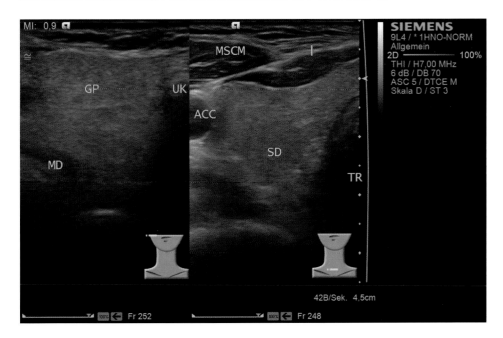

Fig. 9.1 Split screen of the thyroid (SD) and parotid gland (GP) on the left. Both solid glands show a similar homogeneous hyperechoic pattern of internal echoes. ACC, common carotid artery; MD, digastric muscle; MSCM, sternocleidomastoid muscle; TR, trachea; UK, mandible.

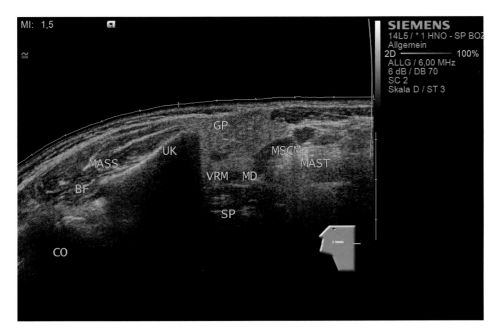

Fig. 9.2 Panoramic view of the parotid bed (GP), left, transverse. The anterior lobes of the parotid gland lie on the masseter muscle (MASS); the anterior border with the oral cavity (CO) can be identified medially as an echogenic margin. More posteriorly it is bordered by the ascending ramus of the mandible (UK) and further posteriorly by the mastoid and sternocleidomastoid muscle (MSCM). The deep lobe of the gland lies in the retromandibular fossa. The posterior belly of the digastric muscle (MD) and retromandibular vein (VR) are situated deep in the gland parenchyma. BF, buccal fat pad; MAST, mastoid; SP, styloid process.

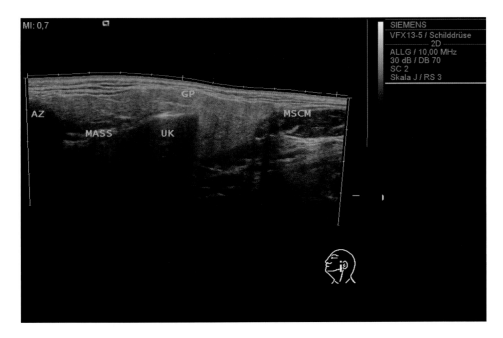

Fig. 9.3 Panoramic view of the parotid bed (GP), left, longitudinal. The zygomatic arch (AZ) forms the cranial border; the sternocleidomastoid muscle (MSCM) flanks the inferior lateral pole caudally. The gland lies medially to the mandible (UK) and the masseter muscle (MASS).

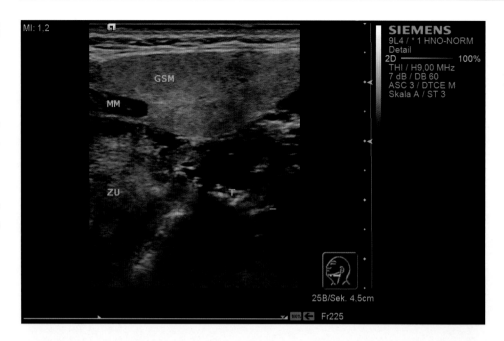

Fig. 9.4 Left transverse view of the submandibular region, showing the left submandibular gland (GSM) in longitudinal section. The anterior extension of the mylohyoid muscle (MM) divides the body of the gland and the uncinate process. The tongue (ZU) and tonsil (T) are immediately adjacent.

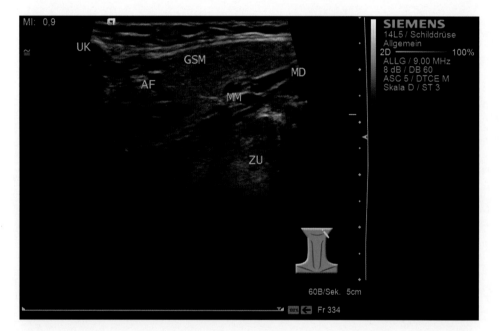

Fig. 9.5 Cross-section of the left submandibular gland (GSM). The probe, however, is held sagittally in the craniocaudal direction. The mylohyoid muscle (MM) and digastric muscle (MD) can be seen clearly. The complete acoustic shadowing of the mandible (UK) forms the cranial/left border of the image. Lying almost immediately adjacent are the tongue (ZU) and tonsillar bed. The muscle fibers of the platysma can be distinguished as a hypoechoic layer, which forms the superficial border. AF, facial artery.

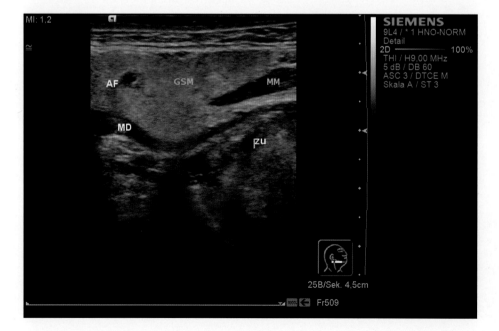

Fig. 9.6 Longitudinal section of the right submandibular gland (GSM). The facial artery (AF) penetrates the posterior part of the gland, while the mylohyoid muscle (MM) tapers off anteriorly in the hilum of the gland. The posterior belly of the digastric muscle (MD) borders the gland at the caudal pole. The immediate vicinity of the oral cavity is clear from the position of the tongue (ZU).

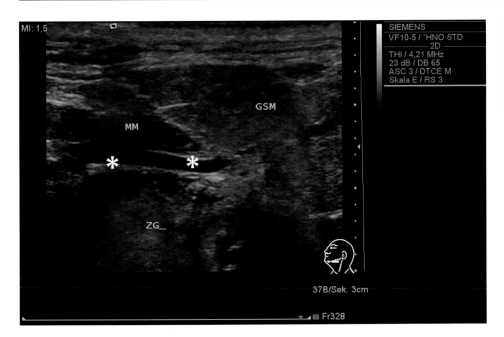

Fig. 9.7 Submandibular region, left, transverse. The parenchymal structure of the submandibular gland (GSM) is unremarkable but shows an anechoic band (asterisk), outlined by an echogenic contour in the hilar region between the mylohyoid muscle (MM) and the tongue (ZG). This was initially suspected to be a **dilated submandibular duct**.

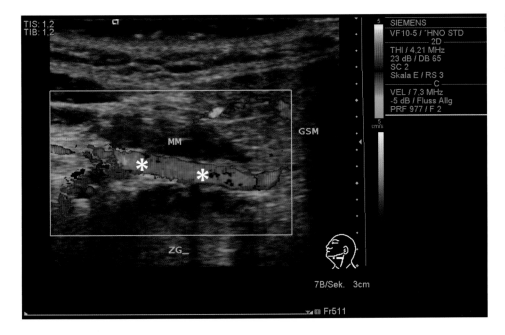

Fig. 9.8 Submandibular region (GSM), left, transverse. After activating the color duplex mode, an artery (asterisk) with clear flow signals can be seen running parallel to the duct. It is very similar in appearance to the duct in the B-mode image. MM, mylohyoid muscle; ZG, tongue.

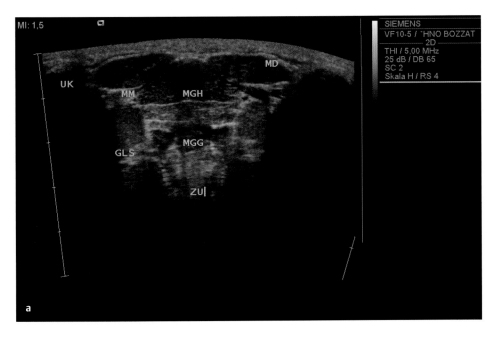

Fig. 9.9a Midline transverse view of the floor of the mouth/mid-tongue. The paired sublingual glands (GLS) lie medial to the inner side of the mandible (UK). The muscles of the floor of the mouth and of the tongue constitute the surrounding structures. MD, digastric muscle; MGG, genioglossus muscle; MGH, geniohyoid muscle; MM, mylohyoid muscle; ZU, tongue.

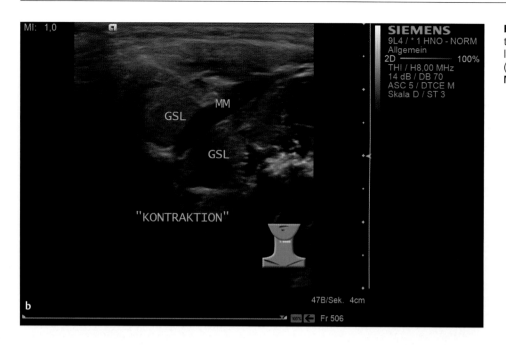

Fig 9.9b Floor of the mouth, paramedian, right, transverse. The right sublingual gland (GSL) is luxated outward through the mylohyoid muscle (MM) by contraction of the tongue. Diagnosis: **Muscular dehiscence of the mylohyoid muscle.**

Inflammatory Changes

Acute Sialadenitis

When the relevant clinical picture calls for further investigation, ultrasonography shows acute sialadenitis as a diffuse enlargement of the entire diseased gland. The organ can usually be distinguished clearly from adjacent structures. The parenchymal pattern appears enlarged, more loosely structured, inhomogeneous, and more hypoechoic than usual (**Figs. 9.10, 9.11, 9.12**; ▶ Video 9.6).

This finding can be attributed to the infection-/inflammation-related increased volume of fluid within the gland. Circumscribed hypoechoic space-occupying lesions can occasionally be seen, providing evidence of an associated inflammatory reaction in the intraglandular lymph nodes. The submandibular gland is the exception here, as no lymph nodes have been described within it. Ultrasonography alone cannot establish whether the parenchymal changes are of bacterial or viral origin. The most common viral agents are paramyxo-, cytomegalo-, coxsackie-, ECHO-. influenza, parainfluenza and human immunodeficiency viruses. For suppurative sialadenitis *Staphhylococcus aureus*, *Streptococcus pneumoniae* and *pyogenes* and *Haemophilius influenzae* are found in many cases. A pus-filled duct can often be demonstrated in suppurative sialadenitis, indicating an obstructive etiology, but it may also occur without any obstruction in patients who are dehydrated (**marantic parotitis**).

Salivary Gland Abscess

Areas of liquefaction appear hypoechoic to anechoic, enclosed by an echogenic wall, with clear distal acoustic enhancement absent of perfusion on color-coded duplex sonography (CCDS) (**Figs. 9.13, 9.14**; ▶ Video 9.7).

Coarse central echoes in the focus of this liquefaction may correspond to necrotic tissue. The palpatoric impression by the ultrasound transducer further undermine a suspected abscess. It is difficult to attribute it to any specific cause (stenosis, calculus) at this stage and it should be investigated further with repeat ultrasound scanning once the acute phase has settled.

Chronic Sialadenitis

The ultrasound appearance of the gland depends significantly on the duration and extent of the infection/inflammation in the parenchyma.

Overall, the echotexture is clearly coarser; the internal echoes appear inhomogeneous, probably as a result of parenchymal fibrosis causing scarring. With advancing functional impairment, the parenchyma becomes more echogenic and shrinks in size. Small cystic areas, consistent with circumscribed duct ectasia, may also appear.

These changes are regularly observed following radiation therapy (**Figs. 9.15, 9.16**) and obstructive sialopathies that have assumed a chronic course (**Fig. 9.17, 9.18, 9.19**).

The various pathogenic causes of chronic sialadenitis cannot be differentiated with certainty with ultrasonography; circumscribed, hypoechoic, clearly defined areas of gland parenchyma may also be histologically consistent with inflammatory foci.

Chronic recurrent juvenile parotitis is a rare condition in childhood and adolescence; and frequently leads to changes in both parotid glands that are visible on ultrasonography (**Fig. 9.20**; ▶ Video 9.8). In the acute stage, the changes are similar to those of acute obstructive sialadenitis. **Chronic recurrent sialadenitis** in adults may look similar to the juvenile form but it is frequently accompanied by visualization of dilated segments of the parotid duct.

A particular type of chronic inflammation in the submandibular gland—**sclerosing sialadenitis (Küttner tumor)**—is often found at the edge of the gland, as a focal hypoechoic, sometimes inhomogeneous lesion within the glandular tissue (**Figs. 9.21, 9.22**).

Ultrasonography of the diseased salivary glands in primary and secondary **Sjögren syndrome** shows the affected glands with an inhomogeneous hypoechoic texture. There are numerous circumscribed hypoechoic lesions that could be either cystic enlargements of the ducts or enlarged intraglandular lymph nodes. The overall appearance is described as "cloudlike" or "leopard skin" (**Figs. 9.23, 9.24, 9.25**; ▶ Video 9.9). With advanced disease, all salivary glands are affected by this **autoimmune sialopathy** and show similar ultrasound changes in the parenchyma.

One particular feature is the presence of intraglandular and cervical lymph nodes, which may indicate the local development of a **MALT lymphoma** (**Fig. 9.26**; ▶ Video 9.10).

> **Pearls and Pitfalls**
>
> Sjögren syndrome, chronic recurrent juvenile parotitis and sarcoidosis present similar images on ultrasound. Diagnosis can be confirmed by clinical presentation and age of the patient.

Epithelioid cell sialadenitis (Heerfordt syndrome) is an acute presentation of **sarcoidosis** characterized by an enlarged gland with an echogenic internal structure, studded with multiple enlarged lymph nodes—corresponding to the hypoechoic areas seen on ultrasonography (**Fig. 9.27**). Strong irregular perfusion is found on CCDS (**Fig. 9.28**). Whenever the condition is accompanied by enlarged cervical lymph nodes, these also show strong hilar perfusion (see also Chapter 6, **Figs 6.3** and **6.7**).

Enlarged Lymph Nodes

Ultrasonography usually shows multiple hypoechoic lesions lying within an unremarkable gland parenchyma. These lesions do not exhibit a marked distal acoustic enhancement. As a rule, the central hyperechoic structure ("hilar sign") can be identified clearly in inflammatory lymph nodes. Furthermore, a hilar/central perfusion pattern is indicative of an inflammatory origin (**Fig. 9.29**).

In the salivary glands, too, ultrasonography does not provide any definitive evidence of benign or malignant lesions in the differential diagnosis of lymph node enlargement. With respect to ultrasound examination, it is also not possible to differentiate with certainty between reactive lymphadenitis, lymphoma, and metastatic growth within the gland, but there are several morphological features (**Fig. 9.30, 9.31, 9.32, 9.33, 9.34**; ▶ Videos 9.11, 9.12, 9.13).

On the other hand, ultrasonography makes it very easy to assess whether a lesion is situated within the gland tissue or lying caudally in an "extracapsular" position (**Fig. 9.35**). In the differentiation between benign and malignant lesions the same criteria apply as in Chapter 6 (p. 58).

Salivary Gland Cysts

As a rule, congenital and acquired salivary gland cysts are filled with more or less serous secretions. On this basis, they meet the typical ultrasound criteria for cystic structures: hypoechoic space-occupying lesions, with clearly defined margins and typical distal enhancement (**Figs. 9.36, 9.37, 9.38**; ▶ Video 9.14). The more viscous the cyst contents, the more echogenic is the ultrasound appearance. Intrinsic perfusion is not found in cysts, but can be demonstrated in solid tumors with cystic components. A special form of salivary gland cyst, the ranula, is described in Chapter 8 (p. 99).

Lymphoepithelial cysts, associated with HIV infection, should also be considered if there is a relevant medical history and ultrasonography shows cystic space-occupying lesions in both parotid glands (**Figs. 9.39, 9.40**).

Sialolithiasis and Obstructive Disease

The classic sonographic criterion for a stone (calculus) is a dense echo with clear distal acoustic shadowing (direct signs of a stone) (**Figs. 9.41, 9.42**).

While distal acoustic shadowing can routinely be demonstrated, the dense echo is sometimes not absolutely clear or cannot be seen at all. A further indirect sign of a salivary stone is the buildup of secretions in the salivary duct (in the absence of a demonstrable calculus). Because of the great difference in impedance, stones in the major salivary glands can certainly be seen on ultrasonography once they have reached ~2 mm in size. The view of small stones lying very anteriorly in the floor of the mouth, which is restricted by the shadow of the mandible, can be improved by tilting the probe (**Figs. 9.43, 9.44**; ▶ Video 9.15). Differential diagnostic thought must be given to phlebolith, atherosclerosis, calcified lymph node, scar formation, malignant tumor, foreign body, arteriovenous malformation and hemangioma.

In considering treatment options, determination of the precise location of the salivary stone (intra- or extraglandular, intraductal) is extremely important. Ultrasound-guided palpation of the stone may be helpful in pinpointing its precise position (**Fig. 9.45**).

> **Pearls and Pitfalls**
>
> While about 90% of the stones in the parotid gland are found in the middle and distal segments of the duct, two-thirds of those in the submandibular gland lie in the hilar region of the gland.

Differentiation of a salivary stone from an **obstructive stenosing sialodochitis** can be difficult in some cases when, as mentioned previously, there are only indirect signs of obstruction (**Figs. 9.46, 9.47**; ▶ Video 9.16).

Further investigation with **sialendoscopy** can be helpful in reaching an assessment of a stone in the duct system by direct visualization. If there is a relevant past medical history, duct dilatation may also be caused by stenosis, for example following a previously performed duct incision.

With the appropriate medical history, the oral administration of ascorbic acid may be very helpful in the initial ultrasound differentiation between stenosis and sialolithiasis (**Figs. 9.48, 9.49**). For this purpose, we use ascorbic acid in powder form, which is distributed throughout the oral cavity. The stimulated production of saliva causes maximum expansion of the obstructed duct system within 60 seconds, allowing improved ultrasound imaging.

> **Pearls and Pitfalls**
>
> Ascorbic acid powder should be at hand in every ultrasound laboratory.

> **Pearls and Pitfalls**
>
> In examining the duct system of the salivary glands and fistulas, the ultrasound probe should be applied with as little pressure as possible, to avoid closing the duct by compression.

With optimal ultrasound guidance, interventional procedures, such as needle biopsy, endoscopic stone removal or stenting for drainage of the salivary duct, can be undertaken in addition to the assessment of the success of lithotripsy (**Figs. 9.50, 9.51, 9.52, 9.53, 9.54, 9.55**; ▶ Videos 9.17, 9.18, 9.19, 9.20, 9.21). The advantage of ultrasonography in this case is the use of these procedures as "inline" procedures; that is to say, performed during the intervention by an assistant. The initial diagnostic ultrasonography allows precise topographical treatment planning.

Sialadenosis

Sialadenosis, often of unknown etiology, may affect all the major salivary glands simultaneously. Ultrasonography shows the affected glands to be diffusely enlarged and not clearly distinguishable from surrounding structures (**Figs. 9.56, 9.57**). The echotexture is uniformly dense. No areas suspicious of tumor are to be seen in sialadenosis. We frequently find parotid gland enlargement in patients suffering from eating disorders such as bulimia.

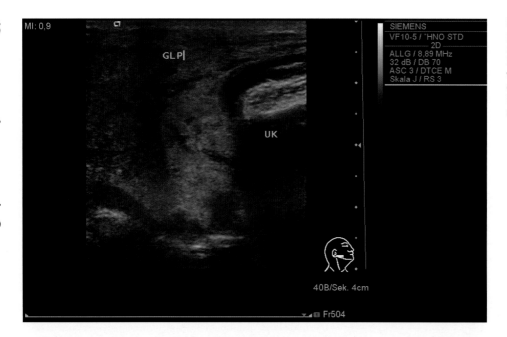

Fig. 9.10 Parotid, transverse, right. The gland parenchyma (GLP) is clearly enlarged in size. It is more loosely structured with a central star-shaped hypoechoic area. The hypoechoid region correlates with dilated interstitial lymphatic spaces. No dilatation of the duct can be seen. UK, mandible. Diagnosis: **Rubella virus infection (mumps) with right-sided sialadenitis of the parotid**.

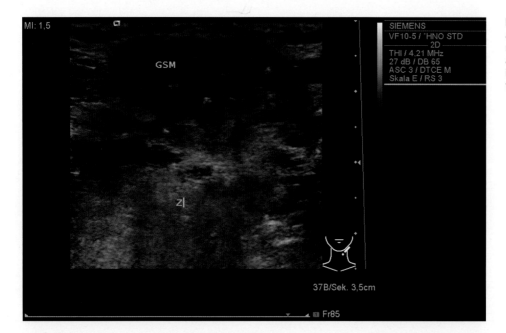

Fig. 9.11 Submandibular region, left, oblique. The acutely enlarged gland (GSM) is hypoechoic and more loosely structured than on the other side, and its margins are not clearly defined. There is an inhomogeneous echotexture within the gland. Z, tongue. Diagnosis: **Acute viral sialadenitis**.

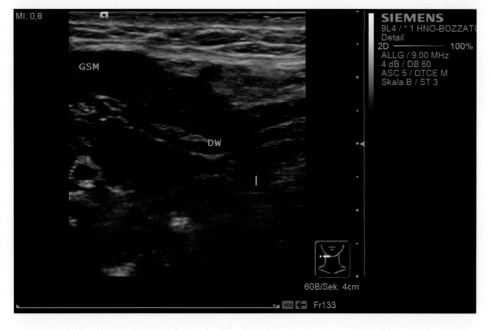

Fig. 9.12 Submandibular region, right, transverse. The acutely enlarged gland (GSM) is hypoechoic, with the swollen parenchyma poorly demarcated from the muscles of the floor of the mouth. The submandibular (Wharton) duct (DW) is filled with purulent secretions and is therefore clearly visible along its path. Diagnosis: **Acute bacterial sialadenitis**.

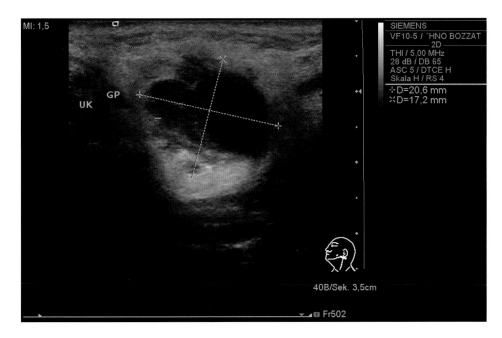

Fig. 9.13 Parotid gland, left, transverse. The clinical picture is one of acute infection. A hypoechoic zone with a central anechoic area can be seen in the middle of the gland (GP). The abnormal area shows distal acoustic enhancement, indicating abscess formation. Sonographic palpation demonstrates the liquid contents as "sludge." UK, mandible. Diagnosis: **Abscess of the parotid gland**.

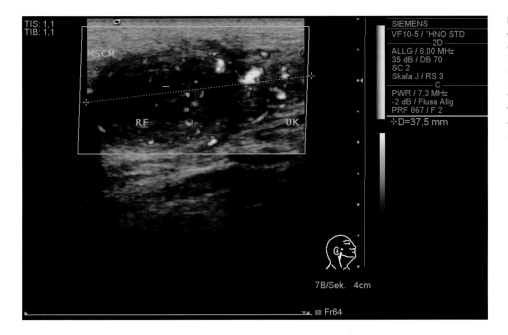

Fig. 9.14 Parotid gland, right, oblique. In the oblique or longitudinal view, the abscess can be delineated further. Caudally, the hypoechoic zone is inhomogeneously demarcated. Sonographic palpation demonstrates the liquid contents as "sludge." Color duplex sonography shows that the liquid anechoic area is not perfused, while the vascularity of the surrounding glandular tissue is good. UK, mandible. Diagnosis: **Abscess of the parotid gland**.

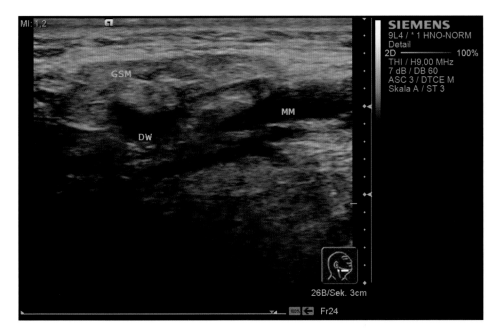

Fig. 9.15 Submandibular region, right, transverse. After radiation therapy, the right submandibular gland (GSM) is reduced in size and has undergone echogenic changes. In the middle, there is sickle-shaped ectasia of the Wharton duct (DW). MM, mylohyoid muscle. Diagnosis: **Chronic sialadenitis after radiotherapy**.

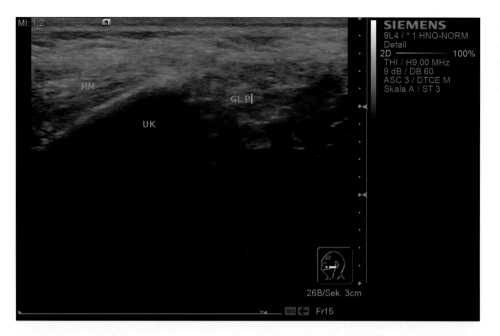

Fig. 9.16 Parotid gland, left, transverse. After radiation therapy, the compact gland parenchyma (GLP) is inhomogeneous, with hypoechoic changes and overall reduction in size. MM, master muscle; UK, mandible. Diagnosis: **Chronic sialadenitis after radiotherapy**.

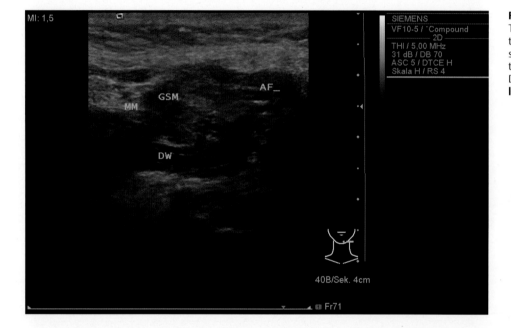

Fig. 9.17 Submandibular region, left, transverse. The submandibular gland (GSM) has a hypoechoic texture and is reduced in size. The obstructed submandibular duct (DW) runs anteriorly on the mylohyoid muscle (MM). AF, facial artery. Diagnosis: **Chronic sialadenitis after long-lasting obstruction**.

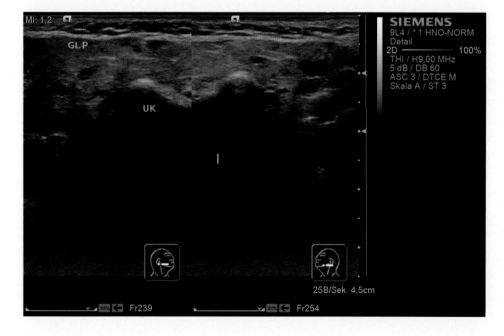

Fig. 9.18 Split screen—parotid region on both sides, transverse. The gland parenchyma (GLP) is hypoechoic and studded with intraglandular nodular lesions. UK, mandible. Diagnosis: **Chronic sialadenitis after long-lasting obstruction**.

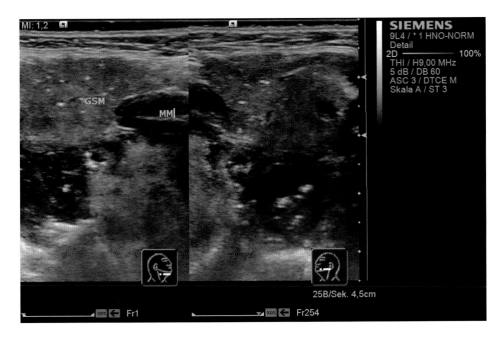

Fig. 9.19 Split screen—submandibular glands on both sides, transverse. In this case of chronic recurrent sialadenitis, the gland parenchyma bilateral (GSM) is compact, echogenic and studded with punctate echoes. MM, mylohyoid muscle. Diagnosis: **Sclerosing sialadenitis after long-lasting obstruction**.

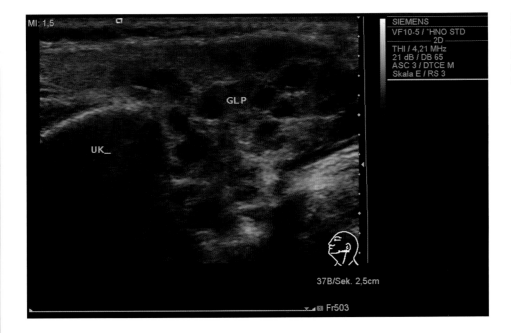

Fig. 9.20 Chronic recurrent juvenile parotitis in a 12-year-old boy. The lateral parts of the gland (GLP) are hypoechoic in a loose cloudlike structure, consistent with the clinically easily observed swelling in the parotid region. Stasis in the duct is not routinely present between episodes.

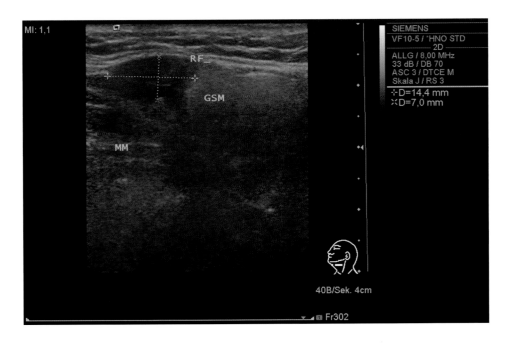

Fig. 9.21 Submandibular region, left, transverse. Within the encapsulated structure of the submandibular gland (GSM) is an oval, hypoechoic, space-occupying lesion (RF). Central dense echoes may be mistaken for the central hyperechoic structure ("hilar sign") of a lymph node. MM, mylohyoid muscle. Diagnosis: **Sclerosing sialadenitis**.

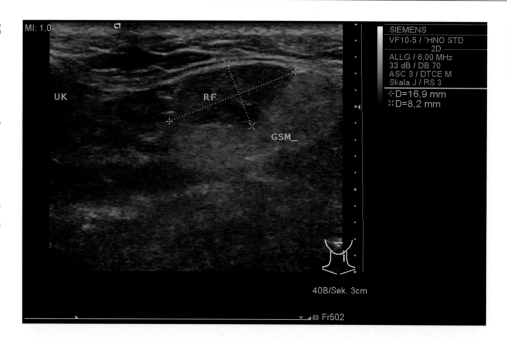

Fig. 9.22 Submandibular region, left, longitudinal. The hypoechoic and well-demarcated process (RF) within the gland tissue (GSM) can be seen more easily in the cross-section of the gland. UK, mandible. Diagnosis: **Sclerosing sialadenitis**.

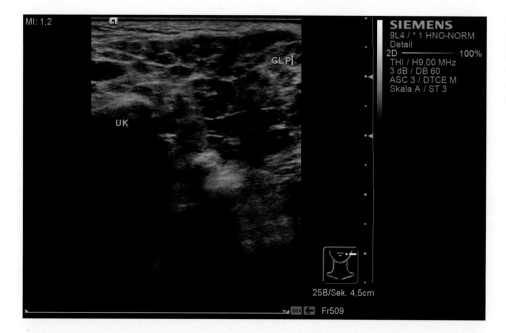

Fig. 9.23 Parotid gland, left, transverse. The parotid gland (GLP) is swollen with a "cloudlike" structure due to hypoechoic lesions. The size of the gland changes with time and acuteness of the inflammation; it may be reduced, enlarged, or normal. UK, mandible. Diagnosis: **Sjögren syndrome**.

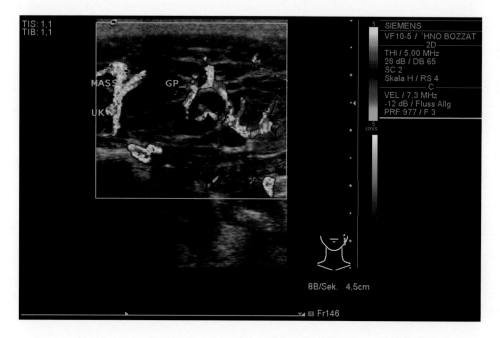

Fig. 9.24 Parotid gland, left, longitudinal. The parotid gland (GP) is swollen by hypoechoic lesions. Imaging of the enlarged gland in color duplex mode shows strong perfusion of the tissue lying between the lesions. MASS, masseter muscle; UK, mandible. Diagnosis: **Sjögren syndrome**.

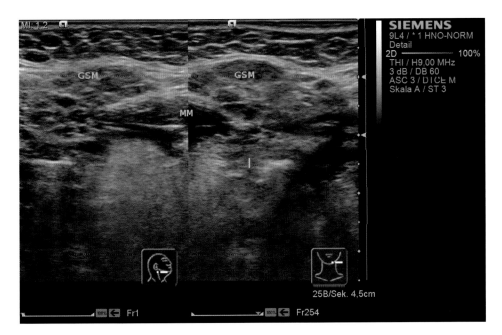

Fig. 9.25 Split screen—both sides, submandibular region, transverse. The submandibular glands (GSM) appear to have a patchy "cloudlike" structure due to hypoechoic lesions. The size of the gland changes with time and according to the acuteness of the inflammation; it may be reduced, enlarged, or normal. MM, mylohyoid muscle. Diagnosis: **Sjögren syndrome**.

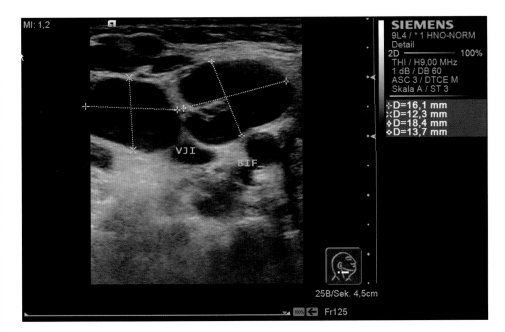

Fig. 9.26 Cervical, right, transverse. New lymph nodes appearing in the right side of the neck in a known case of primary Sjögren syndrome; the nodes are well demarcated with hypoechogenic internal echoes. A few of the many, sometimes conglomerate, nodes show a clear central hyperechoic structure ("hilar sign"). VJI, internal jugular vein; BIF, carotid bifurcation. Diagnosis: **Sjögren syndrome with MALT lymphoma**.

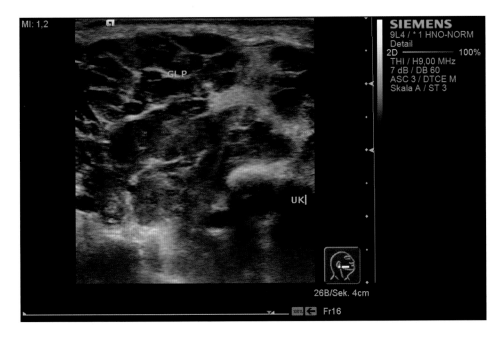

Fig. 9.27 Parotid region, right, transverse. The gland (GLP) is hypoechoic with a loose "cloudlike" structure and ill-defined margins. Clearly defined hypoechoic oval structures can be seen within the lesion. Several salivary glands are usually involved in the acute stage. UK, mandible. Diagnosis: **Sarcoidosis**.

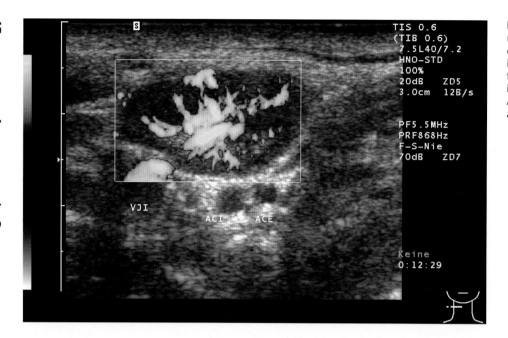

Fig. 9.28 Neck, right, transverse. An oval lymph node with slightly inhomogeneous internal echotexture, lying on the carotid bifurcation in level III, shows very strong hilar perfusion; together with the parenchymal changes seen in the parotid gland, this suggests **sarcoidosis**. ACE, external carotid artery; ACI, internal carotid artery; VJI, internal jugular vein.

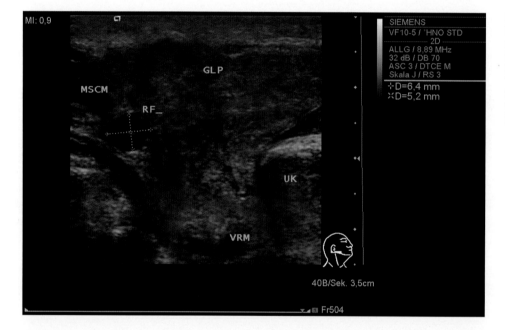

Fig. 9.29 Parotid gland, caudal, right. A round lesion with a central hyperechoic structure ("hilar sign") can be seen lying within the hypoechoic, loosely structured glandular tissue at the anterior border of the sternocleidomastoid muscle (MSCM). The gland (GLP) itself is diffusely enlarged owing to mumps (epidemic parotitis). UK, mandible; VRM, retromandibular vein. Diagnosis: **Enlarged lymph nodes in epidemic parotitis**.

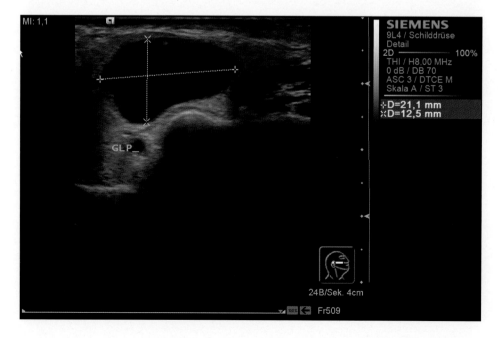

Fig. 9.30 Parotid gland, right, transverse. A solitary, clearly defined, irregular, hypoechoic space-occupying lesion, without a hilar sign, but showing distal acoustic enhancement, can be seen in the middle of the right pretragal parotid gland (GLP). Thus, initial indications are that this is a **cyst**, but further characterization is necessary.

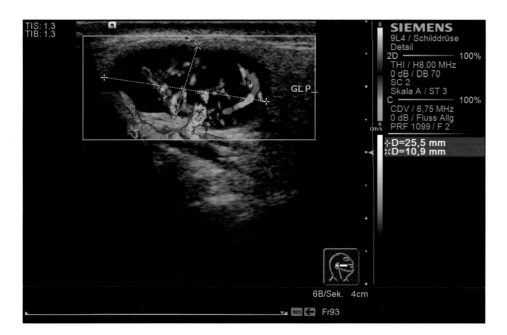

Fig. 9.31 Parotid gland, right, transverse. Color duplex sonography shows very strong central perfusion (see **Fig. 9.30**). Histology confirmed **Hodgkin lymphoma**.

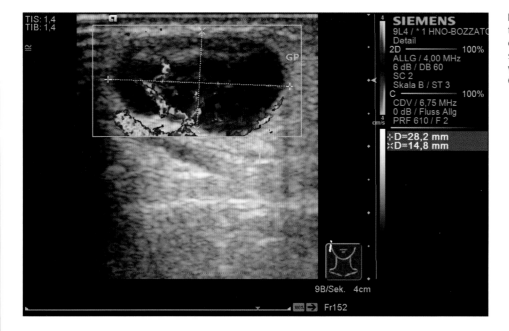

Fig. 9.32 Parotid region, right, longitudinal. At the lateral pole of the parotid gland (GP), a space-occupying lesion, thought to be a lymph node, shows abnormal inhomogeneous internal echoes with a very strong decentralized perfusion on CCDS. Histology showed a **malignant lymphoma**.

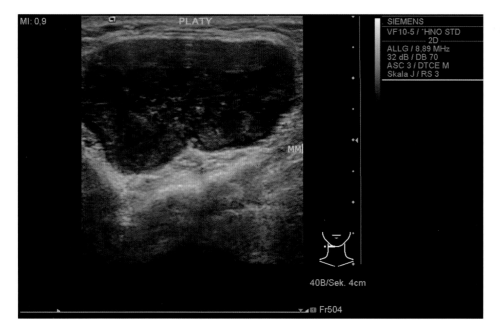

Fig. 9.33 Submandibular region, right, transverse. A rapidly growing tumor (**mantle cell lymphoma**) with lobulated contours in level IB has clearly defined margins and an inhomogeneous hypoechoic texture. MM, mylohyoid muscle; PLATY, platysma.

II Sonographic Anatomy and Pathology

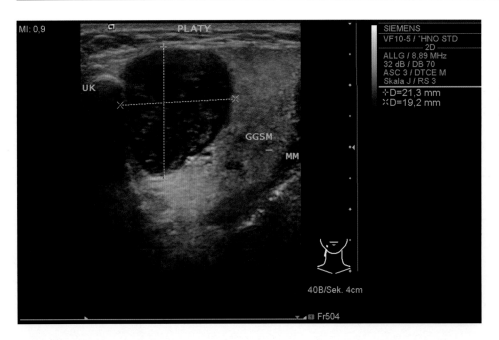

Fig. 9.34 Submandibular region, right, longitudinal. The **mantle cell lymphoma** lies on the mandible (UK) and pushes the gland caudally. Dynamic examination shows that the tumor can be moved over the tissues of the submandibular gland (GGSM). With the lack of any clear distinction from the gland, the differential diagnosis includes an adenoma of the submandibular gland. MM, mylohyoid muscle, PLATY, platysma.

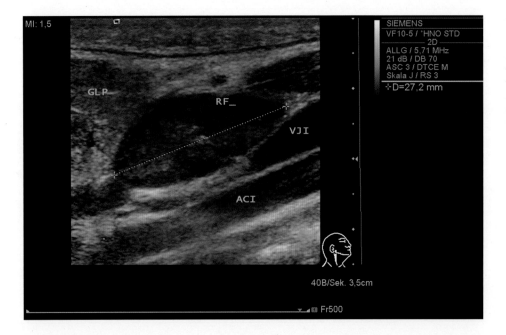

Fig. 9.35 Parotid region, right, longitudinal. A lymph node (RF) is visible at the inferior pole of the parotid gland (GLP), which could not be definitively classified as being intra- or extraglandular in the transverse view. The longitudinal view shows the separation from gland tissue. Immediately adjacent are the internal jugular vein (VJI) and internal carotid artery (ACI). Diagnosis: **Extracapsular lymph node**.

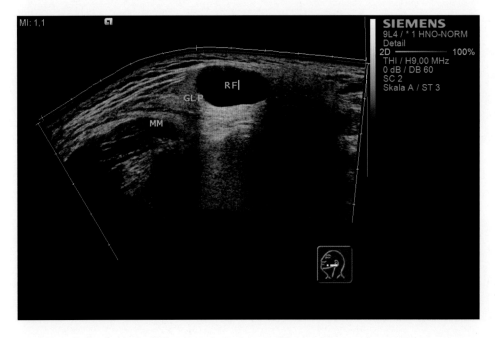

Fig. 9.36 Panoramic transverse view of left parotid region. In the middle of the gland (GLP) lies an anechoic, clearly defined oval space-occupying lesion (RF) with distal acoustic enhancement and the typical appearance of a cyst. CCDS is very helpful in the differential diagnosis, to exclude intrinsic perfusion and substantiate the suspicion of a cyst. MM, masseter muscle. Diagnosis: **Parotid gland cyst**.

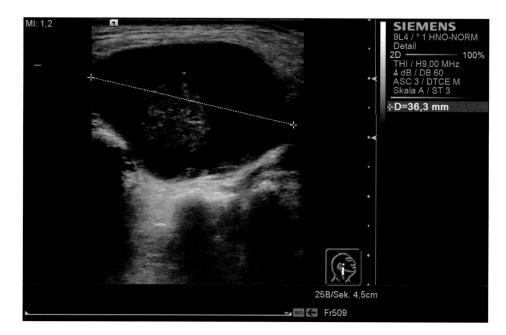

Fig. 9.37 Parotid gland, right, longitudinal. A remarkable feature of this cyst is a central echogenic structure, which moves freely inside it on palpation with the probe. No signs of intrinsic perfusion can be seen on CCDS here either. Diagnosis: **Parotid gland cyst**.

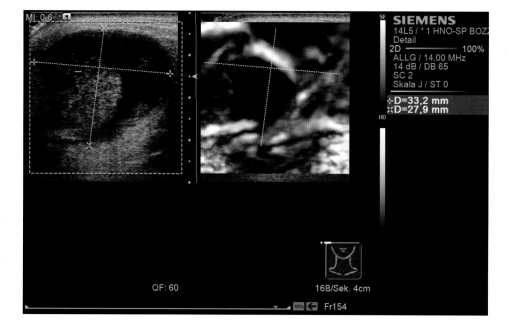

Fig. 9.38 Parotid gland, right, longitudinal. Using ultrasound elastography, the cyst shows a characteristic "bull's eye" pattern, seen here as white horizontal stripes. Diagnosis: **Parotid gland cyst**.

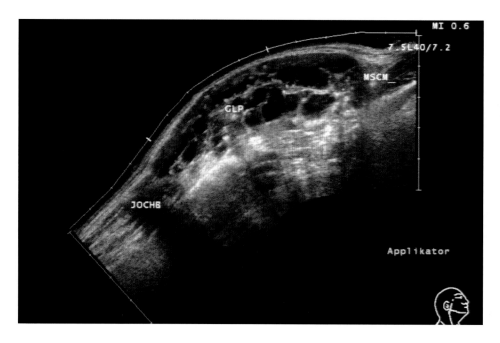

Fig. 9.39 Parotid gland, right, longitudinal, panoramic view. The parenchyma of the gland (GLP) is marbled with multiple anechoic changes, extending from the zygomatic arch (JOCHB) cranially to the sternocleidomastoid muscle caudally. MSCM, sternocleidomastoid muscle. Diagnosis: **Polycystic alteration of the parotid gland in HIV infection**.

II Sonographic Anatomy and Pathology

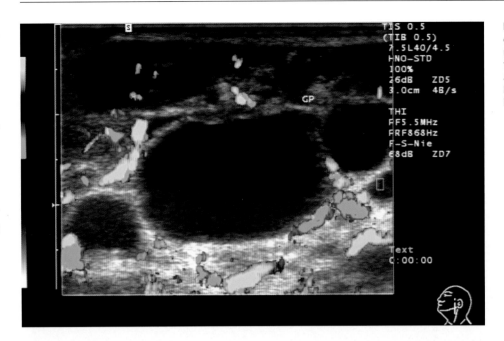

Fig. 9.40 Parotid gland, left, longitudinal. The cystic nature of the enlarged gland (GP) is seen more clearly here; such changes are routinely found bilaterally. CCDS shows that the pericystic areas and septa are hyperperfused. Diagnosis: **Polycystic alteration of the parotid gland in HIV infection.**

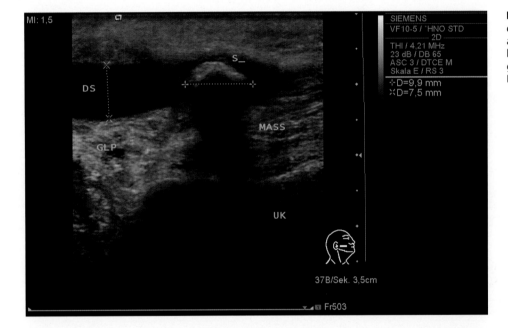

Fig. 9.41 Parotid gland, right, transverse. The dense echo of a salivary gland stone (S) with distal acoustic shadowing obstructs the view of the blocked parotid duct (DS) proximally. GLP, parotid gland; MASS, masseter muscle; UK, mandible. Diagnosis: **Salivary gland stone.**

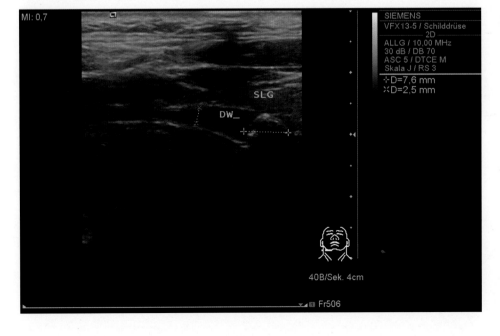

Fig. 9.42 Floor of the mouth, right, transverse oblique. A dense echo with distal acoustic shadowing can be seen at the opening of the duct (DW), causing stasis proximally. SLG, sublingual gland. Diagnosis: **Salivary gland stone.**

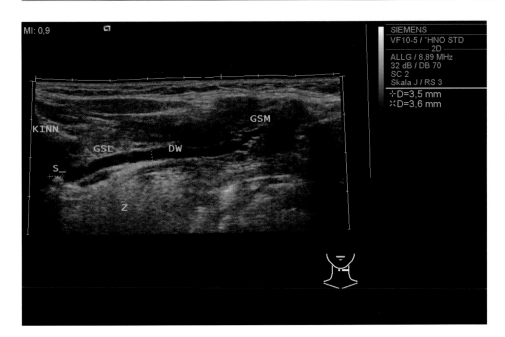

Fig. 9.43 Floor of the mouth, left, transverse oblique. A small stone at the papilla of the submandibular duct (DW). The duct is dilated as far as the hilum of the gland (GSM). The stone (S) is almost hidden by the acoustic shadow of the mandible (KINN). Adjacent organs are the tongue (Z) and sublingual gland (GSL). Diagnosis: **Salivary gland stone**.

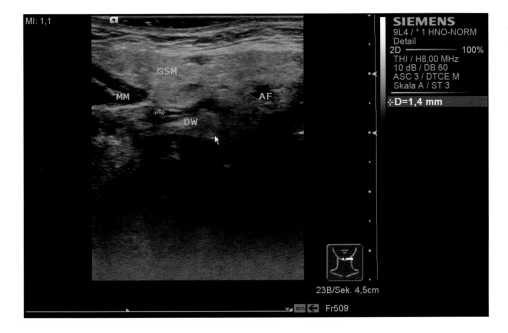

Fig. 9.44 Submandibular region, left, transverse. The hilar stasis in the Wharton duct (DW), in which the mural hypoechoic and echogenic double contour of the wall can be identified easily in the hilum of the gland (GSM). The dense punctate echoes (caliper) measuring 1.4 mm can only be made out with difficulty. AF, facial artery; MM, mylohyoid muscle. Diagnosis: **Salivary gland stone**.

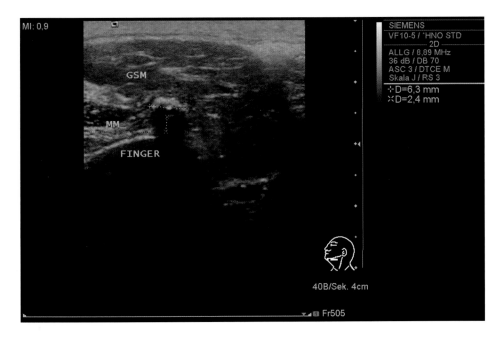

Fig. 9.45 Submandibular gland, left, longitudinal. A hyperechoic stone with acoustic shadowing (marked with the caliper) can be seen in the hilum of the gland (GSM). In the oral cavity, the examiner's palpating finger can be seen as a hyperechoic band (FINGER) on the mylohyoid muscle (MM). Diagnosis: **Salivary gland stone**.

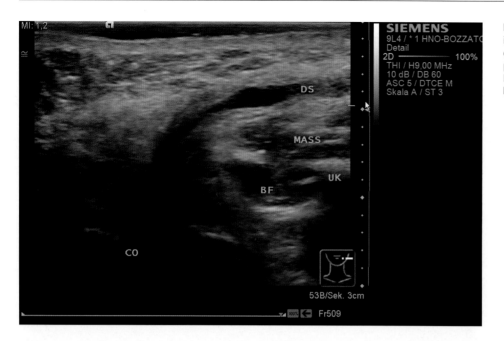

Fig. 9.46 Parotid gland, left, transverse. There is inflammatory narrowing at the papilla in the oral cavity (CO); this is causing stasis in the proximal parotid duct (DS). BF, buccal fat pad; MASS, masseter muscle; UK, mandible. Diagnosis: **Parotid duct stenosis**.

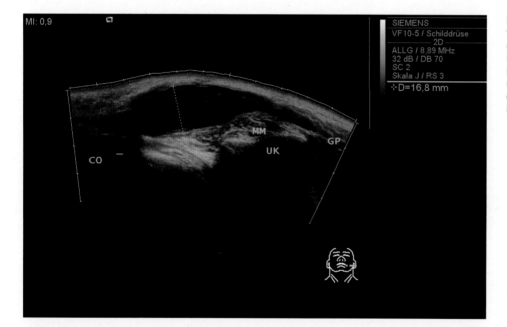

Fig. 9.47 Panoramic view of parotid gland, left, transverse. Scarring leading to stenosis at the opening of the duct following iatrogenic injury in the oral cavity (CO). The fibrosed narrowing is causing proximal stasis in the parotid duct, measuring up to 17 mm maximum. GP, parotid gland; MM, masseter muscle; UK, mandible. Diagnosis: **Parotid duct stenosis**.

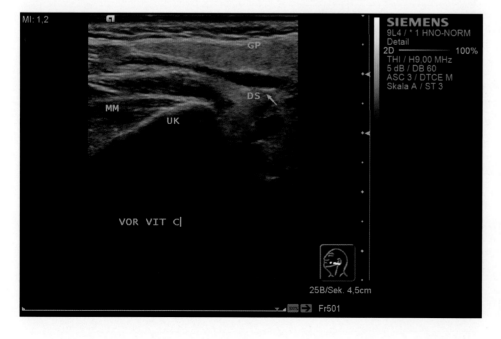

Fig. 9.48 Parotid gland, left, transverse. **Obstructive sialopathy** of the parotid gland (GP, arrow) showing a dilated hilar segment of the duct (DS). MM, masseter muscle; UK, mandible.

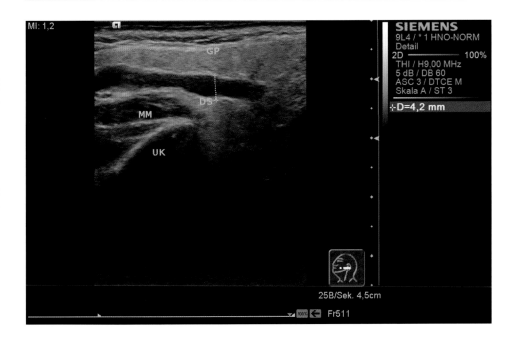

Fig. 9.49 Parotid gland, left, transverse. Sixty seconds **after the administration of ascorbic acid powder**, the stimulated saliva production has visibly dilated the efferent duct, which can be tracked as far as the **stenosis** at the opening of the duct. DS, parotid duct; GP, parotid gland; MM, masseter muscle; UK, mandible.

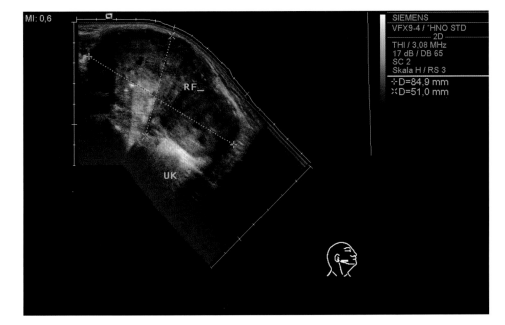

Fig. 9.50 Panoramic view of parotid gland, right, transverse. A mass (RF) suspected of being malignant in a 92-year-old woman is lying on the mandible (UK). It was decided that a core needle biopsy should be performed because of the critical considerations for surgery. Diagnosis: **Parotid metastasis of breast cancer**.

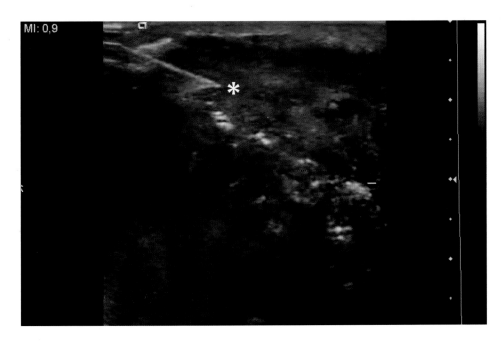

Fig. 9.51 Parotid gland, right, transverse. Biopsy using a Bard Magnum core-needle biopsy gun. The hyperechoic tip (asterisk) of the needle can be seen to the left of the image and is being inserted into the tumor parallel to the longitudinal axis of the probe.

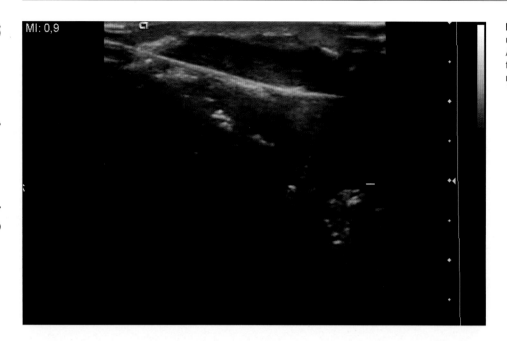

Fig. 9.52 Parotid gland, right, transverse. Biopsy using a Bard Magnum core-needle biopsy gun. Activating the gun advances the needle trough to remove a core of tissue, which is immediately retracted into the needle.

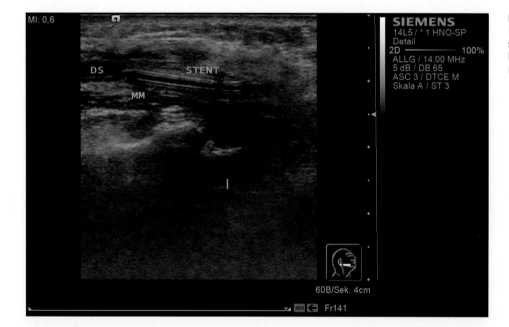

Fig. 9.53 Parotid gland, right, transverse. Following **sialendoscopy and dilation of the stenosis due to scarring**, a silicone stent (STENT) has been inserted into the parotid duct (DS). MM, masseter muscle.

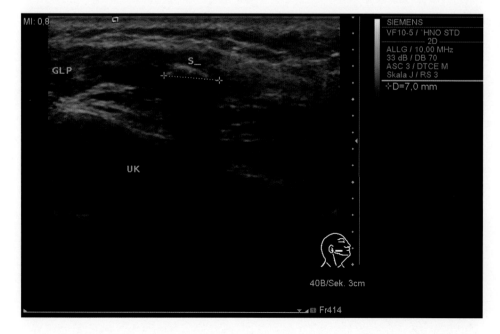

Fig. 9.54 Parotid gland, right, transverse. The right parotid gland measures 7 mm (caliper) **before fragmentation (lithotripsy)** of the salivary stone (S). GLP, parotid gland; UK, mandible.

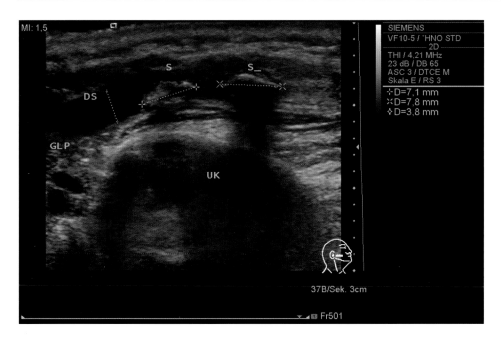

Fig. 9.55 Parotid gland, right, transverse. **After treatment, two fragments (S, S) can now be seen**, which, in part, have measurements greater than the original stone. Fragmentation (lithotripsy) of a stone makes its structure less compact, which may cause an apparent increase in size. DS, parotid (Stensen) duct; GLP, parotid gland; UK, mandible.

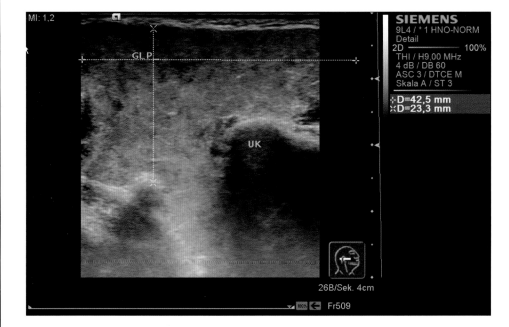

Fig. 9.56 View of the parotid region, right, transverse. The gland (GLP) is echogenic and enlarged, showing distal acoustic shadowing. The underlying tissues or structures cannot be clearly seen. UK, mandible. Diagnosis: **Sialadenosis of the parotid gland**.

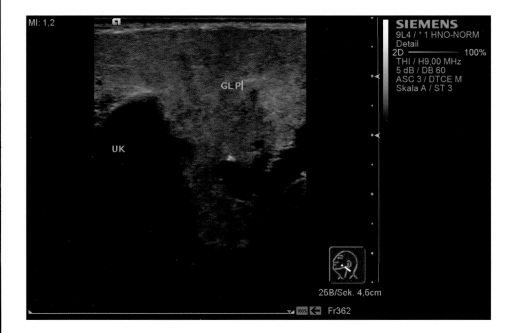

Fig. 9.57 Parotid gland, left, transverse. Diffuse enlargement in a 29-yeard-old female suffering from bulimia. An enlargement was also seen in both submandibular glands. Diagnosis. **Sialadenosis of the left parotid gland**.

Benign Tumors

A characteristic feature of a **benign salivary gland tumor** is the clearly defined margin separating it from adjacent salivary gland tissue.

Angiomas show features of a tumor, but their sonographic morphology with respect to perfusion, sonographic palpation, and borders is heterogeneous (**Fig. 9.58**; ▶ Video 9.22).

Pleomorphic adenomas routinely show a homogeneous, hypoechoic pattern. Nevertheless, inhomogeneous structures with solid and possibly cystic elements may occasionally be seen. Distal acoustic enhancement is the rule (**Fig. 9.59**). The contour is usually oval or lobulated (**Fig. 9.60**; ▶ Video 9.23). Color duplex sonography does not give any characteristic picture (**Figs. 9.61, 9.62**; ▶ Video 9.24).

Like pleomorphic adenomas, **adenomas (e.g., Warthin tumors/ adenolymphomas)** may appear homogeneous and hypoechoic on ultrasonography. However, if it contains a large number of cystic structures, a **Warthin tumor** may also appear almost anechoic with focal distal acoustic enhancement. The tumor is well demarcated from the surrounding gland tissue (**Figs. 9.63, 9.64, 9.65**). Occasionally, septa may be demonstrated between the different tumor elements, which often contain numerous vascular structures.

The presence of multilocular lesions and of bilateral solid space-occupying lesions, in the parotid gland in particular, provides evidence of a **Warthin tumor** (**Figs. 9.66, 9.67, 9.68**; ▶ Videos 9.25, 9.26).

Other, less common, benign tumors of the salivary glands (e.g., **basal cell adenoma**, **oncocytoma**, **sebaceous adenoma**) also show similar uncharacteristic sonographic morphological criteria (**Figs. 9.69, 9.70, 9.71**).

Ultrasonography alone is not sufficient to differentiate the various benign tumors of the salivary glands with a high degree of certainty, but analysis of typical features allows for a primary assessment and timing of the type of surgery.

Pearls and Pitfalls

Acutely inflamed adenomas (especially adenolymphoma) with ill-defined margins, hyperperfusion, and a rapid increase in size can be very difficult to distinguish from a malignant process.

Because nerves are not easily demonstrated on ultrasound examination, it is not possible to determine the precise relationship of a parotid tumor to the facial nerve. The retromandibular vein may, however, be used as a starting point. As a rule, a space-occupying lesion located superficially to the vein lies above the nerve compartment. If, on comparing the two sides, it is seen that the vein is pushed deeper into the underlying tissue, it can be assumed that the tumor is at least in direct contact with the marginal mandibular branch of the facial nerve.

Owing to their superficial component, the demonstration of parapharyngeal "**iceberg tumors**" is not a problem (**Figs. 9.72, 9.73a,b**). However, their extension beneath the ascending ramus of the mandible means that MRI may be required to determine their precise position and size.

An intraglandular **lipoma** has a characteristic rippled echogenicity. It usually has irregular contours, but is distinct from the remaining salivary gland tissue (**Fig. 9.74**). These benign changes typically have a very soft consistency on sonographic palpation.

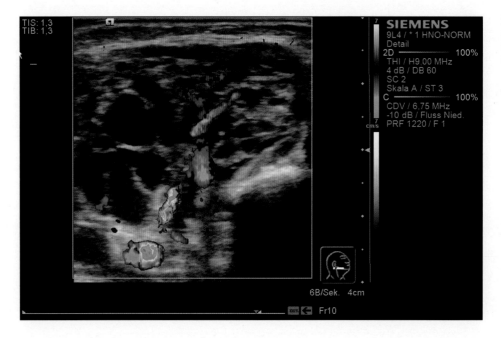

Fig. 9.58 Parotid gland, right, transverse. **Cavernous hemangioma**. The caudal glandular tissue is marbled with macrocystic changes, seen to have strong (venous) perfusion on CCDS.

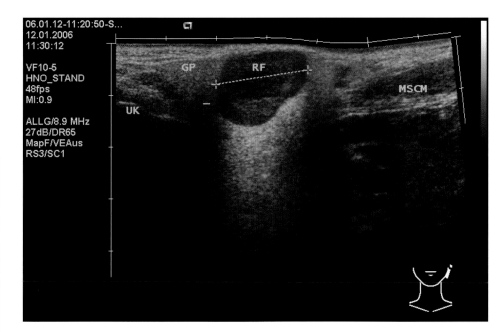

Fig. 9.59 Panoramic view of the parotid gland, left, transverse. A clearly defined lobulated pleomorphic adenoma (RF) lies in the middle of the gland; it is well demarcated and shows distal acoustic enhancement. CCDS provides no clear evidence of perfusion. UK, mandible; MSCM, sternocleidomastoid muscle. Diagnosis: **Pleomorphic adenoma**.

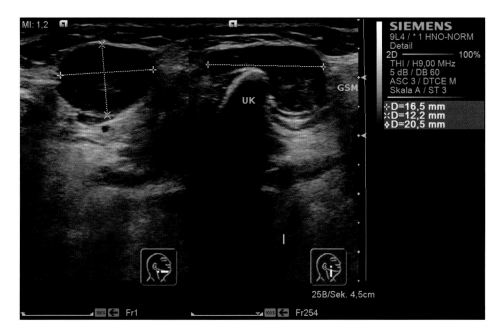

Fig. 9.60 Split screen—submandibular region, right. An oval hypoechoic pleomorphic adenoma of the submandibular gland (GSM) has clearly defined contours with soft echogenic internal echoes. A particular feature of this tumor is its fingerlike extension over the edge of the horizontal ramus of the mandible (UK). Diagnosis: **Pleomorphic adenoma**.

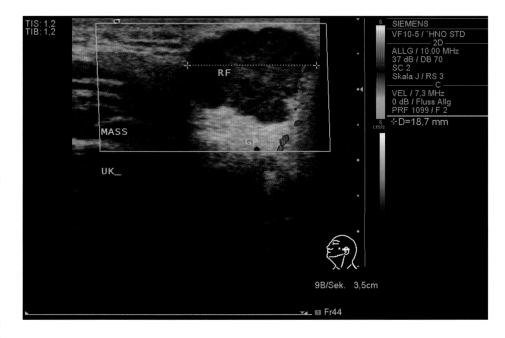

Fig. 9.61 Parotid gland, left, transverse. A lobulated pleomorphic adenoma (RF) lies in the middle of the gland; it is well demarcated and shows distal acoustic enhancement. CCDS provides no clear evidence of perfusion. MASS, masseter muscle; UK, mandible. Diagnosis: **Pleomorphic adenoma**.

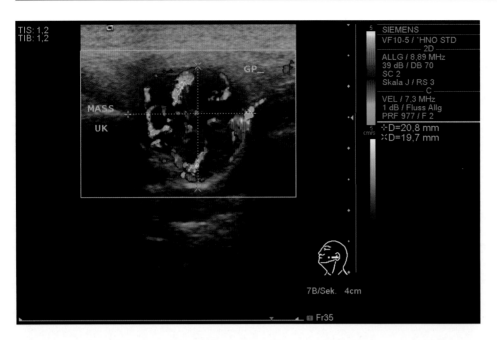

Fig. 9.62 Parotid gland, left, transverse. The rounded, lobulated pleomorphic adenoma seen here lies in the middle of the gland; it is well demarcated and shows distal acoustic enhancement. CCDS provides no clear evidence of perfusion. GP, parotid gland; MASS, masseter muscle; UK, mandible. Diagnosis: **Pleomorphic adenoma**.

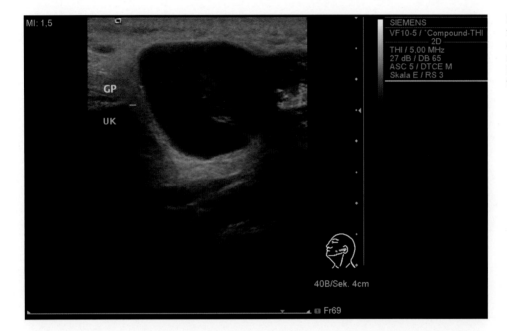

Fig. 9.63 Warthin tumor, parotid gland, left, transverse. A rounded oval, well-defined space-occupying lesion seen in the parotid gland (GP) shows a hypoechoic texture with central echogenic internal echoes. UK, mandible. Diagnosis: **Warthin tumor**.

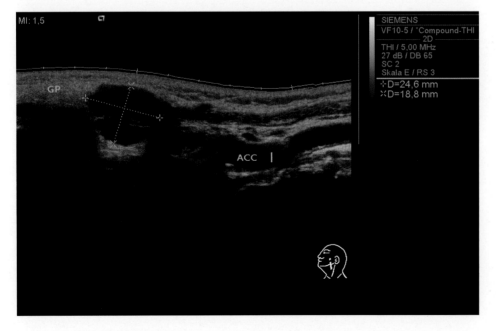

Fig. 9.64 Warthin tumor in parotid gland, left, longitudinal, panoramic view. The tumor is located in the lower pole of the gland (GP). The central echogenic internal echoes can also be seen in the longitudinal view. ACC, common carotid artery.

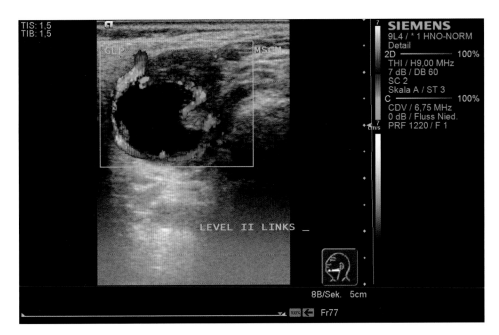

Fig. 9.65 Warthin tumor in parotid gland, left, transverse view of superior pole and transition to level II. The round, well-defined space-occupying lesion seen here in the parotid gland (GLP) has irregular margins around an anechoic zone and pronounced peripheral vascularity. MSCM, sternocleidomastoid muscle.

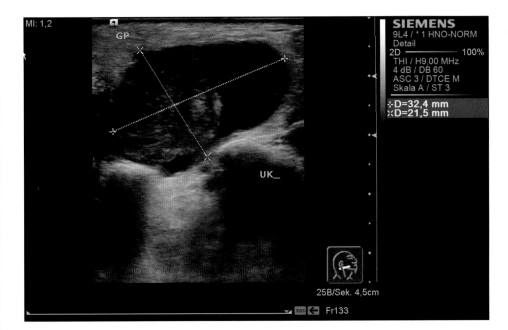

Fig. 9.66 Warthin tumor, parotid region, right, transverse. The well-demarcated space-occupying lesion is hypoechoic with inhomogeneous denser internal echoes. It extends anteriorly over the mandible (UK).

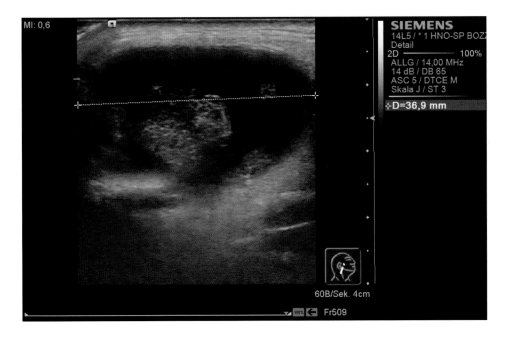

Fig. 9.67 Warthin tumor, parotid region, right, longitudinal. The well-demarcated space-occupying lesion is hypoechoic with inhomogeneous denser internal echoes. The frequently liquid elements of the tumor give rise to distal acoustic enhancement.

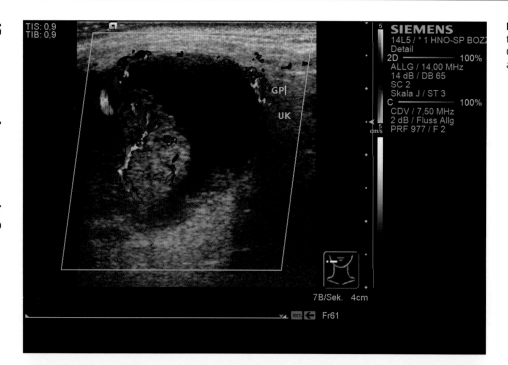

Fig. 9.68 Warthin tumor, parotid region, right, transverse. When there are extensive cystic areas, CCDS helps to differentiate between true cysts and solid tumors. GP, parotid gland; UK, mandible.

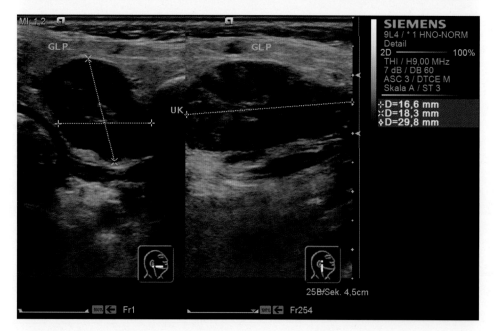

Fig. 9.69 Split screen—**oncocytoma** of the right parotid gland. The image on the left shows an irregular oval space-occupying lesion in the inferior pole of the gland (GLP); sonographic palpation shows that it is mobile at its medial border with the mandible (UK).

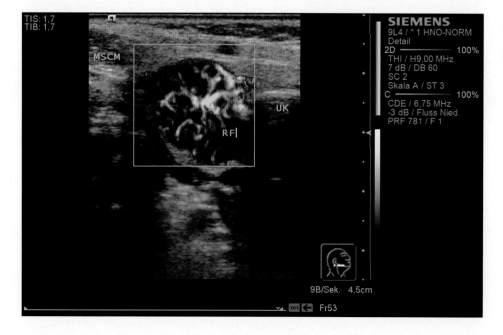

Fig. 9.70 Parotid gland, right, transverse. Power-mode sonography shows very strong central perfusion of the **oncocytoma** (RF). MSCM, sternocleidomastoid muscle; UK, mandible.

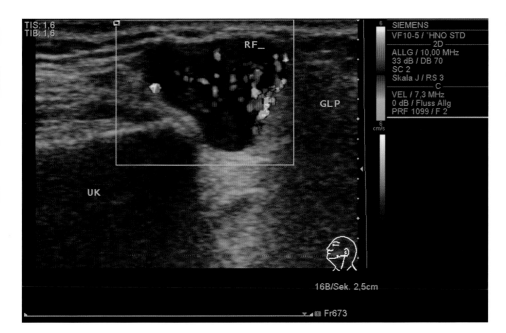

Fig. 9.71 Basal cell adenoma, left, transverse. The well-demarcated polycyclic space-occupying lesion (RF) is diffusely perfused and distinct from the gland (GLP), and shows distal acoustic enhancement. UK, mandible.

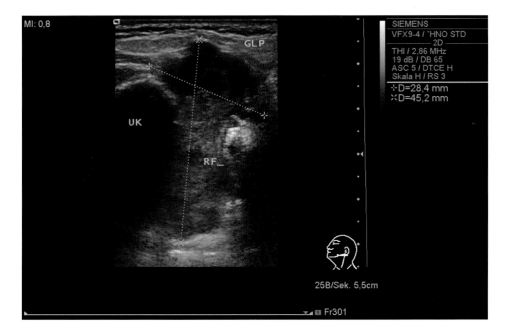

Fig. 9.72a Parotid gland, left, transverse. The iceberg tumor is distinct, polycyclic, and clearly visible even in the deeper tissues (RF). Anteriorly, its extent cannot be determined because of mandibular shadowing (UK). GLP, parotid gland. Diagnosis: **Iceberg tumor of the left parotid gland**.

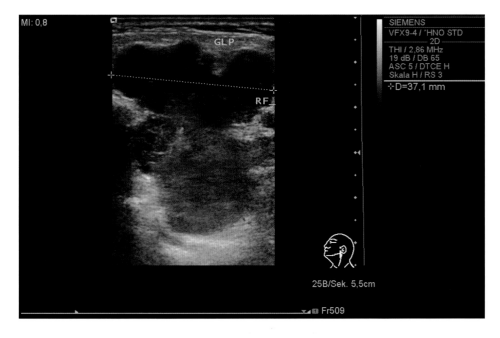

Fig. 9.72b Parotid gland, left, longitudinal. The polycyclic shape of the tumor (RF) is even more visible in the longitudinal view. GLP, parotid gland. Diagnosis: **Iceberg tumor of the left parotid gland**.

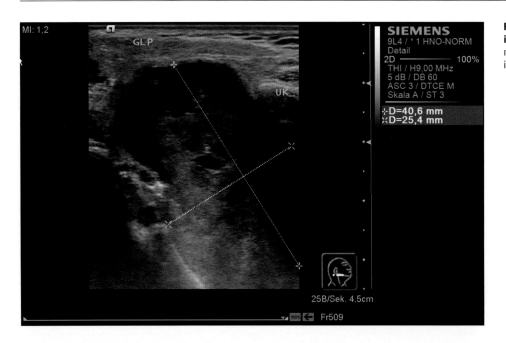

Fig. 9.73a Parotid gland, right, transverse. The **iceberg tumor** is not visible in the anterior and medial extension. Further imaging with MRI or CT is necessary. GLP, parotid gland; UK, mandible.

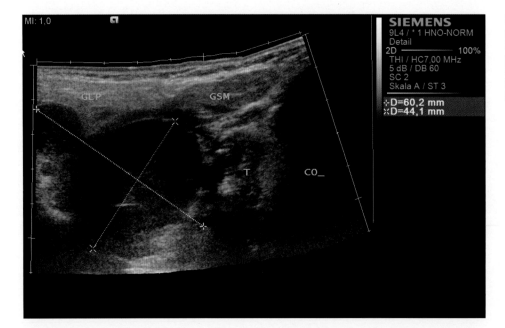

Fig. 9.73b Panoramic image of the parotid gland, right, transverse. The **polycylic iceberg tumor** has its greatest extension in the deep lobe of the gland and touches the tonsillar fossa. In this case, additional imaging is recommended. CO, oral cavity; GLP, parotid gland; GSM, submandibular gland; T, tonsil.

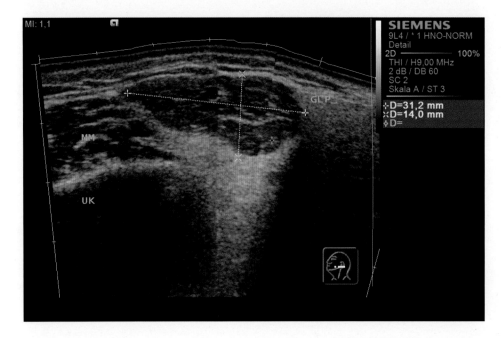

Fig. 9.74 Panoramic view—parotid gland, left, transverse. The hypoechoic space-occupying lesion is oval, with clearly defined margins. It lies superficially and anteriorly in the gland (GLP) and has a striped echogenicity. MASS, masseter muscle; UK, mandible. Diagnosis: **Lipoma**.

Malignant Tumors

Signs of **malignant salivary gland tumors**, irrespective of their histological origin, are ill-defined margins with an inhomogeneous echotexture, nerve involvement, and infiltrative growth into adjacent structures (**Figs. 9.75, 9.76**). Color duplex sonography shows an irregular, sometimes strong, vascular pattern (**Figs. 9.77, 9.78**; ▶ Video 9.27).

> ## Pearls and Pitfalls
>
> As a rule of thumb: the smaller the salivary gland affected by a tumor, the higher the likelihood of malignancy.

In this context, it is absolutely essential to determine the status of the cervical lymph nodes, as finding abnormally configured nodes increases the suspicion of malignancy.

Figures 9.79 and 9.80 compare the sonographic anatomy and macroscopic appearance of a mucoepidermoid carcinoma.

A definitive statement whether the tumor is benign or malignant cannot be made with any certainty, especially in the case of small tumors that do not meet the previously mentioned criteria (**Figs. 9.81, 9.82, 9.84, 9.85, 9.86**, ▶ Video 9.28).

While the presence of facial nerve paralysis is almost certainly evidence of malignant disease, ultrasound examination cannot provide direct evidence of the cranial nerve involvement.

Further diagnostic investigation with CT and/or MRI is essential if the tumor extends to bony structures such as the mandible. skull base, or mastoid.

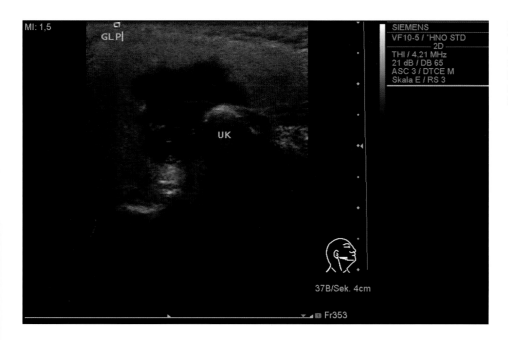

Fig. 9.75 Parotid carcinoma, right, transverse. The position of an **adenoid cystic carcinoma** of the right parotid gland (GLP) can be seen on the mandible (UK). Typical of malignant growth are the ill-defined margins separating the tumor from the adjacent glandular tissue and the inhomogeneous internal echoes.

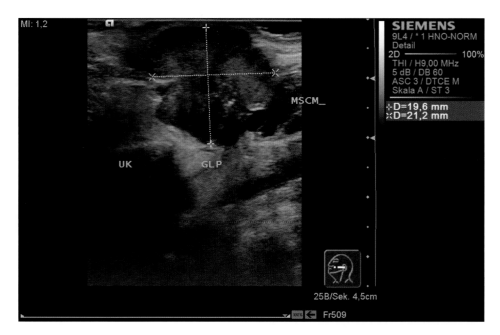

Fig. 9.76 Parotid gland, left, transverse. This **mucoepidermoid carcinoma** of the left parotid gland (GLP) lies very caudally on the anterior border of the sternocleidomastoid muscle (MSCM). Ill-defined margins and an inhomogeneous "turbulent" tissue texture are also indicators of malignant growth. UK, mandible.

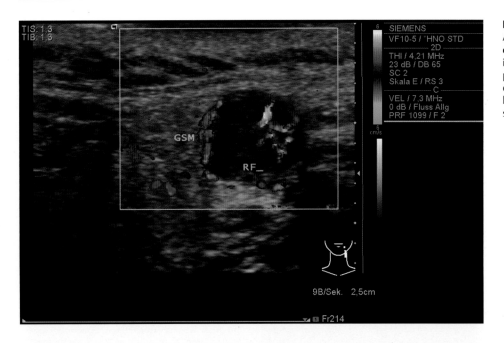

Fig. 9.77 Submandibular region, longitudinal. A round, hypoechoic lesion (RF, **myoepithelial carcinoma**) is lying within the gland. It shows irregular perfusion that is more pronounced in the periphery. Caudally, another hypoechoic space-occupying lesion with a similar echo pattern can be seen outside the gland parenchyma. GSM, submandibular gland.

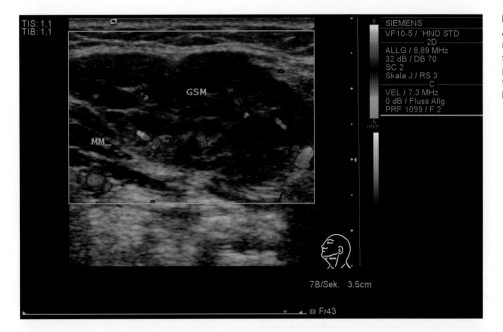

Fig. 9.78 Submandibular region, transverse. As seen in **Fig. 9.77**, the deep lobe of the submandibular gland is enlarged and hypoechoic, showing irregular perfusion. The gland's echo pattern is inhomogeneous; the gland (GSM) is fixed in its bed. MM, mylohyoid muscle. Diagnosis: **Rhabdomyosarcoma**.

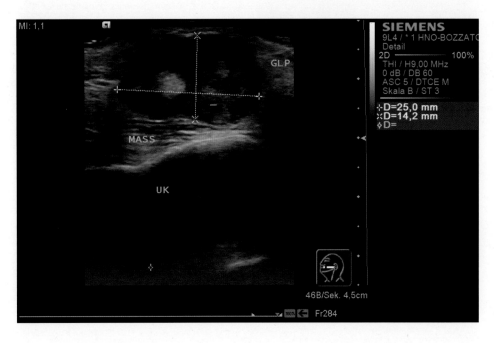

Fig. 9.79 Parotid gland, left, transverse. **Mucoepidermoid carcinoma**. A polycyclic tumor contains areas of greater echogenicity. An interesting incidental finding is the mirror image artifact of the mandible, once again typically found at this anatomical site. GLP, parotid gland; MASS, masseter muscle; UK, mandible.

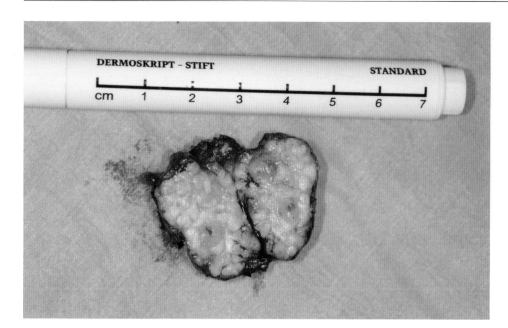

Fig. 9.80 Macroscopic preparation of the lesion shown in **Fig. 9.79**. This view of the tumor allows the precise visualization of the internal texture in comparison. Diagnosis: **Mucoepidermoid carcinoma**.

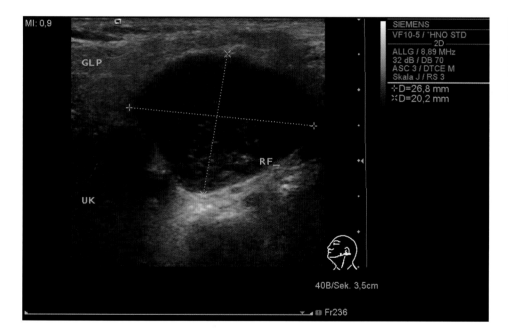

Fig. 9.81 Parotid gland, left, transverse. The hypoechoic space-occupying lesion (RF) is well demarcated from surrounding tissues (GLP) and has a homogeneous internal texture. On histology, however, areas of carcinoma were found within a pleomorphic adenoma. UK, mandible. Diagnosis: **Carcinoma ex pleomorphic adenoma**.

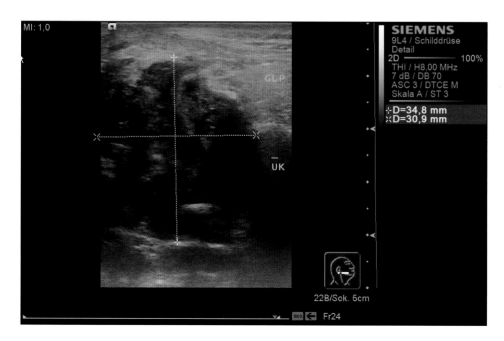

Fig. 9.82 Parotid gland, right, transverse. The space-occupying lesion (caliper), in this case a **mucoepidermoid carcinoma**, is poorly demarcated from the gland (GLP) and has a very inhomogeneous echotexture. UK, mandible.

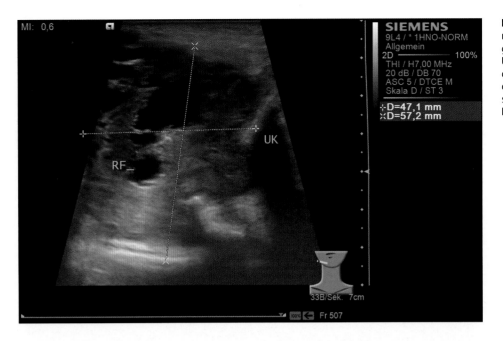

Fig. 9.83 Parotid, right, transverse. A tumor (RF) mesauring 70mm in anteroposterior diameter grew for almost 20 years in this 93-year old male. Ultrasound examination suspected infiltration of the mandible (UK). The contour of the osseous hyperechoic reflex is blurred. The tumor shows intralesional anechoic areas. Diagnosis: **Mucoepidermoid carcinoma.**

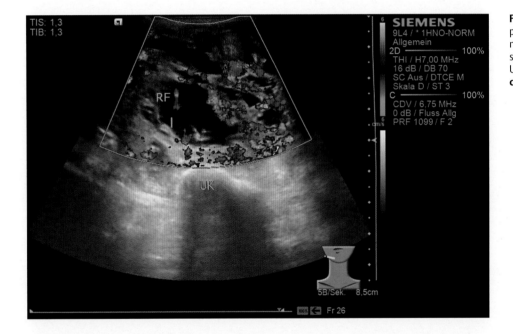

Fig. 9.84 Parotid, right, transverse, CCDS. Same patient as in **Fig. 9.83**. Between the cystic or necrotic anechoic areas, the tumor (RF) shows strong perfusion of the septae in CCDS mode. UK, mandible. Diagnosis: **Mucoepidermoid carcinoma**.

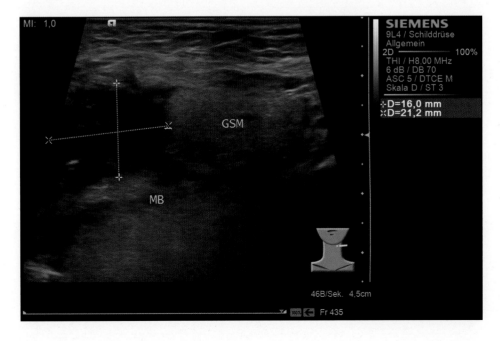

Fig. 9.85 Submandibular region, level 1B, left, transverse. A tumor with ill-defined margins, rapid growth and palpatonic fixated tissue lies in the anterior part of the submandibular gland. Diagnosis: **Adenoidcystic carcinoma.**

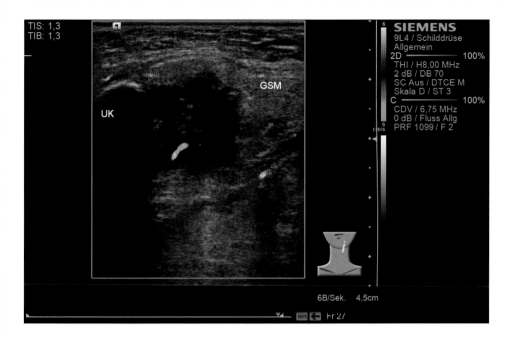

Fig. 9.86 Level 1B, longitudinal, left. Same patient as in **Fig. 9.85**. The tumor extends from the cranial part of the submandibular gland (GSM) up to the medial side of the mandible (UK). Infiltration to the horizontal ramus cannot be excluded. Diagnosis: **Adenoidcystic carcinoma**.

10   Facial Soft Tissues

Anatomy

The hypoechoic structure of the masseter muscle with its pinnate reflection pattern is a primary landmark in the transverse view of the parotid region. The parotid duct (Stensen duct) lies superficially to the muscle but is usually only identifiable as a hypoechoic/anechoic area when it is obstructed (**Fig. 10.1**).

The duct runs anteriorly and medially, traverses the buccal fat pad, and opens into the vestibule of the mouth, opposite the second upper molar, after passing through the (hypoechoic) band of the buccinator muscle (**Fig. 10.2**).

The orbicularis oris muscle and the soft tissues of the lip can be seen anterior to the oral cavity region. These tissues are divided into three layers: a central hypoechoic structure with a more echogenic band in front and behind, corresponding to the anatomical structure of the lips with two layers of subcutaneous tissue and the orbicularis oris muscle (**Fig. 10.3**).

When examining facial structures such as the cartilaginous structures of the auricle, mastoid, or face, ultrasound gel should be applied in sufficient amount to ensure good acoustic conditions.

Anterior to the parotid gland and lying on the ascending ramus of the mandible (echogenic reflection with distal acoustic shadowing), is the masseter muscle with its characteristic pinnate reflection pattern. It can be displayed in the longitudinal and transverse planes, as well as in relaxation and in maximum contraction.

Masseter hypertrophy: Apart from a condition affecting the parotid gland, unilateral swelling of the cheek may be due to hypertrophy of the masseter muscle caused by an occlusal parafunction (**Fig. 10.4**).

The temporomandibular joint is also accessible to ultrasound. The dynamics of the joint can be examined to determine, among other things, any dislocation or disorder of movement (▶ Video 10.1).

Inflammatory Changes

Furuncles and Abscesses

A **furuncle** is an infection of a hair follicle with surrounding tissue reaction; it may occur anywhere on skin with hair. With the typical clinical external picture, ultrasound imaging shows a hypoechoic, star-shaped, loosely structured lesion in the skin (**Fig. 10.5**). The extent of the inflammatory reaction in the deeper tissues can easily be assessed. Anechoic areas with distal acoustic enhancement indicate an abscess (**Fig. 10.6**). Color-coded duplex sonography (CCDS) characterizes the inflammatory hyperperfusion (**Figs. 10.7, 10.8**).

> **Pearls and Pitfalls**
>
> Furuncles above the oral fissure require assessment with Doppler sonography or color duplex imaging of the angular vein. Any signs of venous thrombosis (**Fig. 10.9**) mean that there is a danger of intracranial spread.

Mastoiditis

Retroauricular swelling with a prominent ear on inspection correlates with the ultrasound appearance of a subcutaneous hypoechoic thickening (**Fig. 10.10**). If the ongoing inflamamation breaches the mastoidal osseous cortex the abscess can easily be recognized as a gap in the

continuity of the cortical bone (**Fig. 10.11**). A rapid diagnosis can be made with ultrasonography, especially in children.

Ultrasound examination may be worthwhile in patients, especially children, after lateral skull base surgery such as cochlear implantation and/or for local wound monitoring (**Fig. 10.12**; ▶ Video 10.2).

Preauricular Sinus

Preauricular sinuses and **auditory meatal fistulas** are ectodermal tissue inclusions that can sometimes be assessed on ultrasound imaging with respect to their depth and branching (**Figs. 10.13, 10.14**). When planning the extent of surgery, particular attention must be paid to the possibility of a rare intraparotid extension.

> **Pearls and Pitfalls**
>
> If the fistula can be probed, it may be worth trying a careful instillation of hydrogen peroxide, as a contrast enhancer, to delineate the lesion more clearly in the deeper tissues.

Benign Tumors

Epidermoid cysts or trichilemmal cysts, arising as a result of an obstruction of sebaceous ducts, are ubiquitous on the hair-covered scalp. The adipocytes, fat crystals, and epidermal cells that comprise these lesions generate an inhomogeneous, hypoechoic picture. In the noninflammatory stage, the epidermoid cyst is clearly demarcated from its surroundings and there is often the suggestion of a hypoechoic duct (**Figs. 10.15, 10.16, 10.17**).

As well as an increase in volume, inflammation causes a loss of marginal definition and hyperperfusion. Anechoic areas with distal acoustic enhancement indicate **abscess formation** (**Fig. 10.18**).

Depending on the echotexture, ultrasonography can indirectly determine the consistency of a new lesion. As is the case with cavities filled with viscous mucus, **mucoceles** are firm, elastic, well demarcated, and mobile on sonographic palpation, and display absolutely no intrinsic vascularity (**Fig. 10.19**).

Posttraumatic **hematomas** of the face can be seen as hypoechoic, usually subcutaneous, irregularly defined space-occupying lesions without any signs of intrinsic perfusion (**Fig. 10.20**). Associated with an increasing organization of the hematoma, vascularization can be seen on CCDS over the course of time (**Figs. 10.21, 10.22**).

Solid tumors with visible intrinsic perfusion tend to be hypoechoic or inhomogeneously echoic. To a limited extent, the consistency of a lesion or swelling can also be estimated on the basis of its echogenicity and the findings on sonographic palpation (**Figs. 10.23, 10.24, 10.25**; ▶ Videos 10.3, 10.4).

At first glance, the different types of **vascular malformations** have a similar abnormal ultrasound features in B-mode scans, which makes differentiation more difficult. There is a compressible, loosely structured, honeycomb echo pattern that is partly hypoechoic, partly echogenic (**Figs. 10.26, 10.27**).

Ultrasonography allows the assessment of the extent and depth of these lesions in the relevant structure and adjacent soft tissues. The use of color Doppler ultrasound makes it possible to differentiate vascular malformations from other masses (**Figs. 10.28, 10.29**).

Hemangiomas have a heterogeneous echotexture that is hypoechoic with sinusoidal compartments. The perfused areas of these angiomas are, however, visible on CCDS and measurements can be taken to assess venous and arterial elements (**Figs. 10.30, 10.31, 10.32**). The afferent vessels are branches from the carotid artery territory. Echogenic internal echoes indicate intrinsic venous calcification (phleboliths). Compression with the probe induces an increase in the velocity of the Doppler flow curve.

Lymphangiomas/hygromas, on the other hand, do not produce any color flow or Doppler signals and are easily compressible. Their characteristic feature is a loculated appearance that makes it possible to classify them as macrocystic or microcystic lesions (**Figs. 10.33, 10.34**). With respect to location, most lymphangiomas are found at submandibular, supraclavicular, or parotid sites (see also Chapter 6, p. 75, and Chapter 10, p. 152).

The role of ultrasound-guided fine-needle aspiration biopsies and percutaneous and interstitial laser therapy must be mentioned. It may also be used when injecting sclerotic agents under direct visual.

Malignant Tumors

In dermatology, high-frequency ultrasound probes (18–20 MHz) are used to examine skin lesions. Transducers used in the head and neck from 5 to 14 MHz are nevertheless capable of depicting the majority of skin lesions or tumorous formation. Ultrasonography can be used to assess the extent and the depth of malignant lesions of the facial soft tissues, such as melanomas and **basal cell carcinomas (BCCs)** (**Figs. 10.35, 10.36**). Of course a high proportion of malignant tumors are metastases from squamous cell carcinomas (**Figs. 10.37, 10.38**). The importance of examining the cervical lymph nodes has once again to be emphasized in this context, as they are the site of possible regional metastasis.

Further diagnostic imaging is indicated if the pathological changes are found affecting structures that cannot be reliably assessed with ultrasound, such as bones or the paranasal sinuses.

Pearls and Pitfalls

The relevant draining lymph node stations of the neck must always be examined meticulously if there is any suspicion that the space-occupying lesion is malignant.

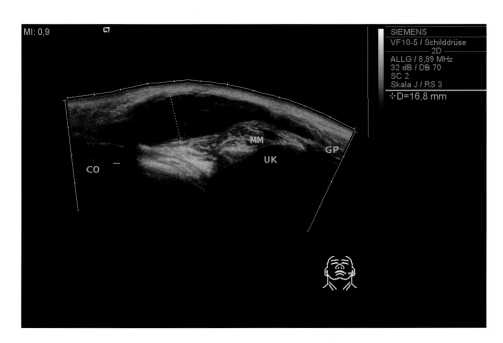

Fig. 10.1 Panoramic view—parotid region, left, transverse. The salivary duct (caliper) is dilated along its entire path from the gland (GP), over the masseter muscle (MM), to its opening into the oral cavity (CO), where it shows stenotic changes. UK, mandible. Diagnosis: **Obstructive sialadenitis**.

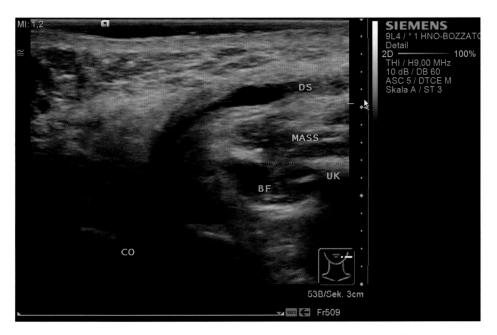

Fig. 10.2 Parotid gland/angle of the mouth, left, anterior transverse. The buccal fat pad (BF) can be identified as a hypoechoic structure with irregular margins located in the region where the duct (DS) of the parotid gland opens into the oral cavity (CO). Lying behind this is the border formed by the masseter muscle (MASS) and the mandible (UK). Diagnosis: **Obstructive sialadenitis.**

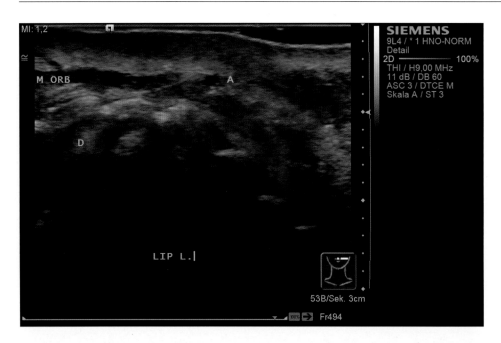

Fig. 10.3 Angle of the mouth/upper lip, left, transverse. The hypoechoic band of the orbicularis oris muscle (M ORB) lies outside the hyperechoic reflections of the teeth (D), which look like cobblestones in relief. At the lateral border is the superior labial artery (A) seen in cross-section.

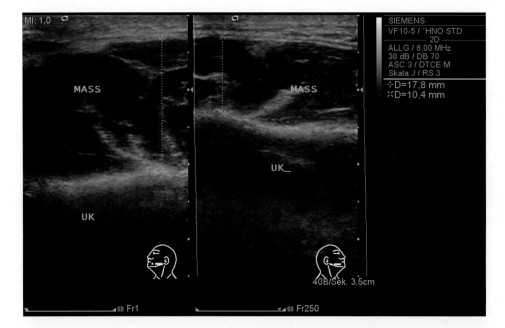

Fig. 10.4 Split screen of the buccal region in the transverse plane. The right masseter muscle (MASS) is clearly thicker than on the other side. UK, horizontal ramus of the mandible. Diagnosis: **Hypertrophy of the left masseter muscle**.

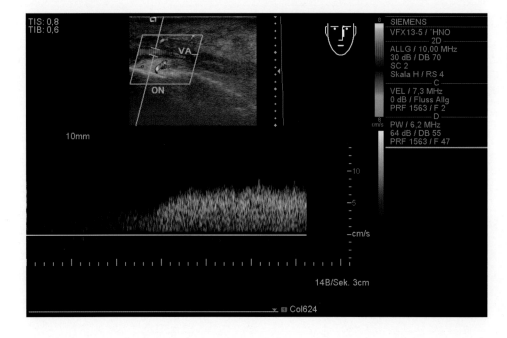

Fig. 10.5 Medial canthus, left, longitudinal, at the nasal bone (ON) in a case of **furunculosis in the medial canthus**. CCDS shows a clear venous Doppler spectrum, and thus rules out any thrombosis. VA, angular vein.

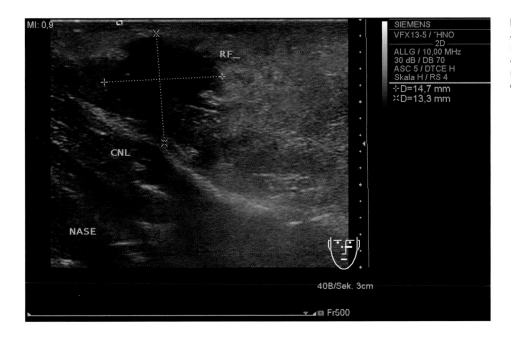

Fig. 10.6 Medial canthus, left, diagonal, with abscess formation (RF) secondary to furunculosis. Hypoechoic tissue thickening with irregular ill-defined margins is seen on the left sidewall of the nose (CNL). NASE, nose. Diagnosis: **Furunculosis of the left medial canthus**.

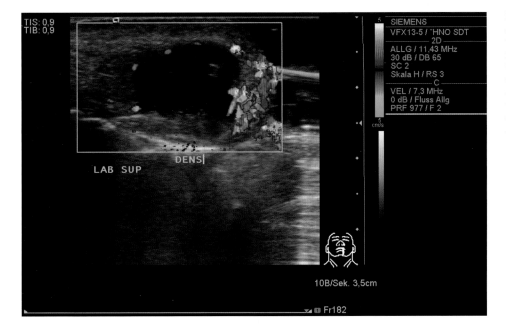

Fig. 10.7 Upper lip, left, longitudinal. In this abscess of the upper lip, a hyperechoic margin forms the border of the inside of the upper lip (LAB SUP) and oral cavity with the tooth lying beneath it (DENS). The lip itself is enlarged and hypoechoic with central anechogenicity. The distal acoustic enhancement typical of an abscess can be seen in the intensified posterior wall echo. The periphery of the abscess is hyperperfused. Diagnosis: **Labial abscess**.

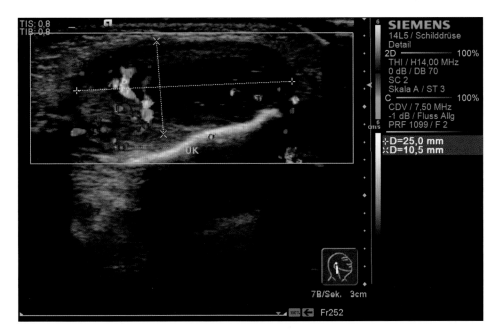

Fig. 10.8 Parotid gland, right, longitudinal, CCDS. The hypoechoic, centrally anechoic swelling in a 2-week-old was first suspected to be an angioma, but the strong peripheral perfusion with no central vascularity was not consistent with this diagnosis. An abscess was confirmed after ultrasound-guided fine-needle aspiration. Diagnosis: **Abscess of the parotid gland and masseter muscle**.

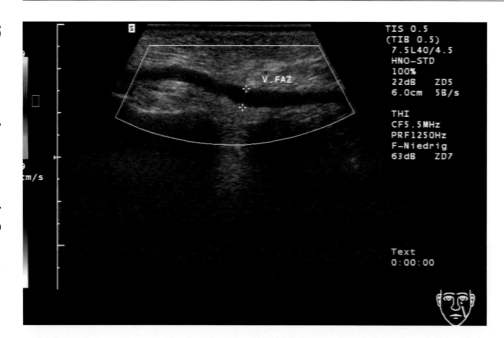

Fig. 10.9 Medial canthus, left, oblique. Thrombosis of the angular vein can be seen in the continuous view of the course of the vein. The lumen of a normal vein, if it can be seen at all, can always be compressed by applying pressure with the probe. Diagnosis: **Thrombosis of the left angular vein.**

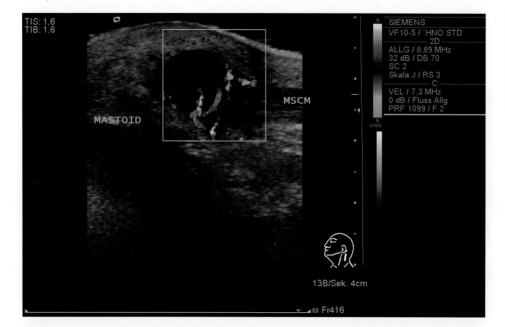

Fig. 10.10 Mastoid, left, longitudinal. The subcutaneous tissue is elevated by a well-demarcated lymph node with a central hyperechoic hilum ("hilar sign") and hilar perfusion, making the ear protrude. This has to be distinguished from an abscess. The mastoid plane (MASTOID) is intact. MSCM, sternocleidomastoid muscle. Diagnosis: **Retroauricular lymphadenitis.**

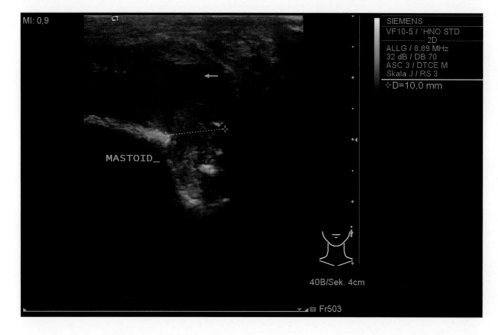

Fig. 10.11 Mastoid, left, longitudinal. The subcutaneous tissue is also thickened by an inflammatory process (arrow). In this case, however, the echogenic contour of the mastoid (MASTOID) is interrupted by the abscess draining to the surface (caliper). Diagnosis: **Acute mastoiditis.**

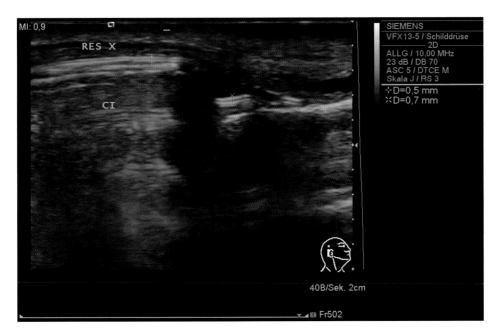

Fig. 10.12 Mastoid plane, right, longitudinal. After a **cochlear implant**, the implant bed shows no signs of hematoma. The cochlear implant (CI) is enclosed in a preshaped hull made out of Resorb X (poly [D,L-lactide] and poly [L-lactide-co-glycolide]) absorbable mesh for osteosynthesis (RES X®, Ethicon, Johnson & Johnson, Norderstedt, Germany), which can be seen clearly in the ultrasound images. The mesh will be absorbed within a few weeks' time.

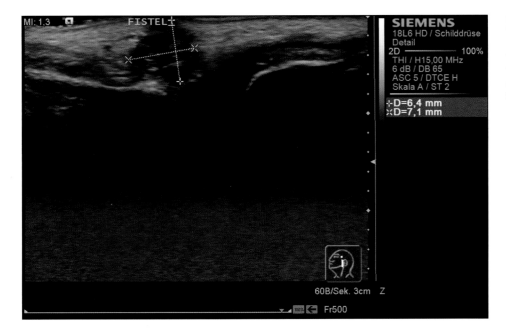

Fig. 10.13 Preauricular region, left, longitudinal. The wavy contour of the outer auricle shows a rounded hypoechoic lesion in the subcutaneous tissues. A connection of the preauricular sinus or fistula (FISTEL) into deeper anatomical regions cannot be distinguished. Diagnosis: **Preauricular sinus.**

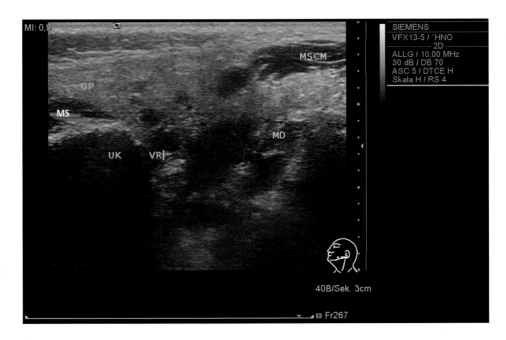

Fig. 10.14 Parotid, left, transverse. **Infected fistula of the auditory passage**. With clinical swelling and trismus, hypoechoic changes can be seen within the glandular tissue of the parotid (GP). These are not restricted to the superficial part of the gland, but are also visible in the deeper regions below the level of the retromandibular vein (VR) and at the digastric muscle (MD). MS, masseter muscle; MSCM, sternocleidomastoid muscle; UK, mandible.

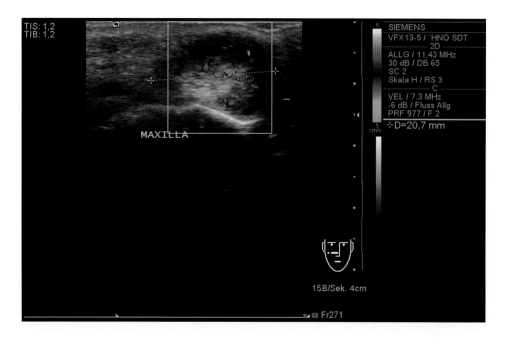

Fig. 10.15 Anterior wall of the maxillary sinus, right, transverse. The epidermoid cyst lying in the subcutaneous tissue appears as a clearly defined hypoechoic space-occupying lesion beneath the skin. The mixed hypoechoic and echogenic components, with some anechoic areas away from the center, are typical of epidermoid cysts. MAXILLA, anterior wall of the maxillary sinus. Diagnosis: **Epidermoid cyst**.

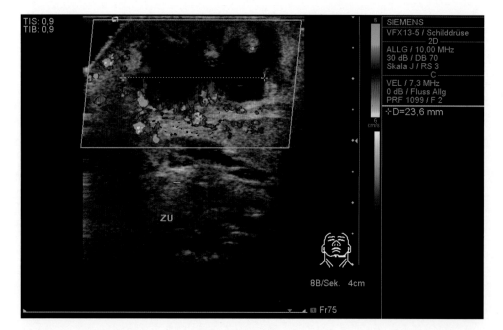

Fig. 10.16 Submandibular region, left, transverse. An **acutely inflamed, enlarged epidermoid cyst** (caliper) can be seen in cross-section as an irregular, inhomogeneous space-occupying lesion immediately next to the epidermis. Inflammatory hyperperfusion can be seen in the surrounding tissue on CCDS. ZU, tongue.

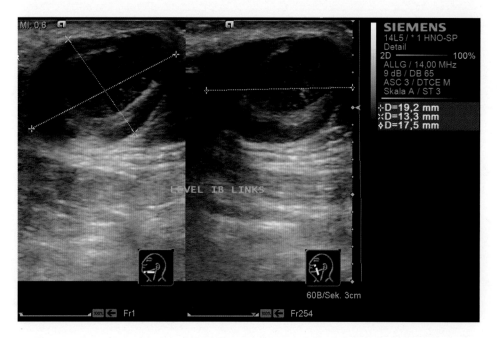

Fig. 10.17 Split screen, submandibular region, left. The **epidermoid cyst** (caliper) can be seen as a rounded, clearly defined space-occupying lesion. The presence of inhomogeneous internal echoes demonstrates the heterogeneous cell contents of the epidermoid cyst.

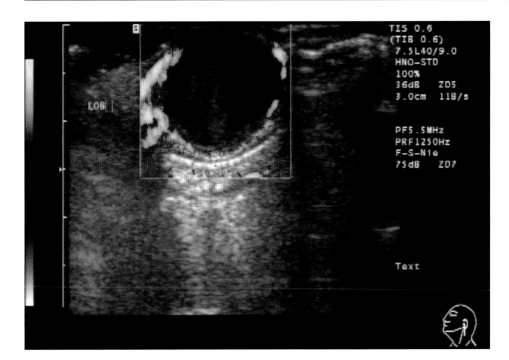

Fig. 10.18 Infra-auricular region/lobe, left, longitudinal. CCDS shows tangential perfusion, but no intrinsic perfusion, of an abscess in the ear lobe (LOB). The lesion is otherwise clearly defined and shows distal acoustic enhancement. Diagnosis: **Ear lobe abscess**.

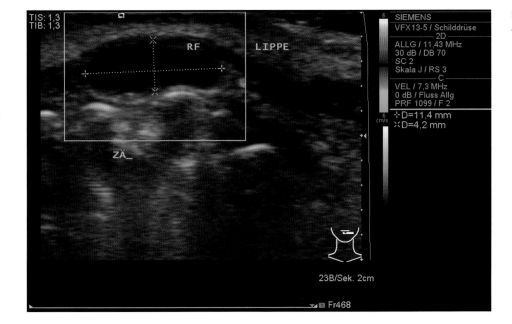

Fig. 10.19 Lower lip, paramedian, left, transverse. A firm, elastic, clearly defined space-occupying lesion (RF) without any intrinsic perfusion can be seen in the lower lip (LIPPE). The teeth (ZÄ) lie directly behind the inner edge of the lesion. Diagnosis: **Mucocele of the lower lip**.

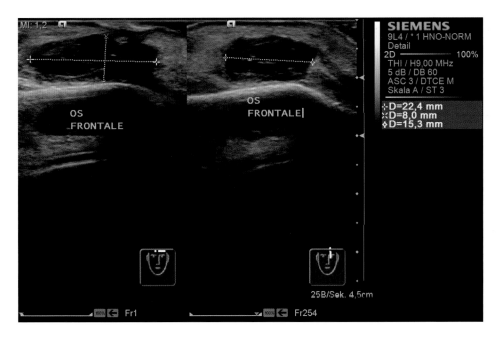

Fig. 10.20 Split screen of a **posttraumatic hematoma** over the frontal bone (OS FRONTALE) on the left. The inhomogeneous space-occupying lesion lies in the subcutaneous tissue and has irregular margins. The echogenic band of the anterior wall of the sinus must be carefully examined to rule out a fracture. Note the space-occupying lesion, with a structure similar to the hematoma, lying beneath the bone; this is a reflection artifact.

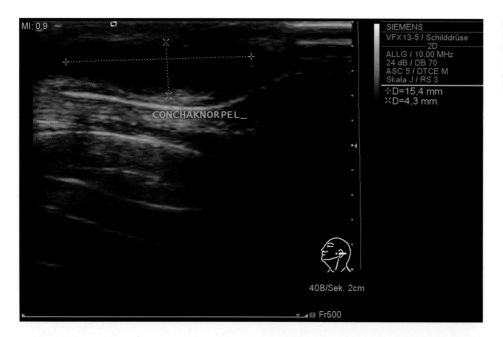

Fig. 10.21 Auricle, left, transverse. Soft-tissue swelling in the cavity of the concha following trauma; the ultrasound examination confirms the picture of a **hematoma of the ear.** The conchal cartilage (CONCHAKNORPEL) lying behind it is intact.

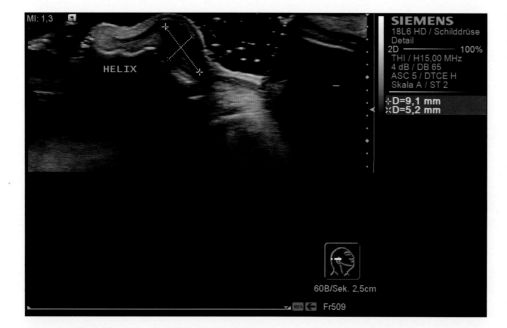

Fig. 10.22 Auricle, right, transverse, cranial. Posterior swelling of the helix (HELIX) following trauma. The **hematoma** (caliper) measures 9 mm × 5 mm on the ultrasound image.

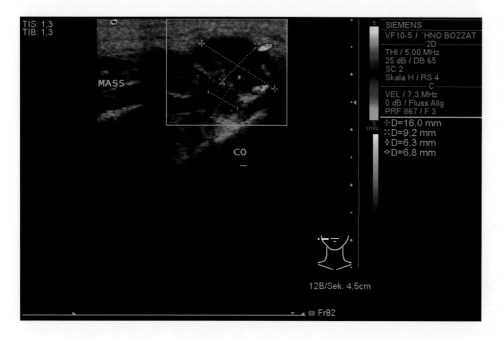

Fig. 10.23 Parotid gland, right, anterior transverse. The solid space-occupying lesion (**pleomorphic adenoma**) in the soft tissues of the right cheek at the anterior border of the masseter muscle (MASS) moves on palpation and is clearly demarcated from the oral cavity (CO). CCDS shows diffuse perfusion of the space-occupying lesion.

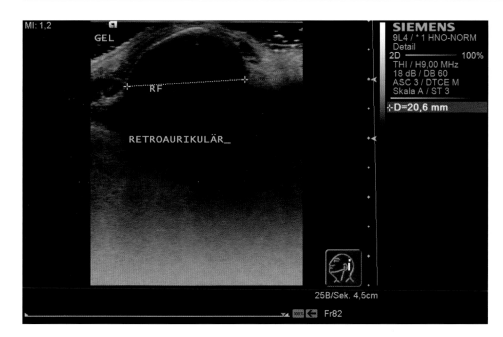

Fig. 10.24 Retroauricular region, left, longitudinal. A **retroauricular osteoma** with an echogenic surface and distal acoustic enhancement, which is indicative of a bony consistency. If the space-occupying lesion is very prominent, sufficient coupling can be obtained only by using a sufficient quantity of ultrasound gel (GEL).

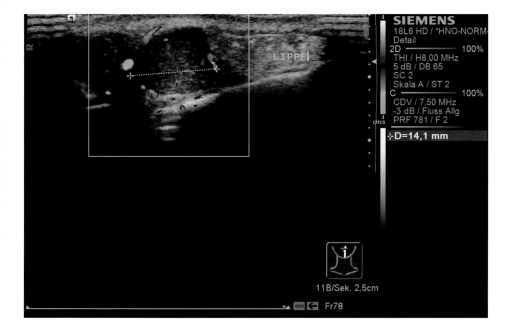

Fig. 10.25 Upper lip, left, longitudinal. A clearly defined rounded, lobulated space-occupying lesion with distal acoustic enhancement (**schwannoma**) can be seen in the soft tissues of the upper lip (LIPPE). CCDS can be used to distinguish it from a cyst; the diffuse perfusion confirms a solid tumor.

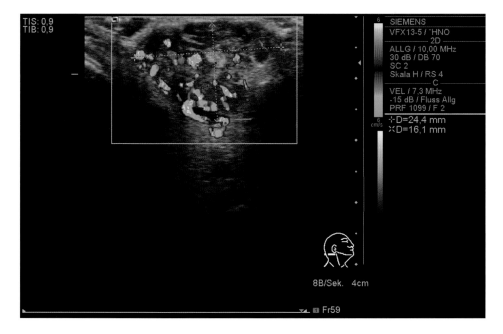

Fig. 10.26 Parotid gland, right, transverse. This **hemangioma** in a 4-month-old appears as a rounded, clearly defined hypoechoic space-occupying lesion with echogenic internal echoes. CCDS shows pronounced diffuse perfusion within the lesion.

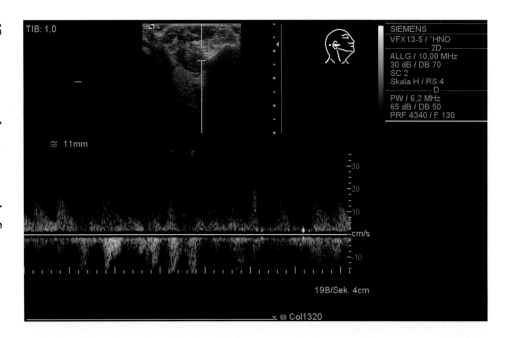

Fig. 10.27 Parotid gland, right, transverse. Doppler flow measurements confirm that the tumor has a mixed arterial and venous supply, consistent with the diagnosis of a **hemangioma** (see **Fig. 10.26**).

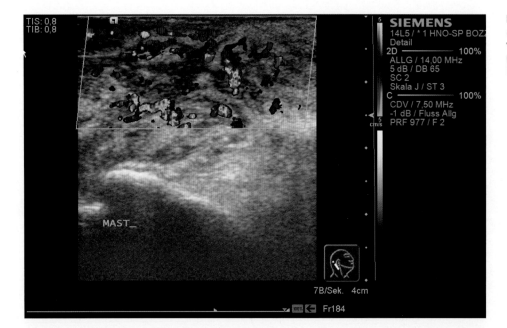

Fig. 10.28 Retroauricular region, right, longitudinal, CCDS. The hypoechoic swelling shows diffuse vascularity that consists in part of arterial and in part of strong venous elements. MAST, mastoid. Diagnosis: **Arteriovenous malformation**.

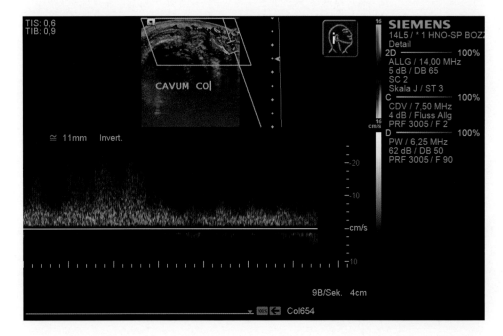

Fig. 10.29 Retroauricular region, right, longitudinal, CCDS, Doppler. The hypoechoic swelling shows diffuse vascularity that consists in part of arterial and in part of strong venous elements (see **Fig. 10.28**). CAVUM CO, mastoid. Diagnosis: **Arteriovenous malformation**.

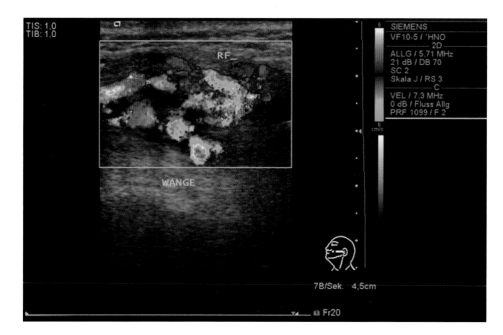

Fig. 10.30 Cheek, left, anterior transverse. CCDS shows mixed vascular perfusion with predominantly venous elements in a hypoechoic space-occupying lesion (RF) in the soft tissues of the cheek (WANGE). Diagnosis: **Arteriovenous malformation**.

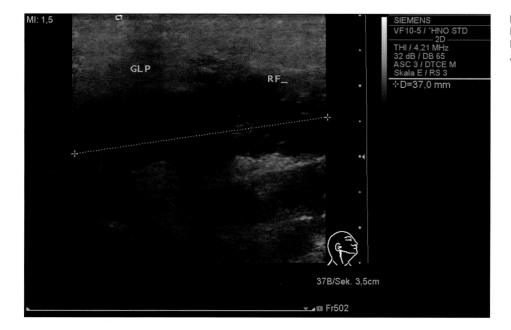

Fig. 10.31 Parotid gland, right, longitudinal. A hypoechoic structure with ill-defined margins can be distinguished between the parotid gland (GLP) and level II. Diagnosis: **Hemangioma**.

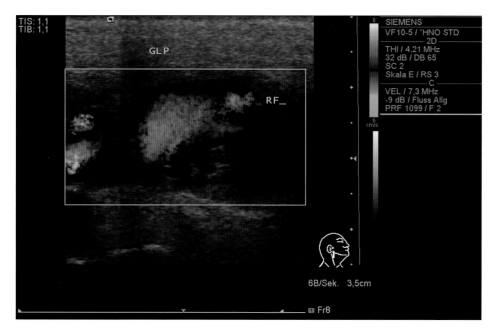

Fig. 10.32 Parotid gland (GLP), right, longitudinal. After additional CCDS, the lesion can be identified as a **hemangioma** (see **Fig. 10.31**).

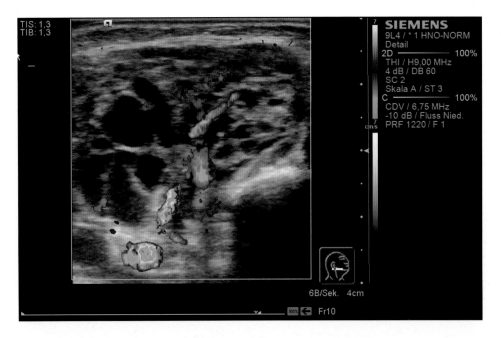

Fig. 10.33 Submandibular region, right, transverse. Submandibular lymphangioma. The **macrocystic lymphatic malformation** is located in the triangle formed between the tongue and the parotid gland. A typical clearly defined lobulated anechoic lesion with distal acoustic enhancement can be seen. Soft echogenic septa may often be found. The septa show strong perfusion.

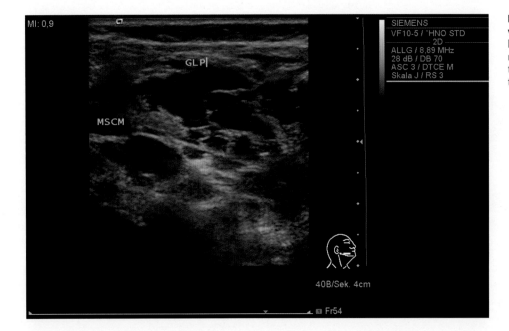

Fig. 10.34 Submandibular region, right, transverse. This **lymphangioma**, seen in cross-section, lies in the immediate vicinity of the sternocleidomastoid muscle (MSCM) and the inferior pole of the parotid gland (GLP). The polycyclic configuration of the angioma is very clear.

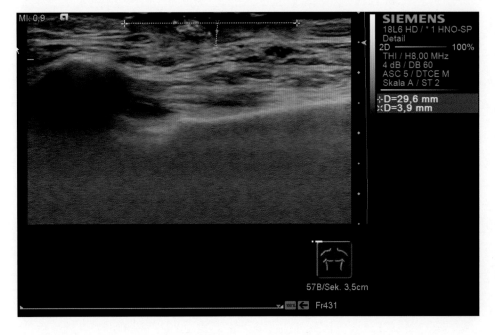

Fig. 10.35 Right cheek, transverse, with basal cell carcinoma. An irregular hypoechoic space-occupying lesion can be distinguished in the skin, extending to a depth of 3.9 mm. The **basal cell carcinoma** (caliper) was removed surgically without difficulty.

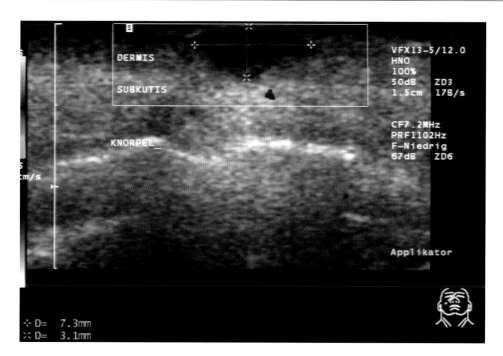

Fig. 10.36 Sidewall of the nose, right, diagonal, with **basal cell carcinoma**. The lesion extends to a depth of 3 mm into the dermis (DERMIS). It does not touch the lateral cartilage (KNORPEL). SUBKUTIS, subcutaneous tissue layer.

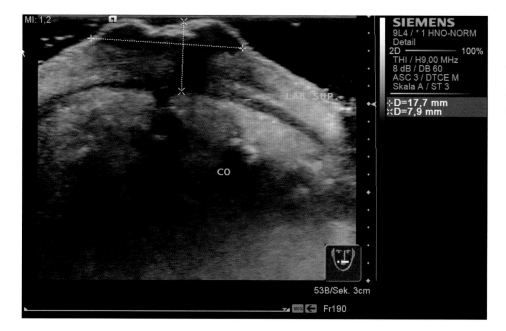

Fig. 10.37 Upper lip, transverse, median, with a **squamous cell carcinoma**. Tissue extension measured in the two planes shown is less than 20 mm, so the tumor is classed as stage T1. This tumor of the upper lip (LAB SUP.) does not reach the orbicularis oris muscle, which curves throughout the upper lip as a hypoechoic band and forms the deep-sited border of the oral cavity (CO).

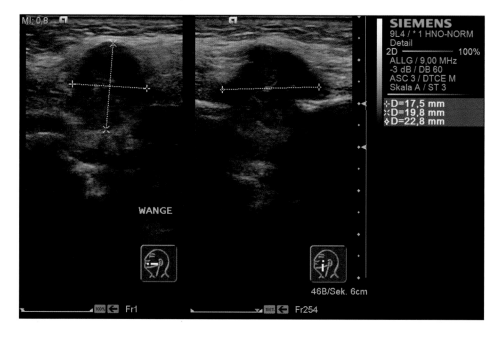

Fig. 10.38 Split screen, buccal region, left, transverse. **Recurrence of a squamous cell carcinoma** of the cheek (WANGE). In the transverse view, the hypoechoic formation seems to lie on the anterior border of the masseter muscle, not far from the oral cavity. In the longitudinal view, however, infiltration of the ascending ramus of the mandible can clearly be seen.

11 Paranasal Sinuses and Midface

Anatomy

Ultrasonography offers a rapid, safe, first-line assessment and is also useful for a preliminary evaluation in cases of trauma. Exposure to ionizing radiation from X-rays can be avoided in both children and pregnant women.

A-mode (amplitude modulation in ultrasound) scanning was previously regularly used. It represents the time required for the ultrasound signal to hit a tissue interface and return the signal to the transducer; the greater the reflection at the tissue interface, the larger the signal amplitude on the screen. However, this mode has been increasingly superseded by B-scan imaging, which has become widely available.

The superficial frontal and maxillary sinuses are usually accessible. The eyeball can be used as a fluid-filled medium that enables the visualization of structures lying behind it as the ethmoid cells and orbit. Of course, normal and pathological structures within the eyeball are also accessible (▶ **Video 11.1**).

Ultrasonography of the nose and sinuses has a few distinct features in comparison with soft-tissue imaging of the neck. Physically, ultrasound waves traverse the anatomical target area (air-filled spaces surrounded by bone) to only a limited extent. In normal maxillary and frontal sinuses, the layers of the cutis (8–10 mm) and the transition from skin to anterior wall of the sinus can be seen, behind which there is usually a total reflection.

Assessment is possible only in the case of pathological conditions, which allow the "posterior wall echoes" to be seen. This usually occurs at a depth of about 40 mm in the maxillary sinus and of 20 mm in the frontal sinus.

The examination of the paranasal sinuses is best carried out with the upper body upright. Additional head positions with hyperextension and anteflexion of the neck may distinguish fluid or effusion from other pathological conditions.

Examination of the maxillary and frontal sinuses is always performed in the transverse and longitudinal planes. It is particularly important to make a comparison of the findings on the right and left side. The starting point of a maxillary sinus examination is at the level of the infraorbital nerve; the frontal sinus examination starts with the

transducer position between the eyebrows. Insonation frequency (as low as possible), penetration depth (±60 mm), and gain (high) should be adjusted beforehand (**Fig. 11.1**).

Inflammatory Changes

Sinusitis

As mentioned above, ultrasound wave transmission in the depths of the sinuses is possible in the presence of an inflammatory process with secretions and mucosal swelling within the lumen of a paranasal sinus (**sinusitis**). If the entire sinus cavity being examined is filled (with pus or mucus) by such a process, the sound is not completely reflected at the anterior wall but is transmitted further to the posterior wall, where it is once again reflected to give a visible "posterior wall echo." The posterior wall of the maxillary sinus has a U- or V-shaped configuration.

Depending on the viscosity of the process inside the lumen it appears hypoechoic to anechoic with sparse isolated internal echoes (**Figs. 11.2, 11.3**). Fluid secretions, if not filling the lumen completely, may become visible by anteflecting the head, and disappear after reclination.

Cysts and **mucoceles** lying against the anterior wall may be seen as rounded space-occupying lesions (**Figs. 11.4, 11.5, 11.6, 11.7**). In the case of an acute exacerbated inflammatory process, destruction of osseous structures is possible and consecutive swelling of neighbouring soft tissue is observed. Structures lying behind air-filled areas are not visible. An isolated process at the posterior wall of the air-filled sinus will escape detection.

Benign Tumors

Benign tumors of the paranasal sinuses, such as **mycetomas** and **adenomas**, are visible on ultrasound images only in isolated cases and are sometimes difficult to distinguish from inflammatory changes

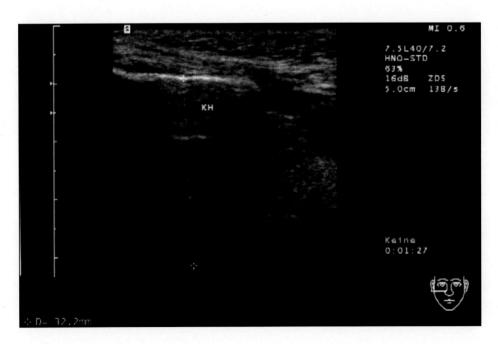

Fig. 11.1 Maxilla, right, transverse. The ultrasound probe is held in the transverse plane beneath the orbit; the image shows the typical normal findings. The first echogenic band can be seen at a depth of 1 cm and forms the border between the anterior maxillary sinus wall and the soft tissue layer. Equidistant below this, but less extensive, are other echogenic reflexes (caliper) in the maxillary sinus (KH). These reflexes are **artifacts** and are generated by multiple-reflection echoes. They should **not be confused with a posterior wall echo**.

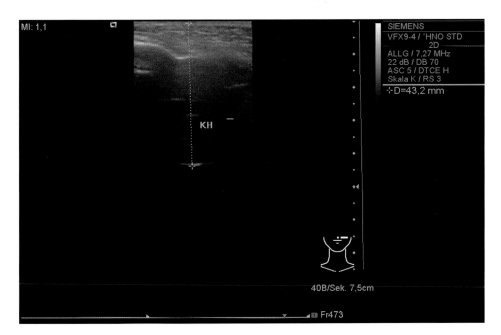

Fig. 11.2 Maxilla, left, transverse. The **posterior wall echo** (KH) can be identified as a clear echogenic band at a depth of 40 mm: the depth at which it is seen (caliper) is decisive for its identification, as this depth corresponds to the anatomical site of the posterior wall. These reflexes are artifacts generated by multiple-reflection echoes. They should not be confused with a posterior wall echo.

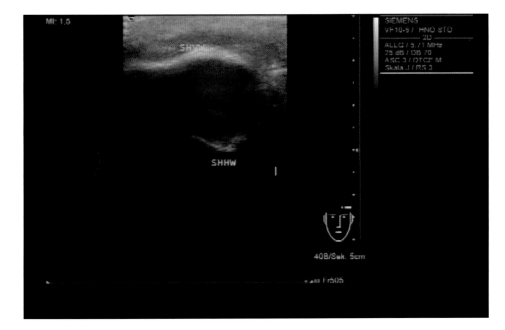

Fig. 11.3 Frontal sinus, left, transverse. Here, a trough-shaped echogenic reflection (SHHW) can be seen at a depth of 20 mm. Like the posterior wall echo of the maxillary sinus, the posterior wall echo of the frontal sinus can be seen in **acute sinusitis**. SHVW, anterior wall of the frontal sinus.

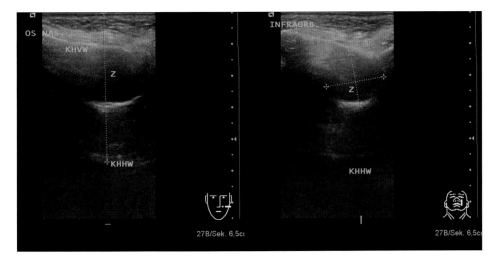

Fig. 11.4 Split screen, maxilla, left. A **cyst** (Z) lying against the anterior wall of the sinus (KHVW) is demarcated as a round hypoechoic structure. As the residual lumen lying behind the cyst is filled with secretion, the posterior wall of the maxillary sinus (KHHW) is visible deeper in the tissues. INFRAORB, infraorbital rim; OS NAS, nasal bone.

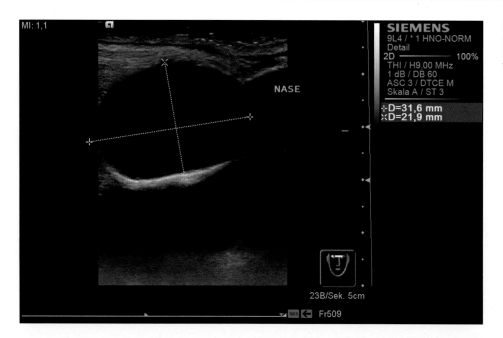

Fig. 11.5 Frontal sinus, right, transverse. The **mucocele in the right frontal sinus**, lying laterally to the nasal bone (NASE), appears as a well-demarcated anechoic structure.

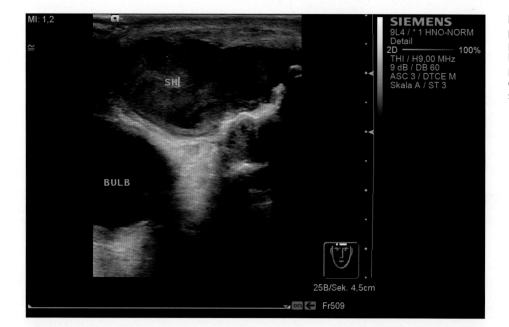

Fig. 11.6 Frontal sinus, right, transverse. A **pyocele of the right frontal sinus** (SH) with purulent contents appears as an irregular lobulated structure with an inhomogeneous echo pattern, lying immediately next to the orbital cavity (BULB). Sonographic palpation shows liquid secretions.

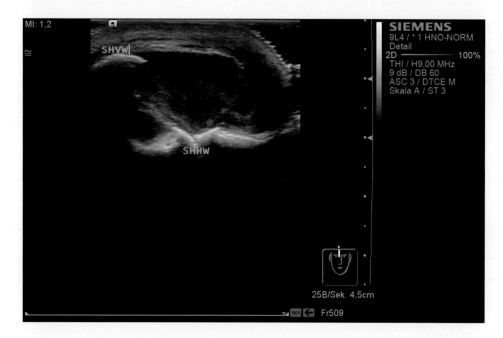

Fig. 11.7 Frontal sinus, right, longitudinal. The **pyocele in the right frontal sinus** has caused a defect in the region of the anterior wall (SHVW) and passage through the skin. The posterior wall (SHHW) is well demonstrated. The three-dimensional extent of the inflammatory changes can be seen.

(**Fig. 11.8**). Multiple inhomogeneous reflecting structures can be seen bordering the anterior wall and possibly extending to the posterior wall of the sinus under examination. Visualization is independent from positioning the head. The usually intense irregular echo pattern distinguishes this finding from the typical echo pattern of an effusion or a mucocele, in which there are rather discrete ultrasound changes on the way from the anterior to the posterior wall. The multiple reflections are therefore the characteristic of a solid mass in the sinus region. An assessment of the histology of the sinunasal lesion is not possible, however.

Malignant Tumors

The ultrasonographic appearance of **malignant tumors** is characterized by their osteodestructive and infiltrative growth into adjacent structures (**Figs. 11.9, 11.10**; ▸ Video 11.2). Disrupted contours and inhomogeneous internal echoes, as well as diffuse irregular perfusion within the space-occupying lesion, may be **substantiate suspicion of malignancy**.

Deeper areas of the paranasal sinus system may become visible after radical surgery of, for example, the frontal sinuses (▸ Videos 11.3, 11.4).

Given the poor prognosis of malignant tumors of, for example, the sinuses, a thorough examination of the cervical lymph nodes is also essential whenever sinunasal cancer is suspected.

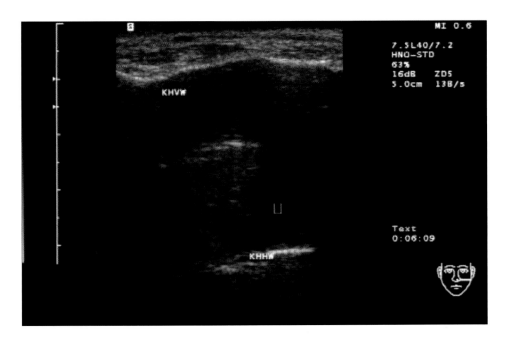

Fig. 11.8 Maxilla, left, transverse. As well as the posterior wall echo (KHHW), a central echogenic structure can be identified in the left maxillary sinus. It must not be confused with the posterior wall echo. Diagnosis: **Mycetoma of the left maxillary sinus**.

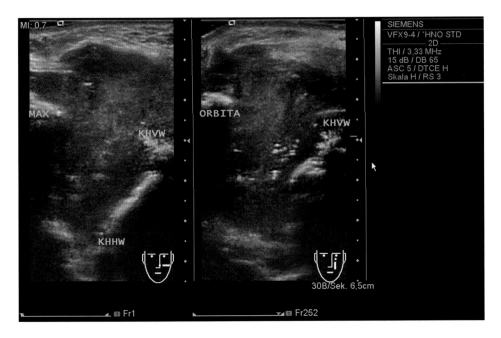

Fig. 11.9 Split screen, maxilla, left. Typical ultrasonographic appearance of an **adenocarcinoma in the left maxillary sinus** (MAX). The anterior wall (KHVW) has been destroyed and the tumor is growing cranially around the inferior orbital margin (ORBITA). The hypoechoic, inhomogeneous tumor fills the lumen of the maxillary sinus completely. Therefore the ultrasound waves reach the posterior wall of the maxillary sinus and a posterior wall echo (KHHW) is visible.

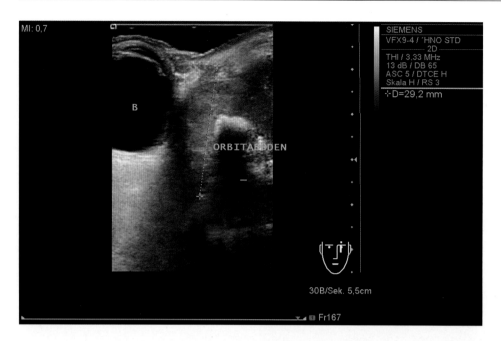

Fig. 11.10 Maxilla, left, longitudinal. The ultrasound scan shows an **adenocarcinoma of the left maxillary sinus**, which has destroyed the orbital floor (ORBITABODEN) and invaded the orbital cavity and lies directly adjacent to the eyeball (B). Infiltration of the periorbital region can be assumed.

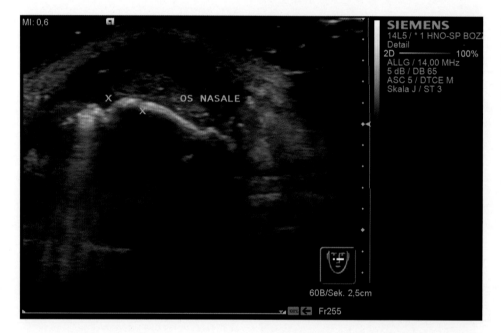

Fig. 11.11 Bridge of the nose, middle third, transverse. The soft tissues immediately below the skin show a half-moon–shaped area of loose hypoechoic structure with the typical appearance of a **hematoma**. The underlying discontinuation of the nasal bone (OS NASALE), which is **fractured in two places** (X, X), cannot be detected clinically as it is masked by the hematoma.

Trauma

B-mode sonography is increasingly being used for an exploratory assessment to demonstrate **fractures of the nasal bone** or mediolateral midface trauma (**Figs. 11.11, 11.12, 11.13**; ▶ Video 11.5). These can be diagnosed with great precision and the success of repositioning can be assessed without causing pain.

Posttraumatic swelling with a hypoechoic extension at the site of bruising is found in hematoma. In fractures a disruption of the visible bone contour is evidentiary for a traumatic dislocation of osseous fragments.

In suspected more complex facial trauma cases, or if there is any cause for doubt, further radiological work-up with computed tomography is compulsory, not least for medicolegal reasons (**Figs. 11.14, 11.15**; ▶ Videos 11.6, 11.7).

Ultrasonography can be used to both assess the success of the repositioning and control the location of the material used for osteosynthesis (**Fig. 11.16**).

Ultrasound assessment is equally helpful in cases where the presence of a **foreign body** is suspected (**Fig. 11.17**). When performing ultrasound foreign bodies are known to have a characteristic echogenicity (usually hyperechoic with distal acoustic attenuation). For radio-opaque foreign bodies, ultrasound can provide additional information for precise localization.

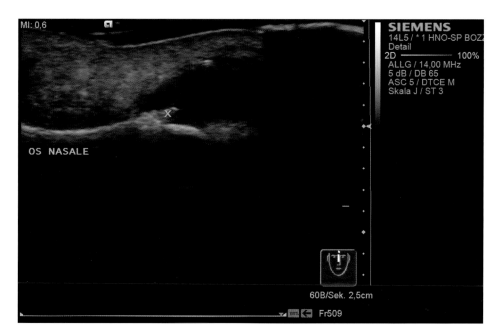

Fig. 11.12 Bridge of the nose, middle third, longitudinal. Discontinuation of the bony contour (X) of the distal part of the nasal bone (OS NASALE) can also be identified beneath the hematoma in the longitudinal plane. This appearance is characteristic of a **fracture**.

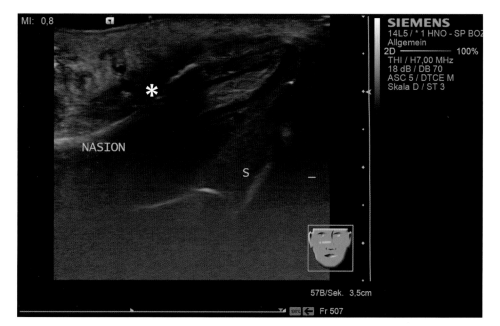

Fig. 11.13 Flank of the nose, middle third, right axial. A dislocated fragment can be seen in this **nasal bone fracture** (asterisk). Distally, the cartilaginous bridge of the nose allows the underlying structures (alar, lateral, and septal cartilages [S]) to be identified.

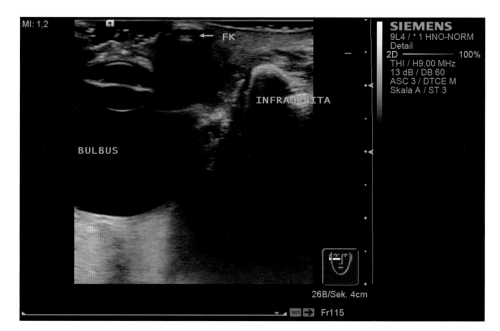

Fig. 11.14 Infraorbital rim, longitudinal oblique. An **orbital margin fracture** with marked dislocation of the infraorbital rim. The craniolateral fragment (FK) is pressing on the eyeball (BULBUS).

II Sonographic Anatomy and Pathology

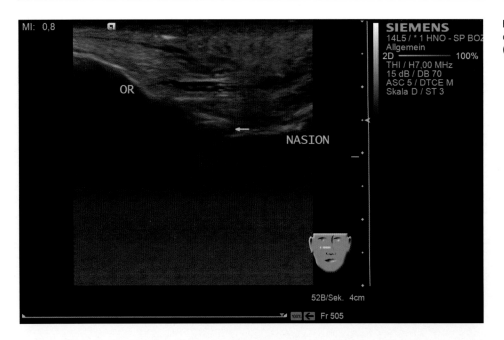

Fig. 11.15 Infraorbital rim, transverse. An inferior orbital rim (OR) **fracture** with marked dislocation (arrow) of the infraorbital margin.

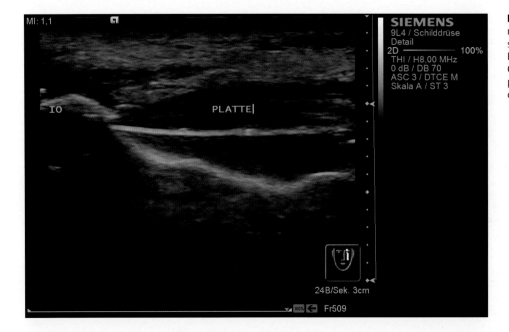

Fig. 11.16 Maxilla, left, longitudinal. Following reconstruction of the anterior wall of the maxillary sinus with a PDS plate (PLATTE) (Poly-P-dioxanon; Ethicon, Johnson & Johnson, Norderstedt, Germany) the ultrasound scan clearly shows the plate covering the anterior wall and confirms its cranial position at the infraorbital margin (IO).

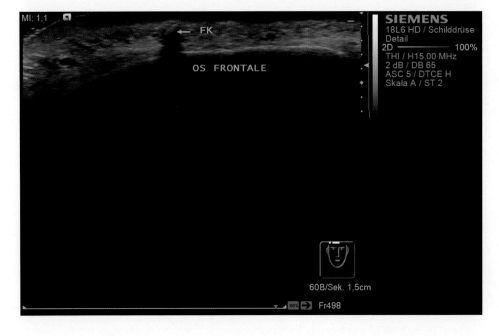

Fig. 11.17 Right frontal sinus, transverse. Following an injury, a **splinter of glass** (FK), seen as a hyperechoic reflection with distal shadowing, can be identified in the subcutaneous soft tissues in front of the sinus (OS FRONTALE).

12 Larynx and Hypopharynx

Anatomy

The larynx and hypopharynx are not always optimally accessible to ultrasound examination because of their anatomical position, with surrounding air-filled spaces and the irregular ossification of the thyroid cartilage found in adults. As a rule, the retropharyngeal space cannot be assessed completely (even when the probe is tilted) because of its location behind the pharynx. In children and adolescents, however, the examination usually gives a complete overview of the structures in this area.

The area should be examined with the patient's head reclined and with sufficient gel applied to even out the irregular contours of the laryngeal prominence. Starting with the acoustic shadowing of the hyoid, the preepiglottic space can be assessed in cross-section (**Fig. 12.1**). In the transverse plane, the epiglottis is visible as a horizontal arching hypoechoic band.

Moving the probe parallel to the midline, the spindle-shaped/oval, hypoechoic, and finely pinnate prelaryngeal muscles, such as the thyrohyoid, sternohyoid, and sternothyroid, can be seen in cross-section. Below these, the tentlike alae of the thyroid cartilage can be seen on both the right and the left (**Figs. 12.2, 12.3**; ▶ Video 12.1). If the cartilage is ossified, its appearance is hyperechoic with distal acoustic shadowing, which may compromise the view of the intrinsic structures of the larynx.

In the endolarynx, it is not always possible to identify the vestibular folds as individual structures with any certainty, as the paraglottic fat and adjacent sinus of Morgagni, with its dense air echoes, may be superimposed (**Fig. 12.4**; ▶ Video 12.2).

On quiet respiration, the vocal cords can be distinguished caudally as echogenic lines converging anteriorly; they oscillate when the patient phonates (▶ Videos 12.3, 12.4).

In their triangular configuration, the arytenoid cartilages can be seen as hypoechoic structures forming the posterior limit of the vocal cords. If conditions are favorable, the epithelial borders of the piriform sinus and the postcricoid region can be identified posterior to the arytenoid cartilage (**Fig. 12.5**; ▶ Video 12.5). The borders of the lateral hypopharyngeal walls extend outward like lips lateral to the caudal thyroid cartilage as a hypoechoic/echogenic double contour.

In adults, it may sometimes be better to examine the larynx unilaterally with the linear array transducer in a paramedian transverse position.

Pearls and Pitfalls

Asking the patient to say quietly a long "heee" establishes the correct positioning of the vocal cord plane for comparison of oscillation on the two sides. The probe has to be readjusted because of the elevation of the larynx with phonation.

Located inferiorly and interrupted by the cricothyroid ligament, the cricoid cartilage, which lies below the thyroid cartilage, and the first tracheal ring can be differentiated (**Figs. 12.6, 12.7**). Only the superficial part of the trachea can be seen on ultrasound imaging: further down, air prevents the structures within the trachea from being demonstrated clearly. The surface of the trachea can easily be identified by its characteristic "rope ladder" appearance.

The cervical esophagus can be identified from its ring-shaped structure and its position, which, anatomically, is immediately to the left of the thyroid gland (**Figs. 12.8, 12.9**; ▶ Video 12.6). Deeper, the esophagus lies on the spine. Osteophytes that narrow the esophageal lumen and cause dysphagia can also be demonstrated on ultrasonography.

Pearls and Pitfalls

Asking the patient to swallow helps to positively identify the esophagus. The mixture of saliva and air can be seen briefly on its way to the stomach as a pathway of mobile hyperechoic "sparkling" echoes the acoustic shadows caused by scattering. The postion of the esophagus usually moves from the left to the right when the patient's head is turned to the right.

Inflammatory Changes

Parapharyngeal and retropharyngeal abscesses are presented in detail in Chapters 6 and 8 (pp. 68–75 and 98).

Benign Tumors

Although laryngoscopy is usually sufficient to diagnose **vocal cord polyps** and **cysts**, anterior lesions can be clearly demonstrated as smooth-walled hypoechoic masses.

Vocal cord paresis obviously remains a laryngoscopic diagnosis, even if it can be seen on ultrasound scanning as asymmetrical movements when comparing the two sides.

Laryngoceles are spaces filled with liquid or mucoid secretions and have to be distinguished from cysts in the neck (**Fig. 12.10**). The detection of a connection between the endolarynx and upper edge of the thyroid cartilage makes the diagnosis easier. Hypoechoic appearance and lack of any intrinsic perfusion undermine the suspicion of a laryngocele, as does the possible enlargement of the lesion with a Valsalva maneuver.

In addition to their detection on laryngoscopy, **vascular malformations** can also be seen on ultrasonography as moderately to strongly perfused space-occupying lesions with inhomogeneous echogenicity and irregular margins (**Figs. 12.11, 12.12**).

Chondromas are rare space-occupying lesions of the thyroid or cricoid cartilages; they can be seen on ultrasound examination as solid thickenings of the cartilage concerned. In the thyroid cartilage, they more often appear as hypoechoic circumscribed swellings with clearly defined margins (**Fig. 12.13**).

A **Zenker diverticulum** or **pharyngeal pouch** can be recognized as a hyperechoic space-occupying lesion with distal acoustic shadowing in the typical site to the left of the thyroid (**Figs. 12.14, 12.15**; ▶ Videos 12.7, 12.8). It may sometimes show spatial enlargement if the sac is filled with debris or secretions. The act of swallowing can also be helpful here, to demonstrate that the space-occupying lesion is associated with the esophagus.

Malignant Tumors

Besides an assessment of the cervical lymph nodes, ultrasound imaging is also recommended for staging the extent of the primary tumor in cases of **laryngeal carcinoma**. While small T1 and T2 tumors can frequently be identified by their anterior extension (▶ Video 12.9), it is particularly easy to differentiate stage T4 tumors by the grade of infiltration of the thyroid cartilage cortex (**Figs. 12.16, 12.17, 12.18**; ▶ Video 12.10).

On ultrasonography, the morphology of a laryngeal malignancy is that of an irregular, ill-defined space-occupying lesion with inhomogeneous echogenicity and irregular perfusion (**Fig. 12.19**). Fixed vocal cords, and therefore stage T3, can be observed in individual cases: when comparing the two sides, a unilateral lack of echogenic movement (oscillation) indicates fixation (▶ Video 12.11). The preepiglottic and paraglottic spaces have to be assessed in both the transverse and longitudinal planes.

Depending on their size and position, **hypopharyngeal carcinomas** can be seen on the lateral wall of the lower third of the thyroid cartilage as ill-defined space-occupying lesions with inhomogeneous echo patterns (**Figs. 12.20, 12.21**; ▶ Videos 12.13, 12.14, 12.15, 12.16).

When examining malignant lesions of the larynx and hypopharynx, particular attention should be paid to any invasion of the vessels, thyroid gland, cervical plexus, and the sternocleidomastoid muscle. Exact sonographic assessment of the tumor dimensions, and visible infiltration of any of the above-mentioned structures, enables the surgical approach to be planned. Further, it may be possible to anticipate the necessity to reconstruct the defect with a regional or microvascular flap. Distinguishing a tumor from the prevertebral fascia, an extension in the retropharyngeal space or the mediastinum may be difficult on ultrasonography alone. It must be emphasized that the anatomy of the larynx and hypopharynx is often altered considerably after cancer surgery and this causes problems in the identification of specific details and landmarks (**Fig. 12.22**; ▶ Video 12.12).

Pearls and Pitfalls

The probe can be used to apply manual pressure on the tumor, to test its consistency/mobility in relation to adjacent structures (sonographic palpation).

If the arytenoid cartilages can be seen clearly, the postcricoid region and the multilayered epithelium of the piriform fossa can also be assessed as such on ultrasound examination.

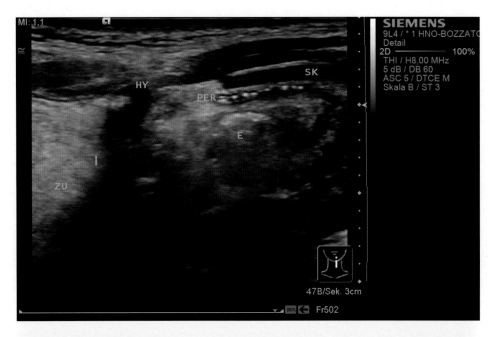

Fig. 12.1 The larynx in the longitudinal plane, with hyperechoic echoes of the epiglottis (E) and the preepiglottic space (PER). The endolarynx, with the thyroid cartilage (SK), lies caudally; the hyoid bone (HY) is seen cranially as an echogenic echo with complete distal acoustic shadowing. ZU, base of the tongue.

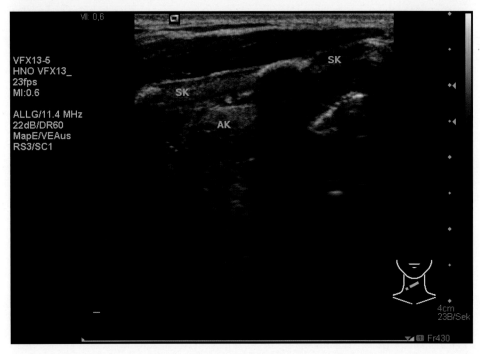

Fig. 12.2 Paramedian, right, transverse oblique view, level VI. The hypoechoic right ala of the thyroid cartilage (SK) shows an echogenic margin (cortex). In the anterior third, there is a hyperechoic area within the cartilage and its distal shadowing hinders the view of the internal structures. The vestibular folds form the anterior echogenic stripes and, depending on the oblique position of the probe, the protuberances of the arytenoid cartilages (AK) and vocal cords can be seen posteriorly. Diagnosis: **Ossification of the right thyroid ala**.

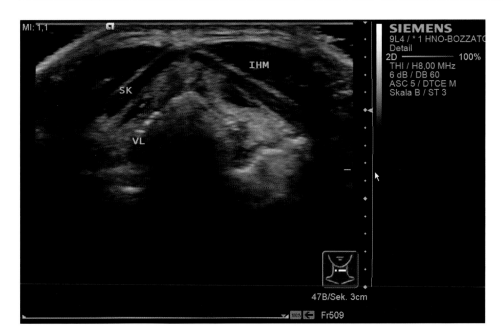

Fig. 12.3 Laryngeal region, transverse. The two thyroid cartilages (SK) can be clearly distinguished as hypoechoic tentlike structures; inside both of these, the vestibular folds (VL) can be seen with irregular dense echoes. IHM, infrahyoid muscles.

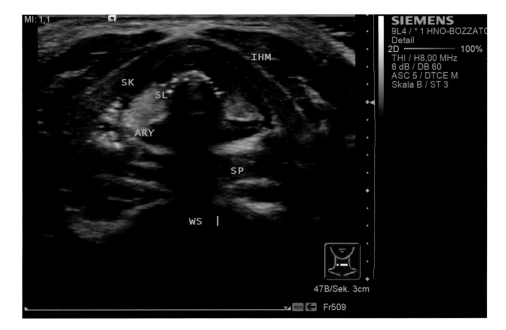

Fig. 12.4 Transverse view of the laryngeal region at a point below the image in **Fig. 12.3**. Hyperechoic punctate echoes can be seen internally, which correspond to the air contained in the sinus of Morgagni. Located posteriorly are the arytenoid cartilage (ARY) and part of the hyperechoic contour of the vocal cords (SL). IHM, infrahyoid muscles; SK, thyroid cartilage; SP, piriform sinus; WS, spine.

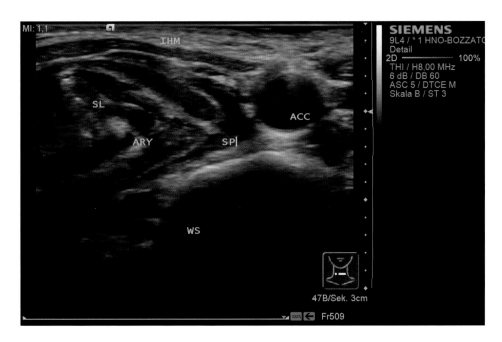

Fig. 12.5 Left laryngeal region, transverse. Here, the endolarynx, with vocal cords (SL) and arytenoid cartilages (ARY), and the infrahyoid muscles (IHM) lying above them can be seen. Projecting laterally to the thyroid cartilage are the left constrictor muscles/left piriform sinus (SP). In immediate anatomical relation to the common carotid artery (ACC) are the vertebral fascia and the vertebral spine (WS).

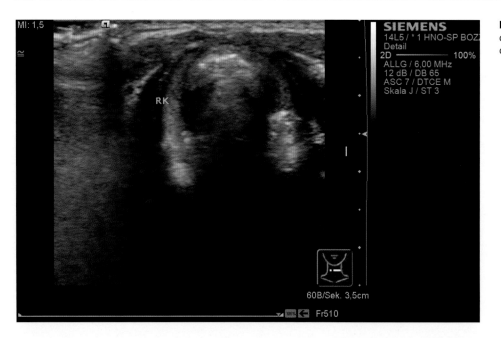

Fig. 12.6 Transverse view at the level of the cricoid cartilage (RK). Lying laterally are the hypoechoic cricothyroid muscles.

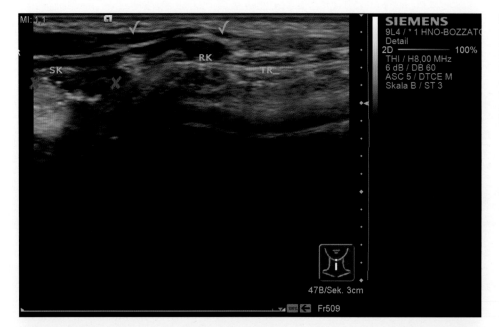

Fig. 12.7 Longitudinal view of the trachea, paramedian, with the hypoechoic thyroid cartilage (SK, red crosses) stretching here from left to right. Appearing oval in cross-section is the cricoid cartilage (RK, green ticks), while, caudally, the smaller hypoechoic cross-sections of the tracheal rings (TR) are recognizable as small oval hypoechoic structures appearing at regular intervals.

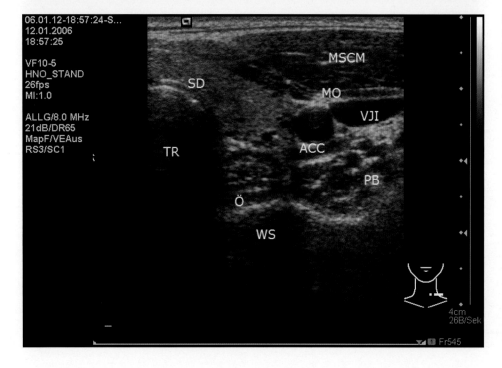

Fig. 12.8 Transverse view, level IV, left. A typical situation in the assessment of the **cervical esophagus** (Ö), which lies near the thyroid gland (SD). Ring-shaped contours show the multilayer structure of the esophageal wall. MO, omohyoid muscle; MSCM; sternocleidomastoid muscle; ACC, common carotid artery; VJI, internal jugular vein; TR, trachea; PB, brachial plexus; WS, spine.

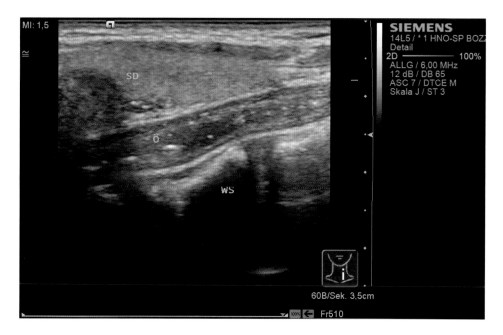

Fig. 12.9 Longitudinal view, left, level IV. The longitudinal view of the **cervical esophagus** (Ö) demonstrates that it lies between the thyroid gland (SD) and the spine (WS); the intervertebral spaces can be seen between the vertebral bodies. Ultrasonography can demonstrate protruding osteophytes in patients with dysphagia. Echogenic and hypoechoic double contours once again show the multilayered structure of the wall.

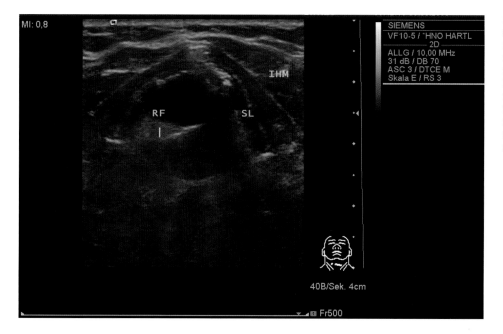

Fig. 12.10 Transverse view, level VI. A hypoechoic space-occupying lesion (RF) lies to the left of the midline within the laryngeal space beneath the thyroid cartilage. The mass has clearly defined margins and there is acoustic enhancement behind it. Note the morphological horizontal mirror image of the lesion deeper in the tissues; this is not a second space-occupying lesion but rather a mirror-image artifact. IHM, infrahyoid muscles; SL, vocal cord. Diagnosis: **Polyp of the right vocal cord**.

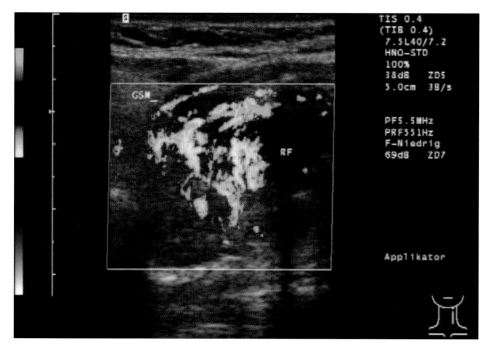

Fig. 12.11 Longitudinal view, left, mid-cervical region. A laryngeal space-occupying lesion (RF), which is cranially separate from the submandibular gland (GSM), demonstrates diffuse strong perfusion on duplex sonography. Diagnosis: **Hemangioma**.

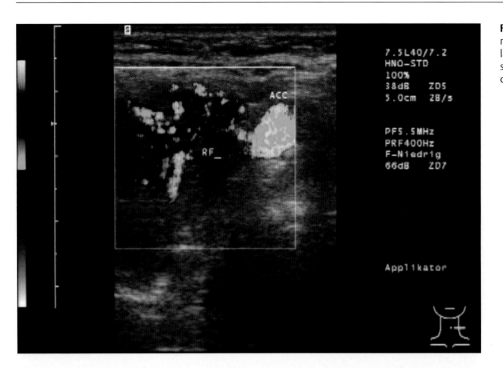

Fig. 12.12 Transverse view, left, mid-cervical region. The space-occupying lesion (RF) extends laterally in the neck to the vascular sheath and is supplied by an afferent branch of the common carotid artery (ACC). Diagnosis: **Hemangioma.**

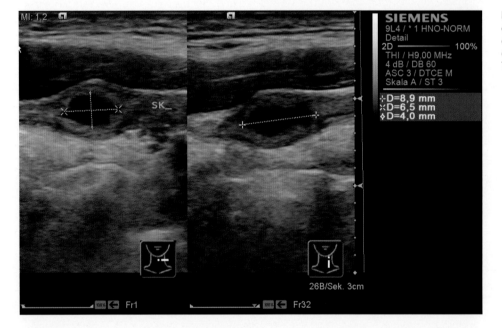

Fig. 12.13 Split screen—laryngeal region. **Chondroma of the ala of the thyroid cartilage**. The center of the ala of the thyroid cartilage (SK) is enlarged and anechoic. The outer cortex is intact. There is usually no perfusion within the lesion.

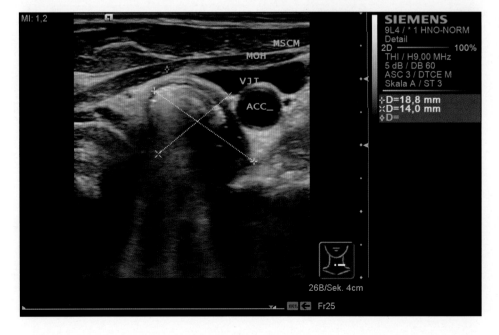

Fig. 12.14 Transverse view, level IV, left. On the omohyoid (MOH) and sternocleidomastoid (MSCM) muscles and lying medial to the common carotid artery (ACC) and the internal jugular vein (VIJ) is a round, echogenic, clearly defined space-occupying lesion that generates irregular echogenic distal artifacts, which are intensified on swallowing. Diagnosis: **Zenker diverticulum.**

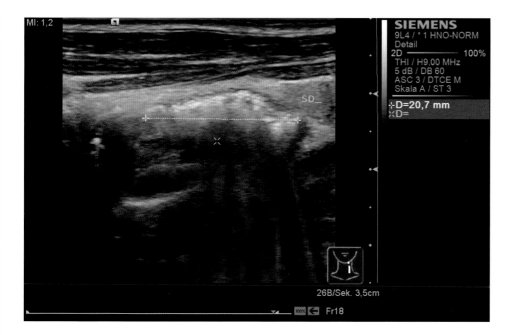

Fig. 12.15 The longitudinal view of the patient in **Fig. 12.14** confirms the suspicion of a **Zenker diverticulum** (points of the caliper), lying in the typical site to the left of the thyroid (SD).

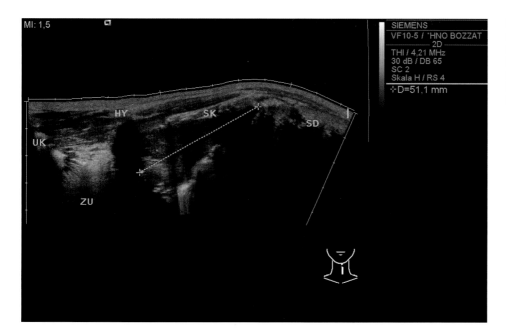

Fig. 12.16 Panoramic view—**cT4 laryngeal carcinoma**. The carcinoma extends from the lower edge of the thyroid cartilage (SK) to the posterior level of the hyoid bone (HY). The mandible (UK) and tongue (ZU) can be seen cranially. In this view, the caudal aspect of the thyroid gland (SD) is not involved.

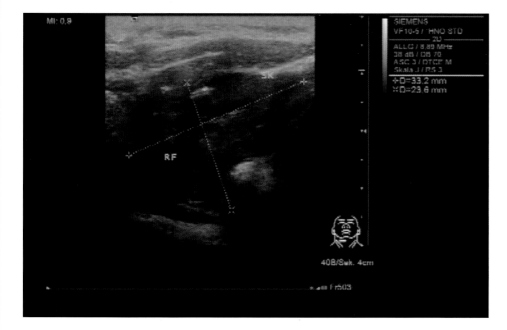

Fig. 12.17 Erosion of the ala of the right thyroid cartilage (SK) by the tumor (RF) can be seen clearly in this right paramedian transverse view. Diagnosis: **cT4 laryngeal carcinoma**.

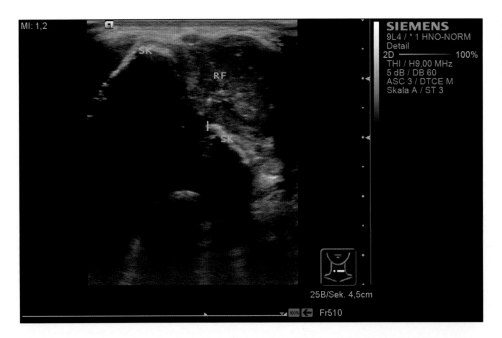

Fig. 12.18 Left transverse view of the larynx with **cT4 laryngeal carcinoma**. To the right of the transverse view, the carcinoma (RF), which is destroying the left ala of the thyroid cartilage (SK), can easily be distinguished as an inhomogeneous hypoechoic lesion.

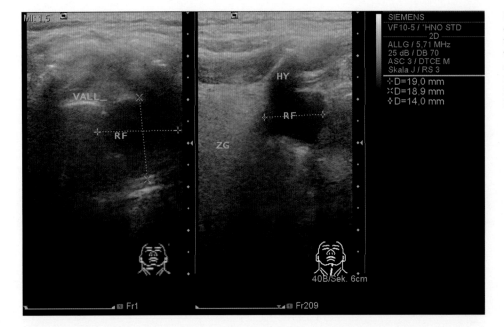

Fig. 12.19 Split screen of a left-sided cT1 **carcinoma of the vallecula**, showing the transverse view on the left and the longitudinal view on the right. There is an irregular, ill-defined, hypoechoic space-occupying lesion (RF), measuring 18 mm × 19 mm × 19 mm, at the inferior/caudal tongue base (ZG, VALL), behind the hyoid bone (HY).

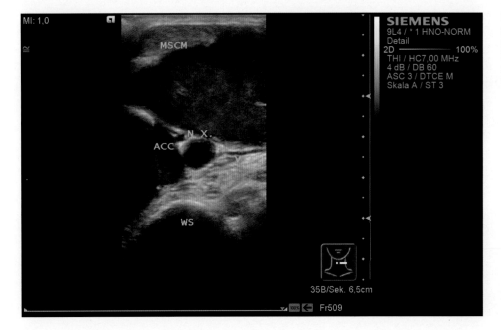

Fig. 12.20 Left transverse view. **Hypopharyngeal carcinoma with infiltrative growth of metastasis in the sternocleidomastoid muscle** (MSCM); the common carotid artery (ACC) and the vagus nerve (N X.) are spared. There is no direct contact with the spine (WS).

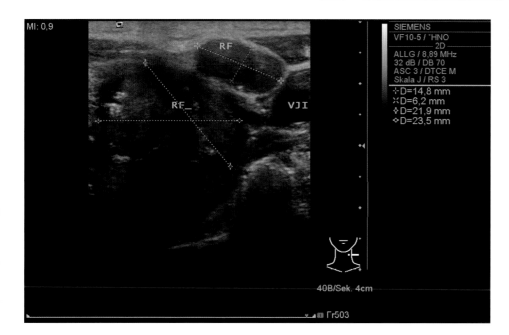

Fig. 12.21 Left transverse view of the neck. A **hypopharyngeal carcinoma** (RF_), with a metastasis lying laterally (RF), shows the inhomogeneous echo pattern of a malignant space-occupying lesion. The internal jugular vein (VJI) is patent and is not compromised by the tumor.

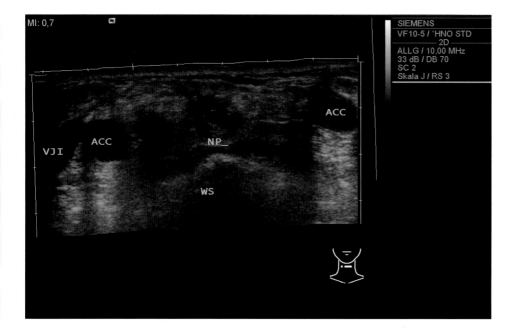

Fig. 12.22 Postoperative midline transverse view. After laryngectomy, the neopharynx (NP) can be identified as a targetlike structure above the spine (WS). The two carotid arteries can also be seen (ACC). VJI, internal jugular vein.

13 Extracranial Vessels

Werner Lang

Introduction

Atherosclerotic lesions of the extracranial arteries are responsible for ischemic strokes in many cases. In Germany, approximately 200 000–300 000 patients suffer from ischemic stroke every year.[1] Ultrasonography has become a routine imaging method because it is a precise non-invasive imaging technique for detecting these lesions. The extracranial carotids are superficial and can be detected precisely by ultrasound. Correct imaging techniques and protocols are necessary, however, to avoid misinterpretation of the images. Ultrasonography must be reliable and reproducible, as it is the primary imaging technique that will lead to consequences for treatment.

There are many important factors to be considered, such as intimal thickness and intimal structure, plaque morphology, and—last, but not least—the grade of stenosis.

Anatomy

The **common carotid artery** (CCA) will be found anterolaterally in the neck medial to the internal jugular vein. In the carotid sheath there are three main structures: the carotid artery, the internal jugular vein, and the vagal nerve. Up to the carotid bifurcation there are no branches; however, sometimes the superior thyroid originates from the CCA. The CCA divides into two branches, the internal carotid artery (ICA) and the external carotid artery (ECA). The location of the carotid bifurcation is at the height of the fourth vertebral body, but this may vary according to individual anatomical proportions (**Fig. 13.1**). Differences may be seen between the right and left bifurcation.

The **external carotid artery** is in many cases the smaller of the two terminal branches of the CCA and it continues anteromedial to the ICA in more than 80% of cases. There may be also a lateral course at the bifurcation, which may lead to a more difficult imaging. The division into its major branches varies considerably. In most cases the division into major branches is seen very well by ultrasound with B-mode

Fig. 13.1 Lateral view at the carotid bifurcation. The common carotid artery is divided into the external and internal carotid arteries.
From Atlas of Anatomy, © Thieme 2008; illustration by Karl Wesker.

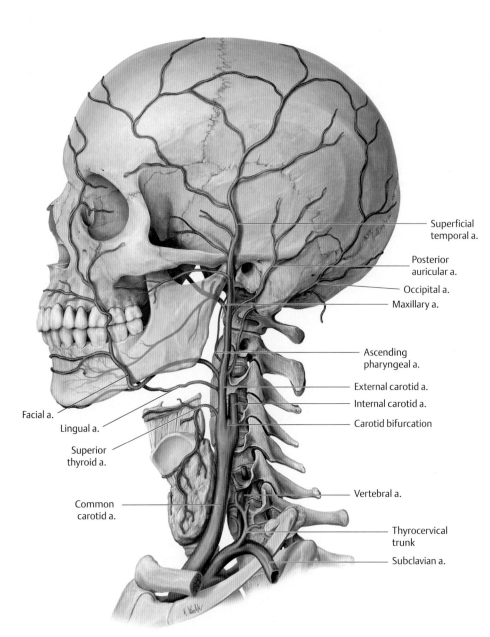

Superficial temporal a.

Posterior auricular a.

Occipital a.

Maxillary a.

Ascending pharyngeal a.

External carotid a.

Internal carotid a.

Carotid bifurcation

Facial a.

Lingual a.

Superior thyroid a.

Vertebral a.

Common carotid a.

Thyrocervical trunk

Subclavian a.

imaging. The ICA will not demonstrate a comparable division, which is a very valuable distinguishing feature in B-mode images.

The **internal carotid artery** is larger than the ECA and has no cervical branches. There might be some variants in very rare cases. These are persistent fetal anastomoses between the ICA and vertebrobasilar arteries, for example the proatlantal arteries that correspond with the C1 and C2 segmental arteries.[2,3] The ICA can be divided into four major sections: the cervical, petrous, cavernous, and cerebral sections. Only the cervical part can be examined by extracranial ultrasound imaging. The ICA normally exhibits a small bulb at its origin. This is seen as a small dilatation in B-mode imaging. The ICA normally follows the internal jugular vein to the skull. Its course is straight up to the base, but may also vary and demonstrate minor or major elongations, coilings (360°) and even kinks, preferentially in older people with arterial hypertension (**Fig. 13.2**).

The **vertebral artery** (VA) is the first branch of the subclavian artery (**Fig. 13.3**). In rare cases its origin is the aortic arch. The VA is divided into four segments: the V1 segment (proximal or ostial segment) from the origin to its entry into the transverse canal at the C6 level; the V2 segment (transversal segment) from its entry into the transverse canal at C6 to the transverse foramen of C2; the V3 segment (suboccipital segment) from the transverse foramen of C2 to its dural penetration at the level of the foramen magnum; and the V4 segment (intracranial segment) from its dural penetration to the vertebrobasilar junction. In 40% of cases the vertebral arteries are not equal in diameter. This asymmetry will be seen on B-mode ultrasound. The VA is described as dominant or minor. There are variations in the course of the VA; the level of entry into the transverse canal is important for ultrasonography. From

this point there is discontinuous imaging of the VA due to artifacts of the cervical bones.[4]

The **internal jugular vein** (IJV) begins at the base of the skull at the jugular foramen and joins the subclavian vein to form the brachiocephalic vein. It is a large vein with valves (▶ Video 13.1) close to its end and collects many external branches. It is located at the lateral side of the CCA, but anatomical findings demonstrate a variety of locations in relation to the CCA (anterolateral and lateral) and there is a relationship between weight and internal jugular diameter.[5]

Carotid Arteries

Examination

The position of the patient may be supine or semisupine with the head rotated and hyperextended to the contralateral side of the examiner. The position of the examiner is beside the patient, close to the ultrasound machine, or, alternatively, at the head of the patient. A transducer with a high frequency (at least 7.5 MHz, up to 13 MHz in certain cases) is used to detect the superficial vessels. A high transducer frequency guarantees high-resolution imaging. This is important for plaque imaging methods. In most cases, a linear transducer gives a good visualization of the carotid arteries. In patients with a short neck, a curved-array transducer might be necessary to obtain adequate imaging of the more cranial portions of the ICA. The imaging of the vessel wall is done by high-resolution B-mode imaging.

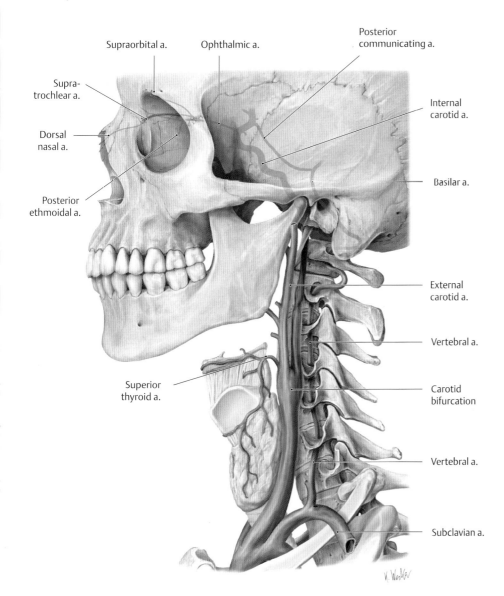

Supraorbital a.   Ophthalmic a.   Posterior communicating a.

Supra-trochlear a.

Dorsal nasal a.

Posterior ethmoidal a.

Superior thyroid a.

Internal carotid a.

Basilar a.

External carotid a.

Vertebral a.

Carotid bifurcation

Vertebral a.

Subclavian a.

Fig. 13.2 Lateral view at the carotid bifurcation. The internal carotid artery goes straight cranially from the carotid bulb. An elongated course, even with coiling, is possible in the extracranial part. From Atlas of Anatomy, © Thieme 2008; illustration by Karl Wesker.

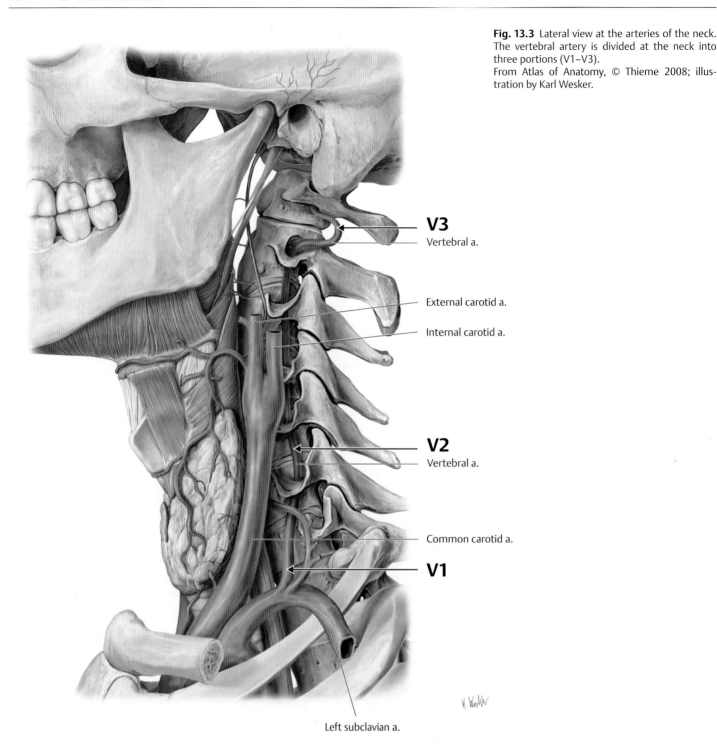

Fig. 13.3 Lateral view at the arteries of the neck. The vertebral artery is divided at the neck into three portions (V1–V3).
From Atlas of Anatomy, © Thieme 2008; illustration by Karl Wesker.

V3
Vertebral a.

External carotid a.

Internal carotid a.

V2
Vertebral a.

Common carotid a.

V1

Left subclavian a.

The longitudinal imaging of the carotid arteries is done in different planes to provide an optimal view of the bifurcation (**Fig. 13.4**). In many cases there are acoustic shadows that prevent exact visualization of the stenosis using only one plane.

Duplex ultrasound combines two-dimensional real-time imaging with Doppler flow analysis to measure blood flow velocities. The method does not directly measure the diameter of the artery or stenotic lesion. Instead, blood flow velocities are used as indicators of the severity of stenosis.[6] The orientation of the cervical vessels is optimal in a transverse section. For longitudinal imaging of the cervical vessels there are three standardized longitudinal projections[1]: positioning of the transducer between the larynx and sternocleidomastoid muscle for sagittal anteroposterior sections[2]; a lateral approach through the sternocleidomastoid muscle; and a posterolateral approach with the transducer behind the sternocleidomastoid muscle.[7] The first step of B-mode imaging is the transverse section and imaging of the vessel wall. The three anatomical layers of the vessel wall (intima, media, and adventitia) are not represented in the B-mode images; B-mode images will not discriminate the intimal layer from the media.

Color Doppler imaging of the arterial circulation is used to demonstrate regions of flow disturbances and abnormal blood flow direction. No measurements are made by color analysis. Pulsed-wave (PW) Doppler is used to perform spectral analysis and measurements of blood flow velocities. The examination of both the ECA and the ICA avoids misinterpretation as comparison of the two spectra will improve the discrimination of the vessels at the carotid bifurcation. All flow measurements are performed in a longitudinal section by PW Doppler. Color Doppler demonstrates regions of stenosis by aliasing. These images are helpful for catching the lesion in the PW mode. If there is suspected occlusion of a carotid artery, a colorless lumen will be seen. Color imaging demonstrates coiling and kinking of vessels by a changeover of color.

PW Doppler is used for flow velocity measurements. All measurements should be obtained with the best possible angulation. The lower

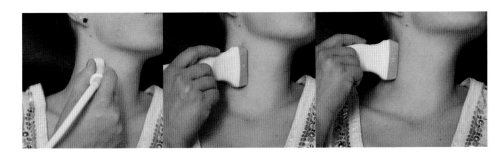

Fig. 13.4 Position of the transducer during examination in the longitudinal view. Left: the sagittal anteroposterior view with the transducer between the larynx and the sternocleidomastoid muscle. Middle: lateral approach through the sternocleidomastoid muscle. Right: posterolateral view with the transducer behind the sternocleidomastoid muscle.

the Doppler angle, the better is the Doppler shift that is achieved. No Doppler shift will be registered with an angle of 90°. The insonation angle should be less than 60° to avoid a critical error in velocity measurements. In many cases angulation below 60° is possible with linear transducers. Especially in patients with a more cranially located bifurcation and a short neck, the insonation angle will be optimized using a curved-array transducer. An insonation angle of 45° is preferred, if possible. The Doppler angle is adjusted to the vector of blood flow, not to the anatomical course of the vessel (**Figs. 13.5, 13.6**). Exact positioning of the sample volume box is necessary to get the optimal signal. To avoid false high velocities, the sample volume box should not be placed in a curved, nondiseased segment.

Normal Imaging

Under normal conditions there is a pulsation of the arteries in B-mode ultrasound. Gentle compression of the neck by the transducer demonstrates a more elliptical shape of the IJV (**Fig. 13.7**; ▶ Video 13.2). In color Doppler mode the transverse view with an angulated transducer demonstrates the different flow characteristics of the internal and external carotid arteries (**Fig. 13.8**; ▶ Video 13.3). The flow characteristics of the ICA are typically a constant flow forward during the systolic and diastolic cycles (**Figs. 13.9, 13.10**; ▶ Video 13.4). The ECA is more pulsatile as a result of a higher peripheral resistance (**Figs. 13.11, 13.12, 13.13**; ▶ Video 13.5). The CCA signal is a "mixture" of both the ECA and the ICA spectra (**Figs. 13.14, 13.15, 13.16, 13.17**; ▶ Videos 13.6, 13.7, 13.8). The anatomical position of the ECA cannot be used to discriminate between the ICA and ECA. There might be misinterpretation of the broad diastolic flow of the ECA in cases of stenosis and occlusion

of the ICA that will form a large collateral flow via the ECA. In case of doubt, a rhythmic tapping of the superficial temporal artery in front of the tragus will give typical alterations in the waveform that can easily be demonstrated in the Doppler spectrum. The carotid bulb shows a typical reverse flow, indicated by a changeover of color from red to blue (**Fig. 13.18**). In color mode a reversed coloration will be seen in some zones of the carotid bulb opposite the ECA.

Intima–Media Thickness

Intima–media thickness (IMT) of extracranial carotid arteries, measured by B-mode sonography, is considered to be a marker of subclinical atherosclerosis. It is a noninvasive and simple B-mode ultrasound examination that can be done very simply. There is a positive correlation between IMT and well-known risk factors of coronary heart disease (CHD). Carotid IMT is a strong predictor of future vascular events.[8]

IMT is measured in the far wall of the CCA. If possible, the internal jugular vein is used to achieve better visualization by amplifying the acoustic signal. The transducer is placed perpendicular to the long axis of the vessel wall of the CCA. The leading-edge method is used to obtain thickness measurements (**Figs. 13.19, 13.20**). The best imaging will be obtained by a high-frequency linear transducer of >10 MHz. Serial IMT measurements should always be performed at the same position, with a distance of ~2 cm to the carotid bifurcation. Only the echogenic layer of the intima and the echo-poor layer of the media are included in the calculation (**Figs. 13.21, 13.22, 13.23**). Imaging should be frozen during the diastolic cycle. Normal values are between 0.5 and 0.7 mm; critical values are 0.9 mm and above.

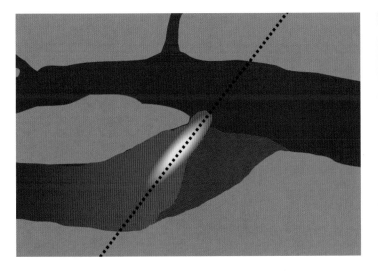

Fig. 13.5 Demonstration of angle correction. The Doppler angle is applied to the vector of blood velocity, which is demonstrated best with color Doppler mode. The bright color visualizes the direction of blood flow in the stenotic region.

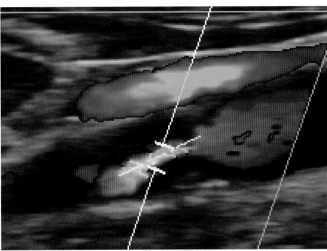

Fig. 13.6 Demonstration of angle correction in color-coded duplex sonography. Note the aliasing in the high-grade stenosis, demonstrating a high velocity. The direction of flow is well demonstrated by color mode.

Atherosclerotic Disease

Plaque Imaging

Many studies have demonstrated that in atherosclerotic lesions the grade of stenosis is important for risk evaluation. However, there is also evidence that the morphology of an atherosclerotic lesion correlates with the risk of stroke. The risk of ipsilateral stroke is much higher in patients with an irregular surface of the plaque (independently of the degree of stenosis) and also in patients with an echogenic lesion.

There have been many attempts to achieve a reliable image of plaque composition by B-mode ultrasound. There are visual scores that have a relatively high degree of subjectivity and even higher intraobserver and interobserver variability. One example is the Gray–Weale classification. An observer can discriminate very well between an overall echogenic plaque and an overall echolucent plaque. The majority of ratings, however, will vary too much to give adequate evidence of plaque components. In contrast to these individual ratings, a more objective method, the GSM scale (GSM = grayscale median), has been introduced. By a somewhat complex procedure, a B-mode image of a carotid plaque is standardized so that the intraluminal blood has a GSM value between 0 and 5. In contrast, fibrous tissue such as the adventitia will be given a reference value between 185 and 195. There is evidence that these "standardized" GSM values correlate with clinical outcomes, such as transient ischemic events or stroke. Despite much effort, fully automated analysis of the plaque components is not yet reliable, the reason being the spatial distribution of the plaque components. The measurement of the GSM offers a median value, which means cumulated information about the plaque (**Fig. 13.24**). The elastin and calcium components have a greater influence on the GSM values than do the lipid components, but it is the lipidic material that is responsible for clinical events rather than the heavily calcified material.[1,9–11]

Exact analysis of the GSM value is dependent on many factors. The most important is the "normalization" of the images; some steps during acquisition of data generate certain errors even in the first steps of standardization. So far, plaque imaging is an emerging technique in carotid ultrasound along with many features to improve imaging (such as contrast-enhanced ultrasound). Despite these reservations, there is a need for a more differentiated approach to assessing plaque stability than grayscale analysis alone.[1]

Automatic plaque analysis has failed so far to provide more reliable images of plaque components than are given by individual rating. The postprocessing methods are standardized, but there is considerable fluctuation in the source data because of the specific settings of the ultrasound machine. For this reason, individual rating of the carotid plaque remains a more practicable method for estimating the risk posed by the plaque (**Figs. 13.25, 13.26**; ▶ Video 13.9). **Table 13.1** (according to Schäberle) summarizes the best-established criteria for characterizing carotid plaque.[7]

Grade of Stenosis

Many randomized trials have shown that there is a correlation between cerebral symptoms and the grade of the stenosis. The criteria for grading ICA and CCA stenosis are brought together in **Table 13.2**. Primary parameters for the grading of stenosis are the presence of a stenotic plaque on B-mode imaging and the peak systolic velocity in the stenosis (**Figs. 13.27, 13.28, 13.29, 13.30, 13.31**; ▶ Video 13.10). In every case with uncertain or contradictory results, secondary (additional) parameters are used: the ICA/CCA ratio and the end-diastolic velocity of the ICA represent such additional parameters. The ICA/CCA ratio is the ratio between the maximum systolic velocity in the CCA and the maximum systolic velocity in the ICA. A high-grade stenosis is regarded as one with an ICA/CCA ratio >4 and an end-diastolic velocity above 100 cm/s. There has been some confusion about the grading of carotid artery stenosis because of the different measurements in the major trials. There is one definition of carotid stenosis in the European Carotid Surgery Trial (ECST), which is different from the grading method used in the North American Symptomatic Carotid Endarterectomy Trial (NASCET). There is a difference of calculated percentages because the percentage of local diameter reduction (according to ECST criteria) is different from the percentage of distal parameter reduction (according to NASCET criteria). Following ECST criteria, the grade of stenosis is in relation to the original lumen; following NASCET criteria it is in relation to the distal lumen. For measurements in a digital subtraction angiogram, NASCET criteria are preferred as it is difficult to get an authentic view of the "local" vessel wall because only the lumen of the vessel is visualized by the contrast medium. The vessel wall, however, is seen by B-mode ultrasound. This is why German ultrasound criteria, for example, follow the local diameter reduction.[12]

There is a consensus that NASCET criteria should be used to describe the grade of carotid artery stenosis. The confusion is about the grade of a carotid stenosis, because an ECST stenosis of 70% can be calculated as 50% by NASCET criteria. There are formulas to interconvert the values: ECST% = 40 + 0.6 × NASCET%, and NASCET% = (ECST − 40)% / 0.6. Examiners should calculate the grade of stenosis with reference to NASCET criteria.

Carotid Artery Occlusion

Especially in symptomatic patients it is very important to differentiate between a near-occlusion and a total occlusion of the ICA. Patients with a near-occlusion may be candidates for revascularization; patients with a total occlusion are definitely not. In any case, ultrasound is not reliable enough and an additional imaging modality such as CT angiography or MR angiography should be used. Several imaging parameters are recommended for optimal discrimination; for example, low wall filter, low pulse repetition frequency, increased gain up to visible background noise, decreased velocity scale lower than 15 cm/s, focal zone at the level of the diseased segment, and increased sample volume gate of more than 2.5 mm. At the point of occlusion there is a typical "to-and-fro" flow pattern at the point of occlusion (**Figs. 13.32, 13.33**; ▶ Video 13.11). When a patent vessel beyond the occluded area is identified, the examiner must determine whether the vessel is a patent ECA or ICA. The tapping maneuver is helpful in recognizing the ECA.[13]

There are three main etiological factors of a carotid artery dissection: spontaneous, traumatic, and as a result of an aortic dissection. The typical finding of a carotid dissection as a result of aortic disease will be in the CCA; however, spontaneous and traumatic dissections will affect the ICA in most cases. In many cases, the origin of the dissection is located cranially in the neck. In some cases the origin is close to the skull. A flapping intimal tear is not seen in every case. This is a result of intramural hemorrhage in some cases with an intimal tear. The false lumen may compress the true lumen by expansion as a result of intramural hemorrhage and thrombosis of the false lumen.

A dissection of the ICA is not visible directly by B-mode ultrasound or color Doppler in every case. However, the partial compression of the true lumen will decrease ICA flow. This can be demonstrated by duplex ultrasound and measurements of the spectrum and flow parameters.

To identify the extent of the dissection, additional examinations such as MRI or MR angiography are required.

Carotid Aneurysm

Extracranial carotid aneurysms are rare. They arise from dissection (pseudoaneurysms), fibromuscular dysplasia, trauma, atherosclerosis, infection, and congenital disorders such as Marfan syndrome. They appear as a pulsatile mass and sometimes as an audible bruit. Intraluminal thrombus may cause intracerebral embolization and stroke. B-mode ultrasound will detect extracranial aneurysms. As a differential diagnosis, a solid or cystic tumor might be seen. Color Doppler mode can be used for visualization of blood flow (**Figs. 13.34, 13.35**; ▶ Video 13.12).

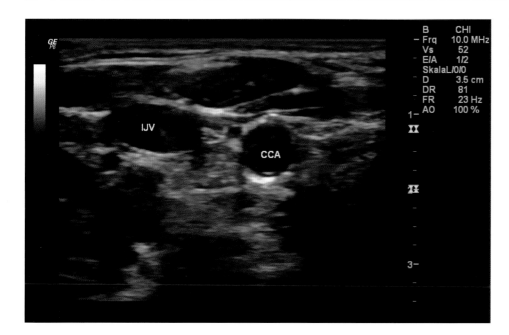

Fig. 13.7 Transverse section of the right neck. See the medial common carotid artery (CCA) and the more lateral, elliptical-shaped internal jugular vein (IJV).

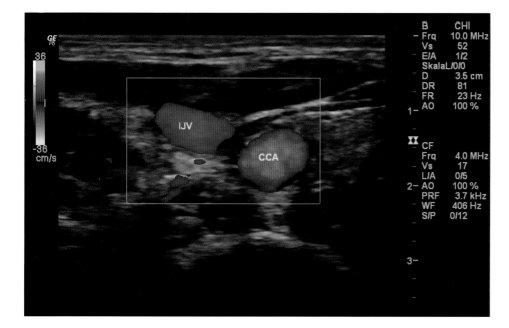

Fig. 13.8 Same cross-section as in **Fig. 13.7**, color Doppler mode. To obtain a proper depiction of color, the transducer should be angled slightly.

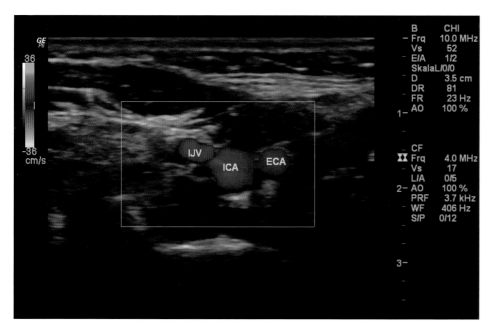

Fig. 13.9 Color Doppler of the carotid bifurcation in a cross-sectional view. The internal carotid artery (ICA) is close to the internal jugular vein (IJV). The diameter of the ICA is larger than that of the external carotid artery (ECA). This is seen in most cases, but it is not a safe parameter with which to discriminate these arteries.

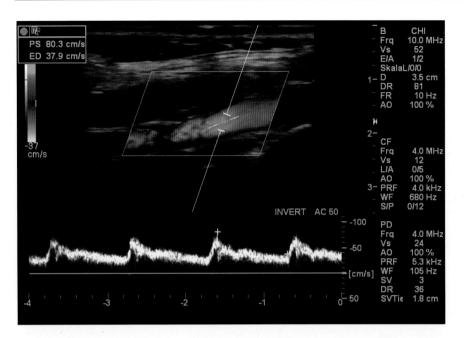

Fig. 13.10 Typical Doppler wave form of the ICA. Notice the large diastolic flow component. The systolic component is less pulsatile than with the ECA.

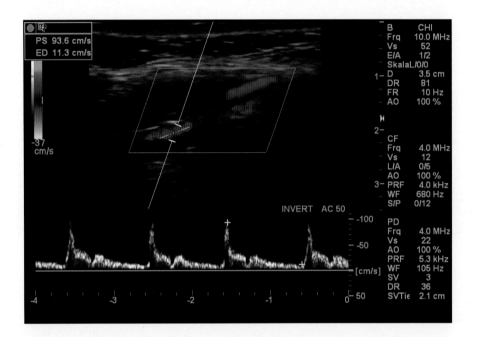

Fig. 13.11 Typical Doppler wave form of the ECA. Notice the more pulsatile Doppler spectrum, in comparison with the ICA (see **Fig. 13.10**).

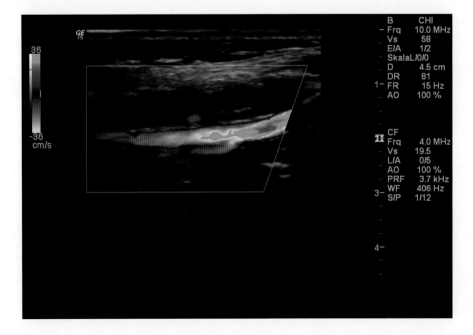

Fig. 13.12 The ECA is divided into several branches; however, heavy calcification may prevent the examiner from detecting the small vessels even with color Doppler. In this image a larger branch of the ECA is visible in color mode. This is a typical sign of the ECA.

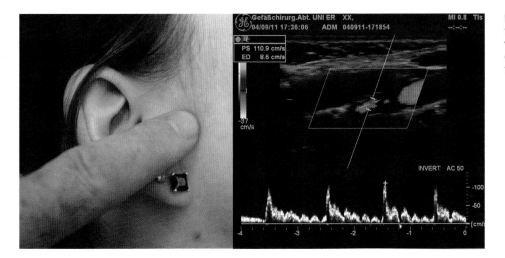

Fig. 13.13 Rhythmic tapping of the superficial temporal artery leads to a pulsation of the ECA waveform. This is to identify the ECA safely, especially in all cases with a similar flow pattern to that of the ICA.

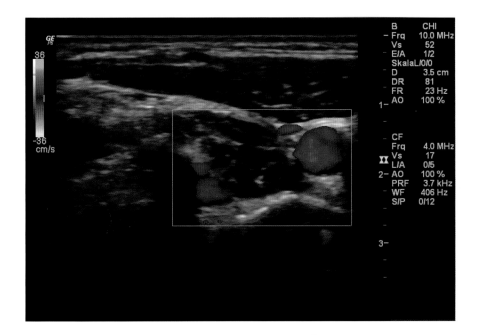

Fig. 13.14 Cross-sectional view demonstrating the proximity of the vertebral artery (left artery) to the CCA (larger vessel with red color at the right side). In contrast to the CCA, the vertebral artery is visible discontinuously due to the transverse processes. In this portion the vertebral artery is visible between two vertebral segments. Note also a small accompanying vein close to the vertebral artery (blue color). The IJV close to the CCA is narrow; in this case there is compression by the transducer.

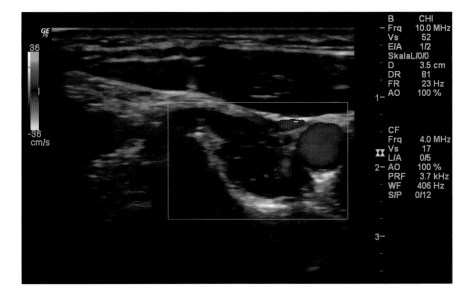

Fig. 13.15 Same view as in **Fig. 13.14**, but the cross-sectional segment is a little more cranial. Thus, the VA is no longer visible owing to acoustic shadows from a transverse process.

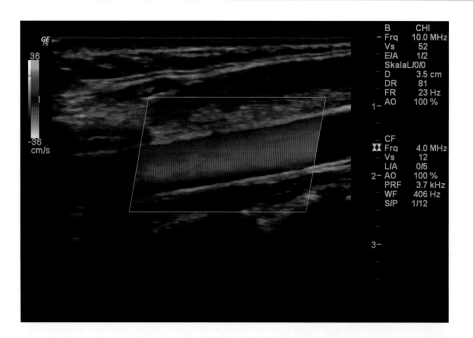

Fig. 13.16 The wall of the CCA is best visualized by B-mode imaging with perpendicular insonation. For color Doppler mode, better visualization is achieved with an angle between the ultrasound beam and the vessel of less than 60°. For this purpose, the transducer should be angled first. Second, electronic beam steering will be helpful, especially with the use of a linear scanner. The homogeneous coloration of the artery demonstrates a normal flow pattern in this picture.

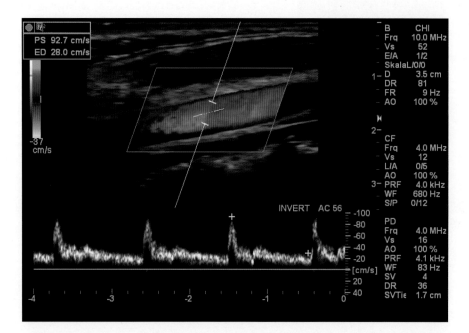

Fig. 13.17 The Doppler signal of the CCA is a "mixture" of the ICA and ECA spectra. There is a typical peak in the waveform, somewhat comparable to the ECA signal, and a remarkable diastolic flow, similar to that of the ICA. The spectrum may vary as a result of high-grade ostial stenosis that cannot be detected by a direct approach.

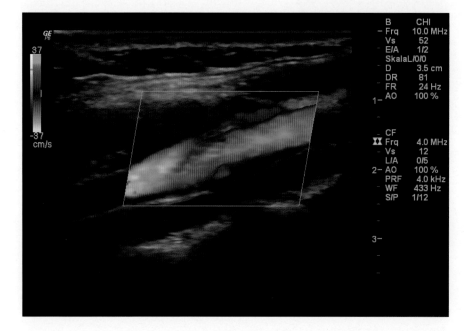

Fig. 13.18 Typical reverse flow at the CCA bulb indicated by a small blue zone at the far wall. The separation zone is located opposite the orifice of the ECA in most cases.

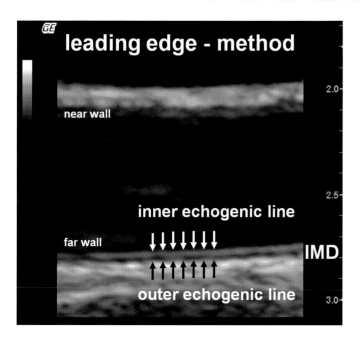

Fig. 13.19 Measurement of the intima–media thickness (IMT) in the CCA using the leading edge method. The longitudinal section of the CCA is visualized in B-mode imaging using perpendicular scanning. Measurements are taken ~2 cm from the carotid bifurcation. There are two echogenic lines; the space between these lines is the intimal layer complex. Normally the IMT is calculated from the mean of three or even more measurements at different locations. See also **Fig. 13.20**.

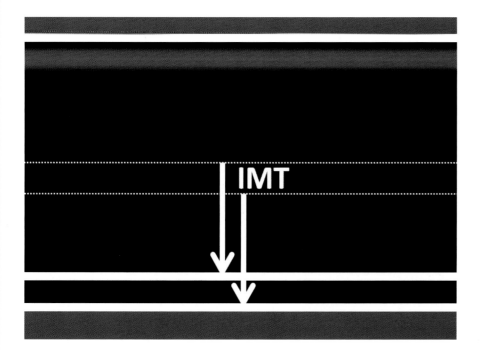

Fig. 13.20 Calculation of the intima–media thickness (IMT). The distance between the inner and outer echogenic line is calculated at the far wall.

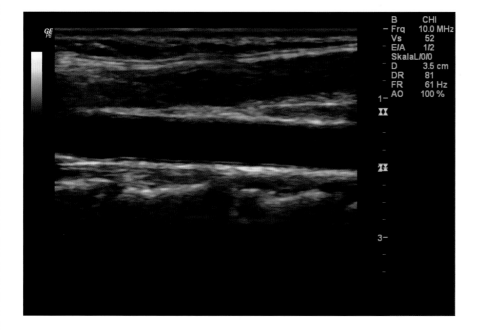

Fig. 13.21 B-mode imaging of the CCA in a longitudinal plane. The intima–media complex is seen at the far wall in relation to the transducer. See also **Fig. 13.22** for a more detailed illustration.

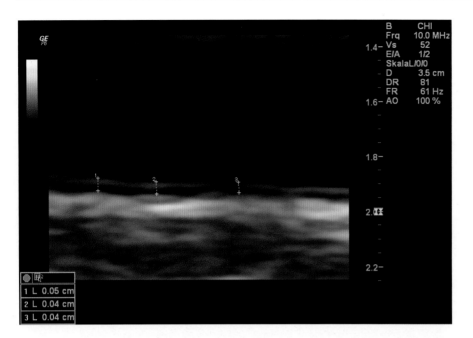

Fig. 13.22 A magnified view of the CCA, with calculation of the intima–media thickness at three different points. The distance to the bifurcation is ~2 cm. The values (from 0.4 to 0.5 mm) are within the normal range.

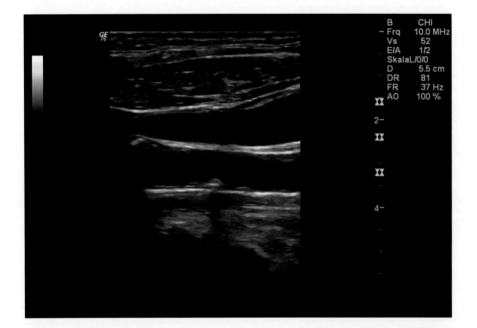

Fig. 13.23 Longitudinal section through the IJV (above) and the CCA. In this case there is a plaque at the far wall that demonstrates atherosclerosis with plaque. In this case, intima–media thickness measurements are uncommon, because there is already a plaque visible.

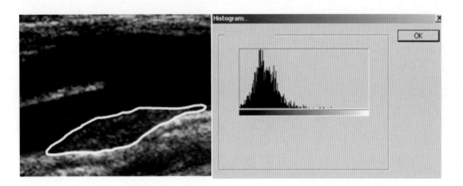

Fig. 13.24 Plaque at the carotid bifurcation with a circular mark. Before calculation of the gray-scale median (GSM), the B-mode picture must be standardized to give a grayscale value between 0 and 5 for blood and between 185 and 195 for the adventitial layer. The circumscribed area is analyzed by Adobe® Photoshop® to produce a median of the grayscale of this area. All values are median of GSM.

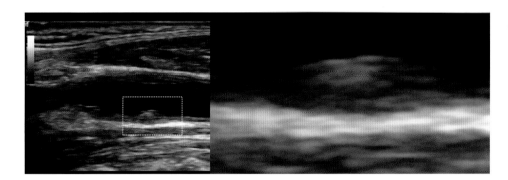

Fig. 13.25 Plaque at the far wall of the ICA. There is a thin fibrous layer with a regular surface. For comparison with an irregular surface, see **Fig. 13.26**.

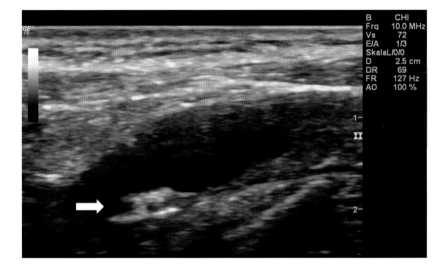

Fig. 13.26 Echogenic plaque with a large ulceration (arrow).

Table 13.1 Established criteria for the characterization of carotid artery plaque, according to Schäberle[7]

Localization	Anterior wall	Posterior wall	
	Caudal	Cranial	
Extension of plaque	Circular	Semicircular	
	Plaque diameter		
Plaque configuration	Concentric	Eccentric	
Plaque surface	Clearly delineated	Poorly delineated	Not delineated
	Smooth	Irregular (0.4–2.0 mm deep)	Ulcer (>2.0 mm deep)
Plaque composition	Homogeneous	Inhomogeneous	
Echogenicity	Echogenic	Echolucent	Cannot be visualized

II Sonographic Anatomy and Pathology

Table 13.2 Grade of stenosis of the ICA

Grade of stenosis (NASCET) (%)		10	20–40	50	60	70	80	90	Occlusion (100)
Grade of stenosis (ECST) (%)		45	50–60	70	75	80	90	95	Occlusion (100)
Main criteria (primary)	B-mode	Evidence							
	Color mode		Evidence						
	Peak systolic velocity (cm/s) at maximum of stenosis			200	250	300	350–400	100–500	
	Peak systolic velocity (cm/s) poststenotic					>50	<50	<30	
	Collaterals (periorbital region)						Evidence	Strong evidence	Strong evidence
Additional criteria (secondary)	Prestenostic reduction of diastolic flow (CCA)						Evidence	Strong evidence	Strong evidence
	Poststenotic flow disturbances								
	End diastolic velocity (cm/s) at maximum of stenosis			<100	<100	>100	>100		
	"Confetti sign" (use low PRF)					Evidence	Evidence		
	ICA/CCA index			≥2	≥2	≥4	≥4		

CCA, common carotid artery; ECST, European Carotid Surgery Trial; ICA, internal carotid artery; NASCET, North American Symptomatic Carotid Endarterectomy Trial; PRF, pulse repetition frequency.

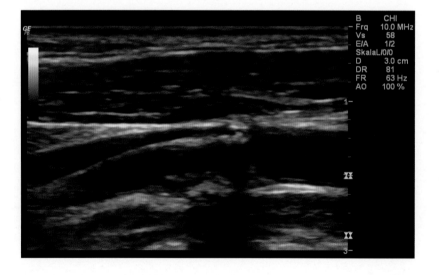

Fig. 13.27 Plaque at the origin of the ICA with some acoustic shadows due to calcification.

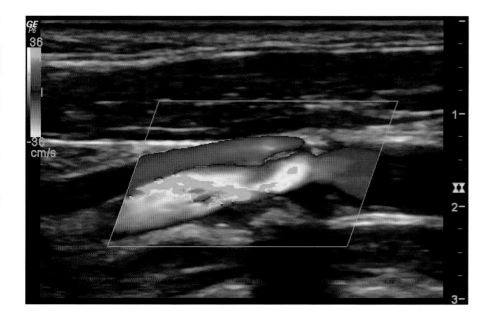

Fig. 13.28 Same view as in **Fig. 13.25**. Color mode with increased flow at the plaque. Aliasing demonstrates a high velocity at the narrowing of the lumen.

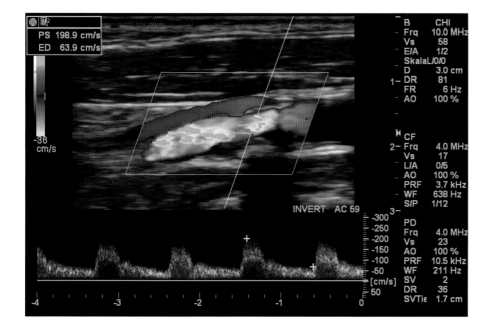

Fig. 13.29 Same as **Fig. 13.26**. The spectrum of the ICA shows an elevated peak systolic velocity. The grade of stenosis is 50%, see **Table 13.2**.

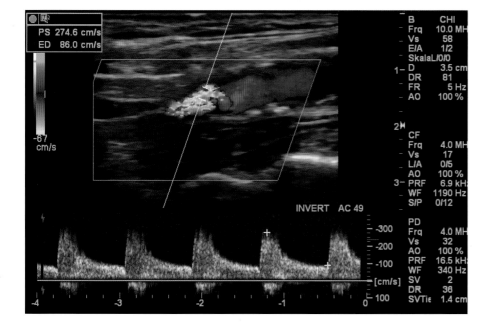

Fig. 13.30 Stenosis of the ICA with a peak systolic velocity of more than 270 cm/s. There is turbulent flow with reverse flow indicated below the zero line.

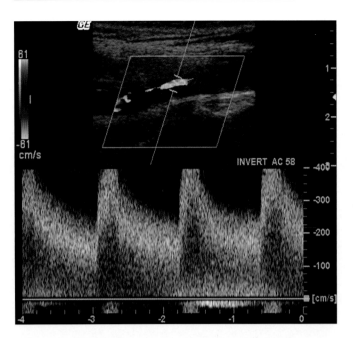

Fig. 13.31 High-grade stenosis of the ICA with a peak systolic velocity above 400 cm/s.

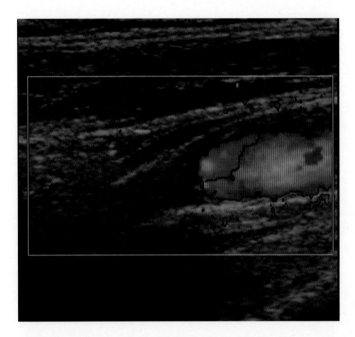

Fig. 13.32 A typical "to-and-fro" flow pattern at the point of occlusion of the ICA at its origin from the CCA. There is flow detection in the CCA with a backward flow at the ICA origin. Look at the color pixel beneath the vessel lumen as a sign of visible background noise.

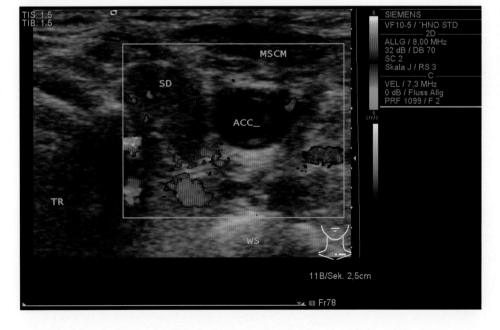

Fig. 13.33 Occlusion of the CCA. The flow detection is enhanced by low pulse repetition frequency (PRF) and high gain to produce visible background noise. In this case echogenic material is also seen in the lumen of the common carotid artery (CCA). SD, thyroid gland; MSCM, sternocleidomastoid muscle.

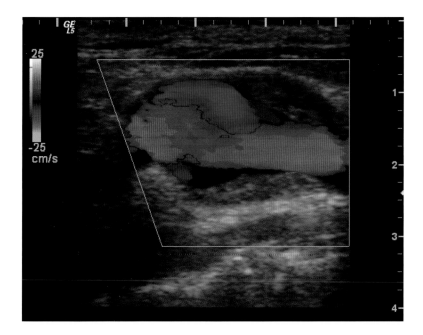

Fig. 13.34 Color Doppler imaging of an extracranial common carotid artery aneurysm after eversion endarterectomy a few years previously. This is a true aneurysm with thrombus formation at the aneurysmal wall.

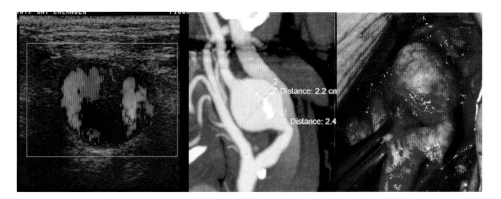

Fig. 13.35 Color Doppler in transverse section of an aneurysm of the ICA. See the CT angiogram in the middle and the intraoperative view on the right.

Vertebral Arteries

Examination

The vertebral artery (VA) can be identified in a longitudinal or transverse section. The sagittal view from the common carotid artery, sweeping the transducer to a more lateral view toward the cervical spine, will give a segmental view of the vertebral artery. Color Doppler mode will visualize the VA better than B-mode alone. The best view of the VA can achieved from the V1 segment from the origin to its entry into the transverse canal at the C6 level (**Figs. 13.36, 13.37;** ▶ Video 13.13) and from the V2-segment (transversal segment) from its entry into the transverse canal at C6 to the transverse foramen of C2 (**Figs. 13.38, 13.39, 13.40;** ▶ Video 13.14). The V3 and the V4 regions are not part of the routine ultrasound examination if the spectral Doppler waveforms in the V1 and V2 segments are normal.

Atherosclerotic Disease

The majority of atherosclerotic lesions of the VA are located close to the origin from the subclavian artery. There is a variety of diameters and peak flow velocities of the VA; thus, there are no calculation tables as there are with ICA disease. The grading of a stenosis of the VA is therefore difficult. Vertebral artery stenosis is suggested when peak systolic velocity at the origin is at least 50% higher than in the more cranial segments. High-grade stenosis is diagnosed when there is a marked increase in peak systolic velocity (peak systolic velocity [PSV] > 150 cm/s).[7]

Subclavian Steal Syndrome

Whereas duplex ultrasound is not accurate enough to detect a focal stenosis in the VA, it is very easy to visualize the direction of blood flow. The flow direction is identical to that in the common carotid artery and the reverse of that in the internal jugular vein. A transverse view of the neck may show flow directions of all three vessels in one frame. In all cases of a strong flow reversal in the VA by subclavian stenosis or occlusion, there is an unequivocal sign of a subclavian steal syndrome (**Figs. 13.41, 13.42**). However, there are some patients who do not show this flow reversal in the VA at rest. The flow reversal will be provoked by arm exercise in these cases.

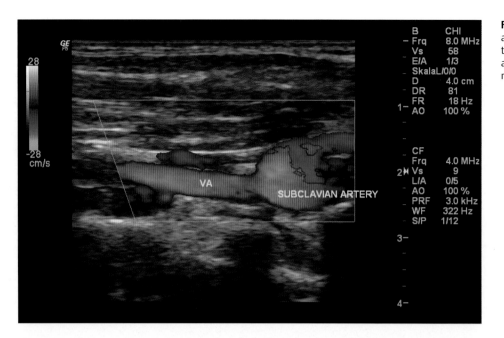

Fig. 13.36 The first segment of the vertebral artery from the origin at the subclavian artery to the C6 level at the cervical spine. Note the right-angled course of the vertebral artery (VA) in reference to its origin.

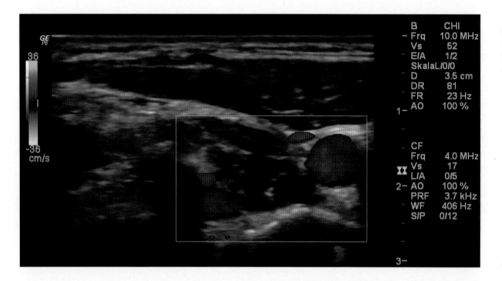

a

Fig. 13.37a,b Segmental view of the right vertebral artery. See the vertebral artery in (a) as a smaller red circle (the larger one is the CCA). In (b), the vertebral artery is not visible due to bony artifacts.

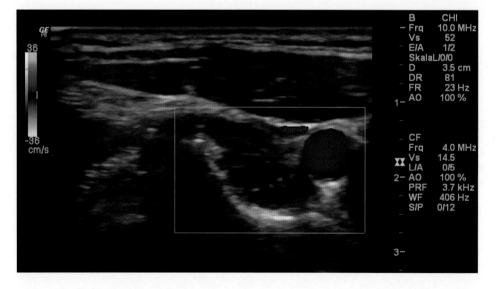

b

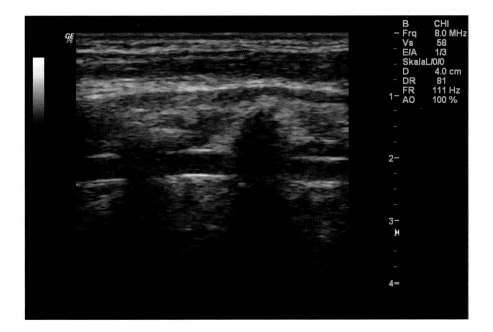

Fig. 13.38 Longitudinal view of the V2 segment of the vertebral artery. See the segmental exposure of the artery due to the bony artifacts of the transverse segments.

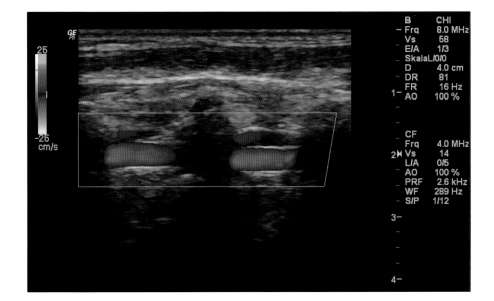

Fig. 13.39 Same frame as in **Fig. 13.38**, additional color Doppler mode. The visualization of the vertebral artery is improved by color imaging.

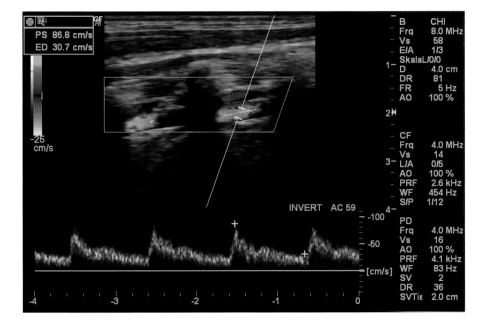

Fig. 13.40 Longitudinal view of the V2 segment of the VA. There is a continuous systolic and diastolic flow in color Doppler imaging.

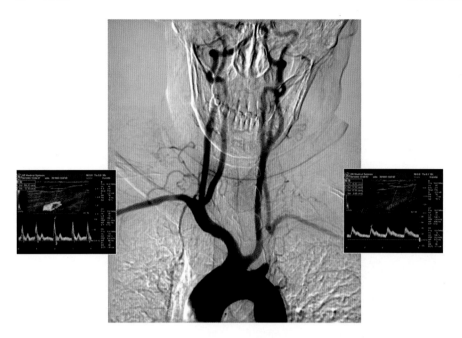

Fig. 13.41 Digital subtraction angiogram of the supra-aortic vessels. There is an occlusion of the left subclavian artery with collateral flow via the left vertebral artery. The Doppler spectrum of the left subclavian artery is flattened in comparison with the right side.

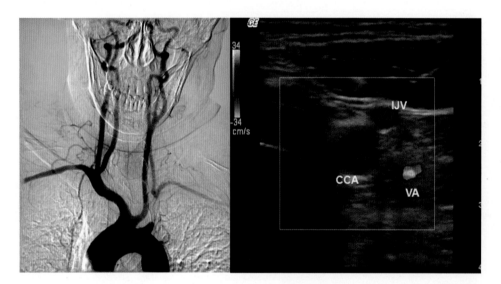

Fig. 13.42 Digital subtraction angiogram of the supra-aortic vessels. Occlusion of the left subclavian artery with collateral flow from the vertebral artery. Flow reversal in the left vertebral artery. The flow reversal is easy to identify on the color-coded transverse section of the neck. CCA, common carotid artery; IJV, internal jugular vein; VA, vertebral artery.

Jugular Veins

Examination

The internal jugular vein is examined with a longitudinal and a transverse view. The transverse view in B-mode is very easy. The IJV may be compressed by gentle pressure with the transducer and will be seen shaped elliptically close to the lateral side of the CCA. For example, the Doppler waveforms can give a hint of a central venous occlusion by thrombosis of the brachiocephalic vein. The rhythm of the cardiac cycle will also not be reflected in case of a compressive tumor outside the vessel wall. The Trendelenburg position of the patient during the examination will improve the filling of the vein.

Thrombosis

A thrombosis of the IJV at the neck, either complete or partial, will be seen with B-mode ultrasound alone (**Fig. 13.43**). The vein cannot be compressed by the pressure exerted with the transducer. In some cases, especially after jugular vein catheters, a partial thrombosis or a small thrombus adherent to the vein wall is seen by B-mode ultrasound. In cases of doubt, color mode will give satisfactory results (▶ Video 13.15). Complications of an IJV thrombosis are rare. Nevertheless, because of the insertion of central venous catheters via the IJV before major surgery in many patients, knowledge of a patent IJV is crucial before puncture. The routine B-mode ultrasound examination of the IJV before a puncture for the implantation of a central venous access catheter may reduce major complications of the procedure by affording a direct view of the target vein.

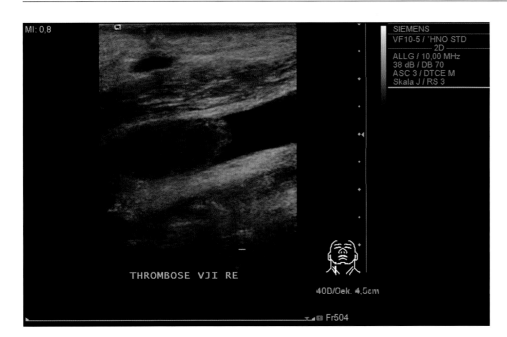

Fig. 13.43 B-mode longitudinal section of the internal jugular vein. Echogenic thrombus in the internal jugular vein.

References

1. Eyding J, Geier B, Staub D. Current strategies and possible perspectives of ultrasonic risk stratification of ischemic stroke in internal carotid artery disease. Ultraschall Med 2011;32(3):267–273

2. Geibprasert S, Pongpech S, Armstrong D, Krings T. Dangerous extracranial–intracranial anastomoses and supply to the cranial nerves: vessels the neurointerventionalist needs to know. AJNR Am J Neuroradiol 2009;30(8):1459–1468

3. Siqueira M, Piske R, Ono M, Marino Júnior R. Cerebellar arteries originating from the internal carotid artery. AJNR Am J Neuroradiol 1993;14(5):1229–1235

4. George B, Cornelius J. Vertebral artery: surgical anatomy. Oper Tech Neurosurg. 2001;4(4):168–181

5. Lamperti M, Caldiroli D, Cortellazzi P, et al. Safety and efficacy of ultrasound assistance during internal jugular vein cannulation in neurosurgical infants. Intensive Care Med 2008;34(11):2100–2105

6. Brott TG, Halperin JL, Abbara S, et al. 2011 ASA/ACCF/AHA/AANN/AANS/ACR/ASNR/CNS/SAIP/SCAI/SIR/SNIS/SVM/SVS guideline on the management of patients with extracranial carotid and vertebral artery disease: executive summary: a report of the American College of Cardiology Foundation/American Heart Association Task Force on practice guidelines, and the American Stroke Association, American Association of Neuroscience Nurses, American Association of Neurological Surgeons, American College of Radiology, American Society of Neuroradiology, Congress of Neurological Surgeons, Society of Atherosclerosis Imaging and Prevention, Society for Cardiovascular Angiography and Interventions, Society of Interventional Radiology, Society of NeuroInter-ventional Surgery, Society for Vascular Medicine, and Society for Vascular Surgery. Stroke 2011;42(8):e420–e463

7. Schäberle W. Extracranial cerebral arteries. In: Schäberle W, ed. Ultrasonography in Vascular Diagnosis. Berlin, Heidelberg: Springer; 2011

8. Lorenz MW, Markus HS, Bots ML, Rosvall M, Sitzer M. Prediction of clinical cardiovascular events with carotid intima–media thickness: a systematic review and meta-analysis. Circulation 2007;115(4):459–467

9. Denzel C, Balzer K, Merhof D, Lang W. 3D cross sectional view to investigate the morphology of internal carotid artery plaques. Is 3D ultrasound superior to 2D ultrasound? Ultraschall Med 2009;30(3):291–296

10. Denzel C, Balzer K, Müller KM, Fellner F, Fellner C, Lang W. Relative value of normalized sonographic in vitro analysis of arteriosclerotic plaques of internal carotid artery. Stroke 2003;34(8):1901–1906

11. Denzel C, Fellner F, Wutke R, Bazler K, Müller KM, Lang W. Ultrasonographic analysis of arteriosclerotic plaques in the internal carotid artery. Eur J Ultrasound 2003;16(3):161–167 Arning C, Widder B, von Reutern GM, Stiegler H, Görtler M. [Revision of DEGUM ultrasound criteria for grading internal carotid artery stenoses and transfer to NASCET measurement]. Ultraschall Med 2010;31(3):251–257

12. Tahmasebpour HR, Buckley AR, Cooperberg PL, Fix CH. Sonographic examination of the carotid arteries. Radiographics 2005;25(6):1561–1575

III Advanced Ultrasound Methods and Outlook

14   Image Processing Methods
Gert Hetzel

The use of advanced computer technology allows for manifold image processing methods which altogether facilitate the identification and evaluation of tissue alterations (**Fig. 14.1**).

The field of view can be extended two-dimensionally—**panoramic imaging**—or three-dimensionally (**3D**) through image processing techniques. Elastic properties of tissue can be determined **beyond the primarily visible (elastography)** and, with the help of high-frequency ultrasound information (ultrasound RF, or radiofrequency, data), the user is able to undertake **sonohistology** (a statistical pattern analysis), detecting information that would not be detectable visually. Mathematical classification algorithms identify characteristic patterns and, with increasing experience, are able to recognize the patterns of specific tissues. The advantage of this procedure is its objectivity. In the following, some innovative procedures will be presented that were introduced to support tissue typing or that have potential as future routine applications.

Panoramic Imaging

While the transducer is manually shifted in the scanning plane, a panoramic image is calculated from the individual overlapping images in real time without additional position detection (**Fig. 14.2**). The calculation is performed from one image to the next, first from two consecutively acquired images, then from the image calculated previously and the image acquired next. For this procedure, each image is subdivided into many small areas. In each section, characteristic properties are identified: These will be searched for in the following image to detect in what way the transducer was shifted and/or rotated. Then the new image will be added to the image already stored (**Figs. 14.3, 14.4, 14.5**).

With this procedure a panoramic image with the high detail and contrast resolution of a single image and a maximum extent of up to 600 mm in length is generated. Different tissue structures can be distinguished more easily if documented in a single image.

The panoramic image is particularly suitable for documenting complete findings, which would not be displayable in single images, and/or enabling a clearer visualization of adjacent structures (**Fig. 14.6**).

Harmonic Imaging; Tissue Harmonic Imaging

In harmonic imaging (tissue harmonic imaging [THI]) the nonlinear parts (such as harmonics) of the ultrasound echo signals returning from the tissue are used for image generation (**Fig. 14.7**).

The THI images appear to be higher in contrast than conventional images, since the tissue structures differ in their behavior with respect to pressure and negative pressure rather than in their acoustic impedance differences, which are the basis for conventional image generation (**Fig. 14.8**).

At first, THI was a by-product of contrast-enhanced ultrasound: The principle of displaying harmonics only was developed to suppress tissue signals and display only contrast medium signals. It was then discovered that harmonics are also created when ultrasound propagates inside the tissue. Owing to the different sound wave velocities of the tissue with pressure and negative pressure, the sound wave deforms depending on tissue characteristics, and harmonic frequency parts are generated. These are utilized for image generation (THI).

Ultrasound system manufacturers offer various methods of separating harmonics from fundamental waves. Basic systems work with high-pass filter technology (narrowband) whereas more advanced systems are equipped with subtraction filters and work with broadband technology (**Fig. 14.9**). The broadband visualization of the harmonic tissue properties through THI leads to particularly clear images free of artifacts (e.g., of the vascular walls; **Fig. 14.10**).

Broadband Harmonic Imaging, Phase Inversion Technique

Broadband harmonic imaging is able to separate harmonic from fundamental image signals in a particularly effective way.

THI includes procedures such as phase inversion (PI) technology. With PI, two transmit pulses of equal shape but different phases (180° = inverted or inverted polarity) are transmitted from the same position of the body. The two ultrasound line echoes are received and digitally interpolated. On in-phase addition of these two line echoes, the unmodified echo parts cancel and echo modifications add up, so that the harmonic frequency parts are available (**Fig. 14.11**).

THI is basically helpful for hard-to-scan patients and increases the rate of patients who can be finally diagnosed using ultrasound.

THI can deliver particularly clear and artifact-free images (e.g., of the vascular walls or in the near field) and will help in assessing distal sound phenomena that are visualized better with the activated mode. However, in the near field, enhanced contrast will lead to a coarse-grained image that may not optimally display the ultrastructure of different tissues (**Figs. 14.12, 14.13, 14.14, 14.15**).

Spatial Compounding

Sectional images are acquired from different directions with spatial compounding procedures (**Fig. 14.16**). The resulting single images are composed into a geometrically correct single image. The advantages are that areas of similar tissue properties are displayed as a more homogeneous area; tissue differences are distinguished more clearly; and curved contours are enhanced and displayed with less angle dependence (compare **Fig. 14.12** with **Fig. 14.17**).

In most cases the result is visually more satisfying. One reason is that the speckle patterns generated by interferences in the tissue are different for different acquisition directions and are blurred in the overlay. The actual tissue structure information stays the same from different directions and adds up. As a result, the image appears smoother and with softer contours. The use of compounding imaging (CI) techniques has clearly proven itself for use in the near field of head and neck soft tissue, with or without THI, and therefore CI should be activated or used as a default preset (**Figs. 14.18, 14.19**).

Three-dimensional Ultrasound Imaging: 3D Image, 4D Image

To acquire data in the three-dimensional dataset for reconstruction, the transducer is moved perpendicularly to the scan plane manually or automatically. The registered volume includes either the B-mode image only and/or the (color-coded) flow information. The calculated and reconstructed volume can be displayed three-dimensionally transparently or with surface rendering, or in maximum intensity projection (MIP) (**Fig. 14.20**). One advantage is the free selection of arbitrary view planes (▶ Video 14.1). Moreover, three-dimensional representations illustrate topography and volume information.

If the rate of the display per second of the 3D volumes is high enough to allow adequate tracking of the volume movement, this is referred to as 4D imaging. Here, time is the fourth dimension and frame sequences acquired in real time are created (▶ Videos 14.2, 14.3).

So far, applications of three-dimensional techniques have not gained acceptance in head and neck ultrasound scanning (**Figs. 14.21, 14.22**; ▶ Video 14.4). Improvement of reconstruction modules and real-time display might bring advantages in the near future, especially in the fields of education and patient information.

Ultrasound Contrast Enhancement

Various procedures are applied for the visualization of contrast media (**Table 14.1**), including in particular interesting approaches for second-generation contrast media with low mechanical index (low-MI) imaging. The user wants to see the contrast medium in clear contrast to the tissue to be able to evaluate the wash-in and presence of the contrast medium.

Initially, filter procedures were used to visualize the contrast medium. The property of contrast medium blisters of showing harmonic frequency vibrations (e.g., twice the excitation frequency: second harmonic) due to excitation by suitable base frequencies was exploited. These "vibration" frequencies are filtered out.

With second-generation contrast media (low-MI), the separation of tissue and contrast medium signals can be substantially improved by using an optimized excitation sequence and sequentially different processing of the received echo signals. This can be done to a point at which the tissue signal is almost totally suppressed and only the contrast medium is visible. One of these special procedures is the **contrast pulse sequence (CPS)** procedure, which is based on the characteristic of the contrast medium blisters (in the excitation frequency band that also includes the base band, the fundamental frequency band) to respond to pressure differences in a nonlinear way.

The signal detected through this procedure is the "nonlinear fundamental" signal. For the nonlinear fundamental signal the difference between tissue and contrast medium is approximately 30 dB higher than for the harmonic signal. This is the basis for the clearer separation of contrast medium and tissue, which means that the tissue can almost be suppressed.

The procedure is based on the principle that a sequence of transmit pulses of different amplitudes and different phasing is transmitted for each ultrasound image line (**Fig. 14.23**; ▶ Video 14.5). Here, too, high demands are put on the controllability of the large number of transmitters of the array elements.

For receiving, procedures similar to phase inversion procedures are used (but taking into account amplitude and accurate phasing). In the

Table 14.1 Contrast enhancement procedures

Filter, harmonic
• Phase modulation, phase inversion (PI), wideband harmonic   — Inverted pulses along a scan line
• Power modulation (PM), harmonic   — Amplitude modulation along a scan line
• Autocorrelation   — Power Doppler, harmonic
• Stimulated acoustic emission (SAE)
• Contrast pulse sequencing (CPS)   — Simultaneous modulation of amplitude and phase

head and neck region, contrast media are used to distinguish between nonperfused and insufficiently perfused masses and to visualize perfusion patterns/angioarchitecture, for example with lymph nodes and vascular diseases. Evaluation of bolus kinetics or the wash-out behavior of a contrast enhancer may also give information on the perfusion characteristics of a tissue region (**Figs. 14.24, 14.25**; ▶ Video 14.6).

"Contrast enhancement" can also be achieved easily using hydrogen peroxide and carefully injecting it into fistulas. The depth extension of ducts is improved in most cases (**Figs. 14.26, 14.27**).

Elastography

Ultrasound elastography is a new application in ultrasound diagnostics and is based on the centuries-old manual palpation method.

In analogy to manual palpation, elastography makes use of the fact that the compressibility of tumor tissue is frequently different from that of healthy tissue, tumor tissue being harder and more solid. This procedure is applied to visualize the viscoelastic characteristics of tissue. In elastographic ultrasound examinations, pressure is applied on the tissue to be examined and the changes in the structures in the image are used for diagnosis (**Fig. 14.28**; ▶ Video 14.7).

In the most basic case of compression elastography, the examiner exerts a slight external pressure on the organ with the ultrasound transducer during the examination. Software will evaluate the slightest tissue shifts between the individual images and show the strain with spatial resolution. Strongly strained regions are soft, while solid regions are not compressible. Differences in tissue elasticity can be visualized, in either grayscale or color-coded grading. Thus, another tissue property can be visualized by ultrasound and can be viewed in addition to the usual morphological image characteristics (**Figs. 14.29, 14.30, 14.31**; ▶ Videos 14.8, 14.9, 14.10, 14.11).

With the **acoustic radiation force impulse (ARFI)** method the pressure is applied through a strong ultrasound pulse with the transducer position unchanged; then the image modifications are evaluated. There are different approaches to this, including quantification through shear wave calculation (**Fig. 14.28**).

Sonohistology

In addition to elastography and contrast enhancement, sonohistology is another approach that tries to provide not only qualitative parameters. In a conventional B-mode image, different grayscale values indicate different types of tissue. This visual analysis and interpretation, however, is done by the sonographer and depends on his or her knowledge and experience. A frequent reproach of ultrasound is the expressed operator dependency. Advanced and computerized approaches such as sonohistology are therefore used to find new objective parameters independent of the examiner. In sonohistology, all of the information of a static image is divided into segments. The volume of data in the segments exceeds by far that used for image generation. Statistical analytic algorithms evaluate the associated tissue characteristics (e.g., attenuation, backscatter, structure) and can learn to identify specific tissue patterns from these. At present this is still a research approach, but one that has shown very promising results in initial pilot studies (**Fig. 14.32**).

Outlook

Ongoing developments show that diagnostic ultrasound and its associated procedures will by no means fall into evolutionary stagnation. One future-oriented approach is referred to as "molecular imaging," meaning the combination of sonographically visualizable particles, such as contrast enhancer blisters, with diagnostic or therapeutic components. These particles can be introduced into tissues under visual control and made to interact there by controlled application ultrasound energy. For example, the sonographic activation of chemotherapeutic substances could revolutionize oncological therapy.

The capabilities of diagnostic ultrasound for identifying and evaluating tissue and vascular changes will continue to be optimized in the future, turning ultrasound imaging in the hands of experienced examiners into the primary imaging modality for the head and neck region.

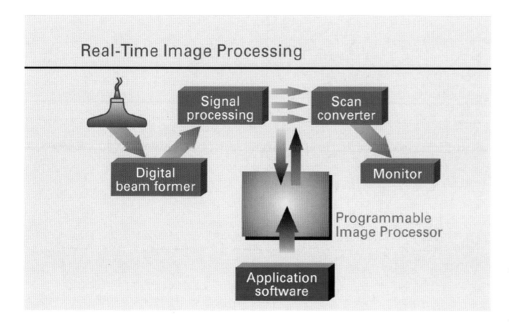

Fig. 14.1 Use of processors for image processing. Real-time image processing. The development of high-speed image processors and their integration into ultrasound systems has contributed to a considerable increase in postprocessing capabilities and paved the way for the application of complex image processing algorithms in new imaging methods. The image processor comprises one or more video processors. Each processor can perform several billion operations per second and has a storage capacity of several hundred images in B-mode, color Doppler mode, or power Doppler mode. In the signal-processing chain of the ultrasound system, the image processor fits between signal preprocessing and the scan converter. Data are transferred either directly after the signal preprocessing or from the scan converter into the local storage of the image processor. The latter can, as can the scan converter, form images or retrieve already stored images and process them. This expansion has gone beyond conventional postprocessing, which is limited to the static allocation of an input-grayscale value to a dedicated output value and to simple filtering procedures. The new image processor is programmable and offers a large number of possibilities for the development of new applications, such as applications for the automatic calculation of contours, adaptive image contrast optimization, and 2D and 3D panoramic imaging. (Courtesy of Siemens AG.)

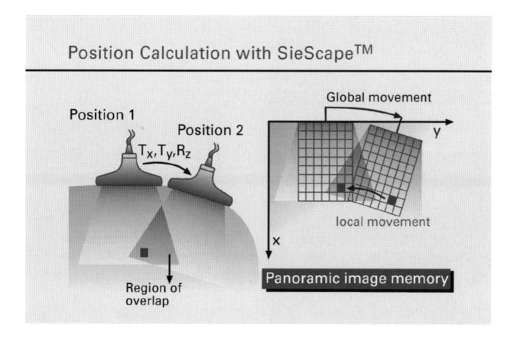

Fig. 14.2 Capture of panoramic image information. The calculation of the transducer's position without the need for position sensors constitutes a special challenge to panoramic imaging (in B-mode) and color panoramic imaging (including power Doppler mode). It is based on the similarity of consecutively scanned single images. To obtain a two-dimensional panoramic image, the transducer is guided freehand across the sectional plane $(x-y)$. The movement from position 1 to position 2 can be described by two translational movements, T_x and T_y, and a rotational movement R_z around the z-axis, perpendicular to the $x-y$ plane. Direct movement of the transducer in the z direction is not allowed. The calculation of T_x, T_y, and R_z utilizes the similarity or equality of the image contents within overlapping regions. The images are first divided into segments and the local movement of the image content is calculated for each segment. The estimated global movement is obtained by analyzing the local movements. It becomes more and more precise through iterative comparison with actual image information and the correction of the parameters of movement, so that the panoramic image can be assembled from the original images. The precision in the acquisition of motion data makes it possible to take the usual measurements over even longer distances. (Courtesy of Siemens AG.)

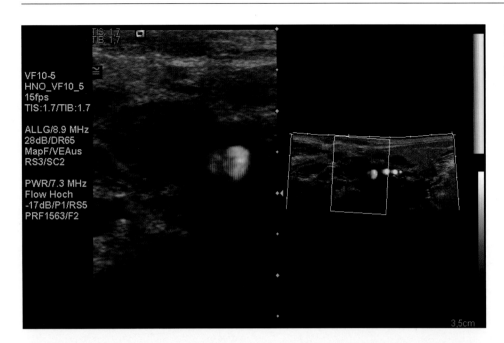

Fig. 14.3 Panoramic image with synchronous use of power Doppler. On the left side is a single image of the tissue segment that was processed to the panoramic display on the right side.

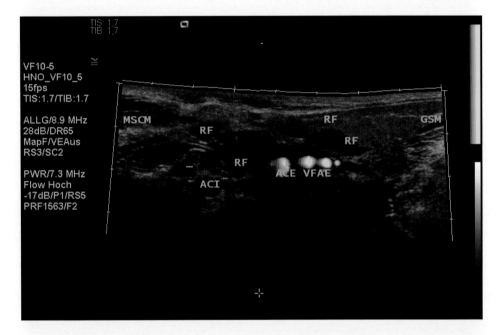

Fig. 14.4 After identification, muscular and vascular structures are visualized in an improved way through topographic coherences, as in this example of the position of lymph nodes relative to glands and vessels. ACE, external carotid artery; ACI, internal carotid artery; GSM, submandibular gland; MSCM, sternocleidomastoid muscle; RF, lymph node; VFAE, facial vein.

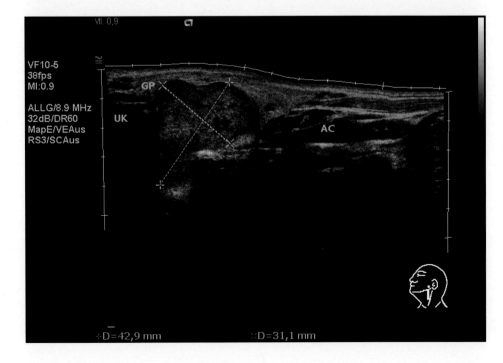

Fig. 14.5 Parotid region, longitudinal. In the panoramic mode the relative position of the tumor (calipers) with respect to the expansion under the horizontal ramus of the mandible (UK) and carotid artery (AC), as well as the caudal position of the gland (GP), is documented. Diagnosis: **Iceberg tumor.**

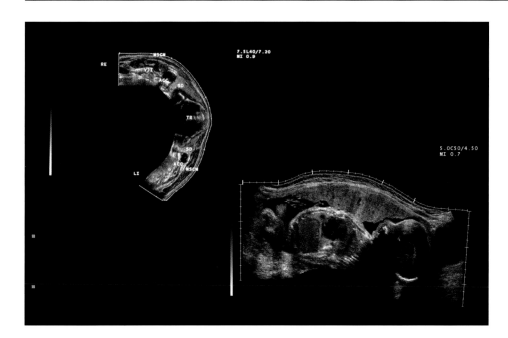

Fig. 14.6 Applications of panoramic imaging. Left side: Transverse panoramic image of the thyroid gland at neck level V. Right side: Longitudinal depiction of a human fetus outlining the contours of the face, trunk, and limbs.

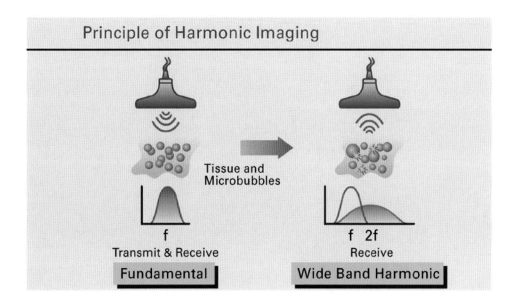

Fig. 14.7 Principle of harmonic imaging. Owing to nonlinear effects that arise when the ultrasound signal propagates within the tissue, or when it is scattered by contrast-enhancing microbubbles, echo signals do not consist only of fundamental frequencies (echo frequency, transmit frequency) but also contain multiples of the transmit frequency (2nd, 3rd, ... harmonics), which are exploited in harmonic imaging. In conventional fundamental imaging, the bandwidth of the echo signal processing corresponds to the bandwidth of the transmit pulse. Harmonic echo signals remain unused. Broadband harmonic imaging, a technique that makes use of the broadband properties of the transducer and processing chain, utilizes the harmonic components of the signal and separates them from the fundamental components. (Courtesy of Siemens AG.)

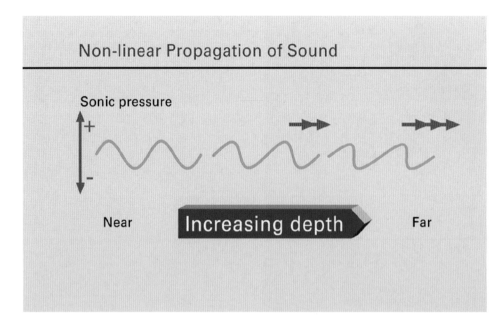

Fig. 14.8 Nonlinear propagation of sound. Rarefactional and compressional pressure influence the propagation of sound in tissue in different ways. At low-pressure amplitudes, the pulse form remains almost unchanged as compression and dilatation have little influence on the sound velocity. The pulse propagation is linear and the pulse's frequency content remains unchanged (apart from the attenuation effect). Conventional B-mode imaging makes use of these linear echo signals (receive frequency, transmit frequency). At higher amplitudes, sound propagation is increasingly nonlinear, as the signals are distorted when penetrating the tissue. When tissue is compressed, the sound velocity increases and the peak of the pressure wave is moved forward. If tissues are stretched, the sound velocity diminishes. This causes the trough of the pressure wave to move more slowly. The effect is cumulative and increases as the penetration depth increases. Owing to these signal distortions, "harmonic frequencies" (for example second or third harmonics) mix with the fundamental frequencies contained in the transmit signal. "Tissue harmonic imaging" utilizes only the harmonic portions of the signal for imaging. (Courtesy of Siemens AG.)

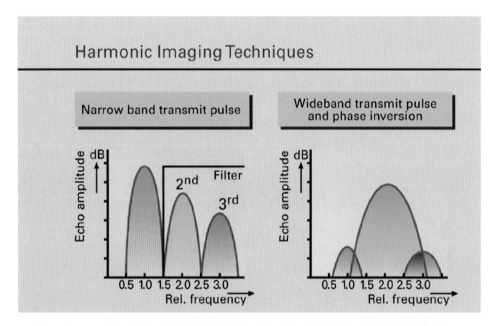

Fig. 14.9 Harmonic imaging: narrow band and broadband procedures. There are two methods of separating fundamental and harmonic echo signals. The frequency-based "second harmonic imaging" separates the harmonic components (mainly the stronger second harmonic frequencies) from the fundamental components using a bandpass filter. To achieve efficient separation, the transmit pulse requires a narrow bandwidth. This technique may reduce both axial and contrast resolution. Wide-band harmonic imaging, in combination with a phase inversion technique, utilizes the full bandwidth of the transducer to gather all the echo signals. Compared with signals from harmonic frequencies, fundamental signals are significantly reduced. There is less overlap and bandpass filters may be selected to be wider. As with B-mode imaging, the bandpass filter can be optimized dynamically to obtain the best image quality at each imaging depth. (Courtesy of Siemens AG.)

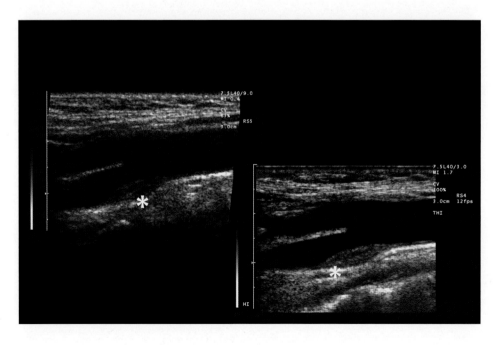

Fig. 14.10 Phase inversion technology: broadband harmonic imaging. Longitudinal view of a common carotid artery. Left: The fundamental B-mode image. Right: After the activation of tissue harmonic imaging there is increased contrast and improved delineation of the hypoechoic atherosclerotic plaque (asterisk). (Courtesy of Siemens AG.)

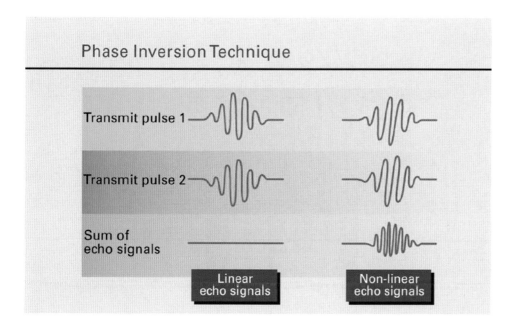

Fig. 14.11 Application of broadband tissue harmonic imaging (THI). Phase inversion. The phase inversion technique, a precondition for wide-band harmonic imaging, is based upon the fully digital signal-processing capacity of ultrasound systems. Two consecutive pulses are transmitted into the body, where, relative to the first pulse, the phase of the second pulse is inverted by 180°. When the returning echo signals of these transmit pulses are added together, the linear fundamental echoes cancel each other out, whereas the nonlinear harmonic echo signals do not. As a result of this addition, the fundamental and odd harmonic components are suppressed whereas the even harmonic ones, especially the second harmonic frequency components, are reinforced. Thus, B-mode images are obtained that show significantly enhanced contrast and spatial resolution. (Courtesy of Siemens AG.)

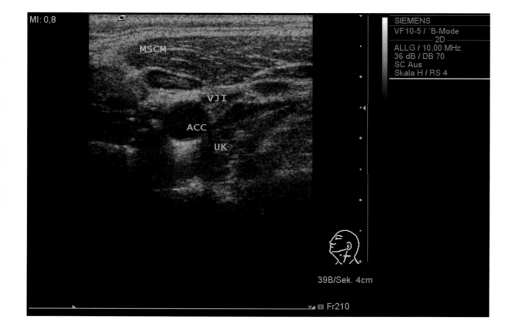

Fig. 14.12 Neck, left, transverse, level IV. In the conventional B-mode image the landmarks such as the common carotid artery (ACC) and the sternocleidomastoid muscle (MSCM) are clearly visible. VJI, internal jugular vein; UK, mandible.

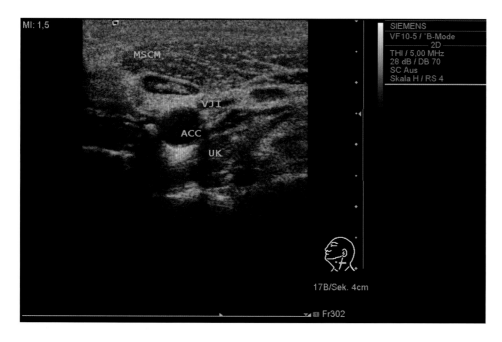

Fig. 14.13 Neck left transverse level IV (same as Fig. 14.12). After activation of the tissue harmonic imaging function, sound phenomena such as tangent artifacts and distal echo enhancement of the common carotid artery (ACC) can be seen more clearly. However, the tissue demarcation of the sternocleidomastoid muscle (MSCM) appears more diffuse. VJI, internal jugular vein; UK, mandible.

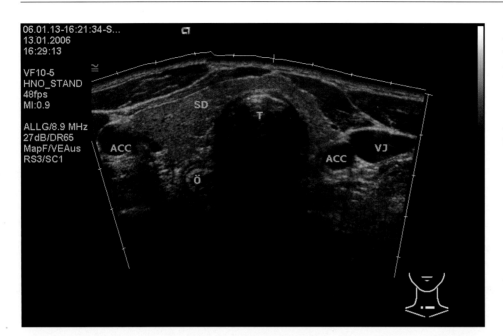

Fig. 14.14 Panoramic image, neck, median transverse. In the **conventional B-mode image** the landmarks such as the common carotid artery (ACC), thyroid gland (SD), and sternocleidomastoid muscle (MSCM) are clearly visible. The right-sided position of the esophagus (Ö) is conspicuous, but can be easily explained by the fact that the patient had his head turned to the left, causing the esophagus to slide to the right. T, trachea; VJ, internal jugular vein.

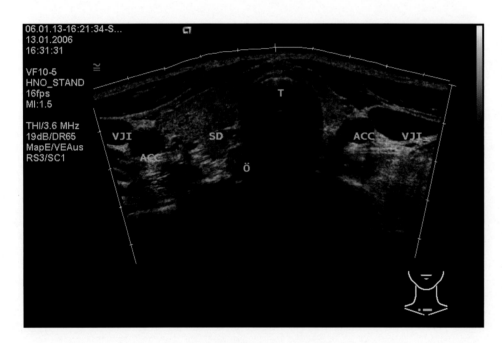

Fig. 14.15 Panoramic image, neck, median transverse (same as **Fig. 14.14**). When displayed in **tissue harmonic imaging** (THI) mode the image appears darker, as only the harmonics are used for image generation. The transmit frequency is reduced to half in THI mode compared with conventional B-scan mode. ACC, common carotid artery; MSCM, sternocleidomastoid muscle; Ö, esophagus; SD, thyroid gland; T, trachea; VJI, internal jugular vein.

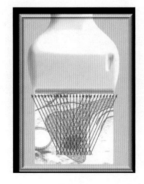

Fig. 14.16 Principle of compound imaging. The spatial compounding approach with different directions for transmitting and receiving. Transmission in one direction (parallel downward), reception from different directions with a fixed transducer position through the use of transducer subapertures. It may also be possible to steer transmission in the same way. (Courtesy of Siemens AG.)

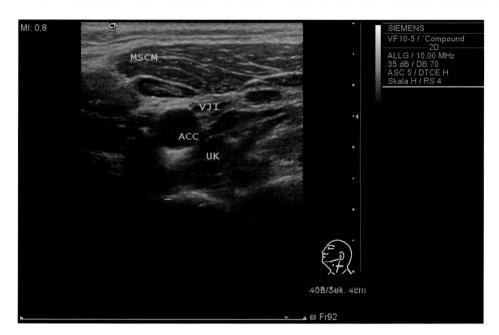

Fig. 14.17 Neck, left, transverse plus **compound imaging**, level IV. This leads to improved tissue visualization. ACC, common carotid artery; MSCM, sternocleidomastoid muscle; VJI, internal jugular vein; UK, mandible.

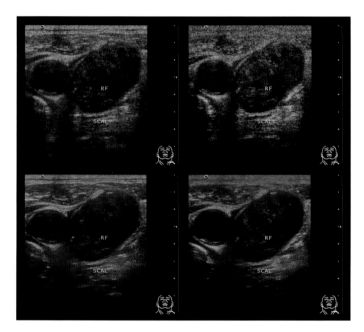

Fig. 14.18 Neck, left, transverse with a **metastasis** in level V. The metastasis (RF) is on the scalene muscle (SCAL). Upper left: transversal B-scan image showing a lymph node without hilar signs in polycyclic configuration. Upper right: corresponding image from THI with slightly better delineation of the node from the surrounding tissue but with coarse-grained tissue display. Lower left: compound imaging (CI) with improved delineation, tissue contrast, and visualization of the internal structure of the mass. Lower right: THI plus CI (THICI) enhances the lymph node internal structure even more.

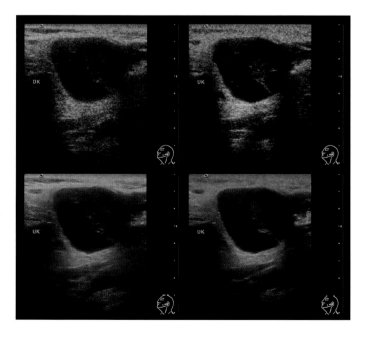

Fig. 14.19 Parotid, left, transverse. A **pleomorphic adenoma** of the parotid gland lies close to the mandible (UK). Upper left: transversal B-scan image through the caudal gland pole with a roundish hypoechoic mass. Upper right: corresponding image from THI with improved contrast of the internal echoes and clearer visualization of the distal acoustic enhancement, but with tissue display more coarse-grained. Lower left: compound imaging (CI) with improved delineation and visualization of the internal structure of the mass. Bottom right: in comparison, there is little enhancement of image quality through the combination of THI and CI (THICI) at the bottom right.

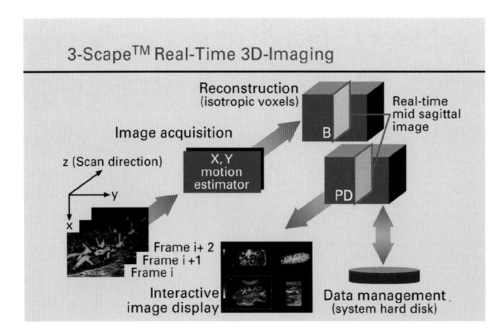

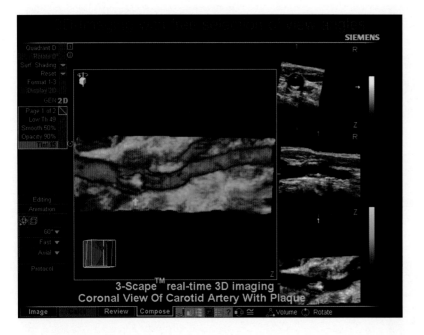

Fig. 14.20 3D/4D imaging. The high performance of the image processor and the motion correction procedures are the key to the acquisition of 3D images in real time. To acquire 3D images in B-mode and power Doppler mode, the transducer is moved freehand parallel to z, i.e., perpendicular to the sectional plane (x–y), or in a rocking motion around the y-axis, or in a rotational motion around the center of the transducer. Position sensors are not required but can be employed for higher geometric accuracy. Algorithms for the registration of the image and motion, based on echo information from adjacent layers, are used to determine the position of the transducer and to align the image data. There then follows the reconstruction of the 3D data, separately for B-mode and power Doppler mode, which enables the usual image postprocessing also at a later time. The 3D datasets contain isotropic voxels in the storage unit, i.e., the size of the smallest information unit is the same in all three directions. By utilizing 3D in real time, the user is in direct control of the quantity and quality of the image data, because during image acquisition a real-time midsagittal panoramic image is obtained on the monitor. Immediately afterward, the user can reconstruct and depict interactively organic and vascular structures, at high resolution and in any orientation. It is also possible to obtain surface- and volume-rendered views (a maximum intensity projection [MIP], for example) from any angle (360°). At the same time, B-mode or power Doppler-mode data can be selectively switched on and off. (Courtesy of Siemens AG.)

Fig. 14.21 Example: carotid artery, application of three-dimensional reconstruction. An atherosclerotic plaque is visualized within the carotid bulb (arrow). (Courtesy of Siemens AG.)

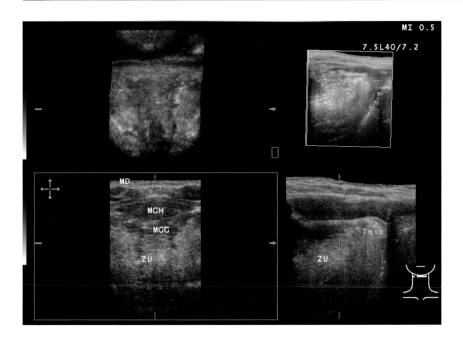

Fig. 14.22 Floor of the mouth, transverse. The dataset of a tongue has been used for three-dimensional reconstruction. Lower left: "Classical" transverse view of the floor of the mouth and the tongue. Lower right: "Classical" corresponding longitudinal view. Upper left: Reconstructed view of the tongue where a "horizontal" plane of the anteroposterior extend of the organ is given The triangular shape of the tongue can be recognized. Upper right: The reconstructed volume of the tongue is displayed with surface rendering. The cube (yellow frame) can be moved and viewed in arbitrary angles, Light and shadow effects enable a plastic impression. MD, diagnostic muscle; MGH, geniohyoid muscle; MGG, genioglossal muscle; ZU, tongue.

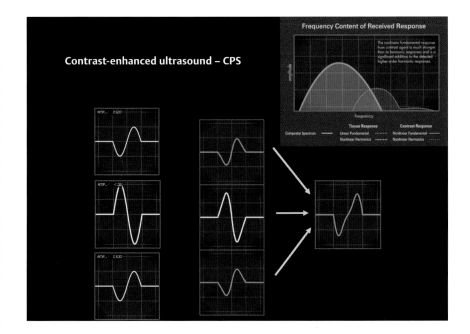

Fig. 14.23 Special contrast pulse sequence (CPS) procedure for contrast imaging to detect and differentiate masses. (Courtesy of Siemens AG.)

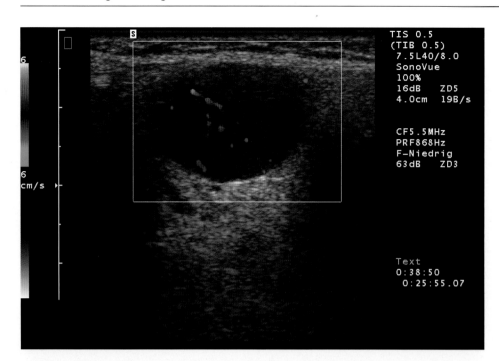

Fig. 14.24 Nodular structure of the left parotid gland. Color-coded duplex sonography (CCDS) shows only weak flow signals. Compare **Fig. 14.25**.

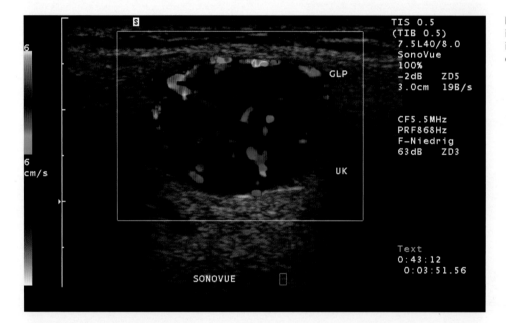

Fig. 14.25 (Compare **Fig. 14.24**.) After administration of a contrast enhancer (SonoVue®), there is clear visualization of the diffuse but peripherally enhanced perfusion pattern.

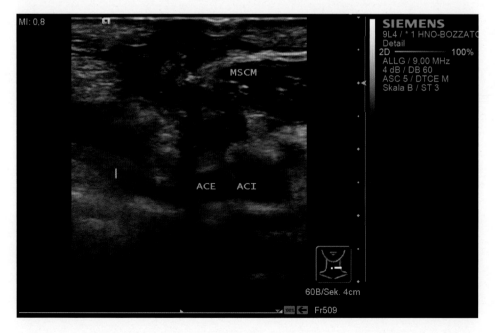

Fig. 14.26 Neck, left, transverse. A **postoperative wound** with hypoechoic blurred contour. The extension of a suspected fistula and its relation to the vessels (internal carotid artery [ACI] and external carotid artery [ACE]) remains unclear. MSCM, sternocleidomastoid muscle. Compare **Fig. 14.27**.

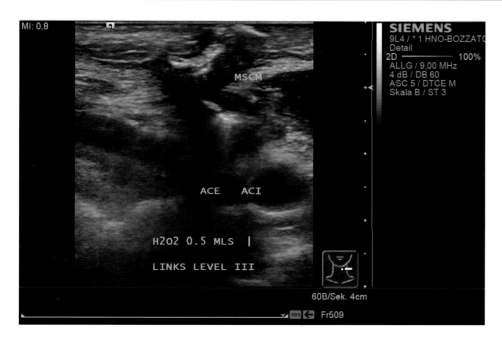

Fig. 14.27 (Compare **Fig. 14.26**.) Neck, left, transverse. After injection of **hydrogen peroxide**, the fistular duct is visible. ACE, external carotid artery; ACI, internal carotid artery; MSCM, sternocleidomastoid muscle.

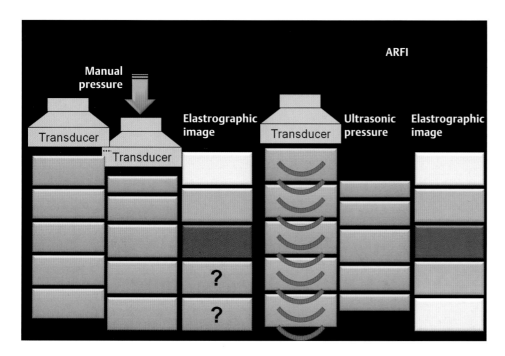

Fig. 14.28 Comparison of compression and acoustic radiation force impulse (ARFI) elastography. (Courtesy of Siemens AG.)

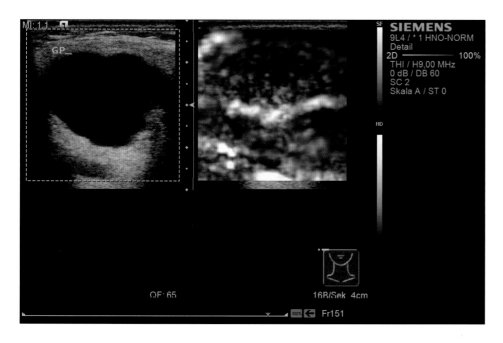

Fig. 14.29 Elastographic display of a **parotid cyst**. The grayscale display of viscoelastic characteristics shows a central horizontal zone (bull's eye). The upper scale at the right side of the image denotes tissue stiffness from bright–soft (SF) towards dark–stiff (HD). QF denotes the **reproducibility** of the measurement influenced by pressure applied by the probe on the skin of the patient.

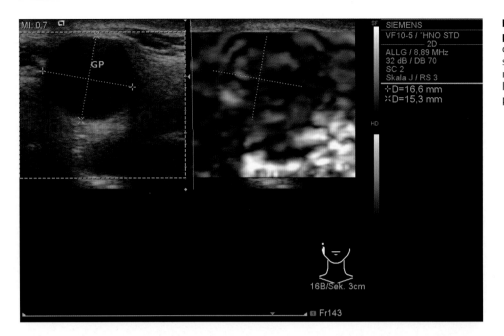

Fig. 14.30 Elastographic display of a **malignant parotid tumor** with grayscale display of viscoelastic characteristics. The garlandlike pattern of stiff and soft tissue parts appears to be characteristic for malignant tumors. Simultaneously seen on the left side is the conventional B-mode view. GP, parotid gland.

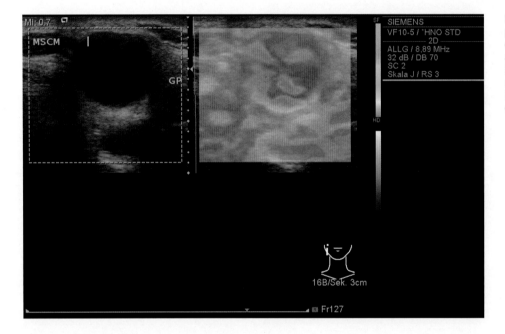

Fig. 14.31 Elastographic display of a **malignant parotid tumor** with color display of viscoelastic characteristics. The garlandlike pattern of stiff and soft tissue (red and green) parts appears to be characteristic for malignant tumors. Simultaneously seen at the left side is the conventional B-mode view. MSCM, sternocleidomastoid muscle; GP, parotid gland.

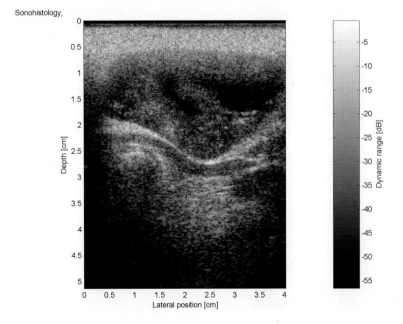

Fig. 14.32 Parotid tumor under sonohistological examination. After image acquisition the high-frequency dataset is analyzed by a range of statistical algorithms to extract specific tissue-characterizing information.

Further Reading

Adibelli ZH, Unal G, Gül E, Uslu F, Koçak U, Abali Y. Differentiation of benign and malignant cervical lymph nodes: value of B-mode and color Doppler sonography. Eur J Radiol 1998;28(3):230–234

Ahuja A, Ying M. Grey-scale sonography in assessment of cervical lymphadenopathy: review of sonographic appearances and features that may help a beginner. Br J Oral Maxillofac Surg 2000;38(5):451–459

Ahuja A, Ying M. An overview of neck node sonography. Invest Radiol 2002;37(6):333–342

Ahuja A, Ying M. Sonography of neck lymph nodes. Part II: abnormal lymph nodes. Clin Radiol 2003;58(5):359–366

Ahuja A, Ying M, Evans R, King W, Metreweli C. The application of ultrasound criteria for malignancy in differentiating tuberculous cervical adenitis from metastatic nasopharyngeal carcinoma. Clin Radiol 1995;50(6):391–395

Ahuja AT, Chow L, Chick W, King W, Metreweli C. Metastatic cervical nodes in papillary carcinoma of the thyroid: ultrasound and histological correlation. Clin Radiol 1995;50(4):229–231

Ahuja A, Ying M, Leung SF, Metreweli C. The sonographic appearance and significance of cervical metastatic nodes following radiotherapy for nasopharyngaeal carcinoma. Clin Radiol 1996;51(10):698–701

Ahuja A, Ying M, Yang WT, Evans R, King W, Metreweli C. The use of sonography in differentiating cervical lymphomatous lymph nodes from cervical metastatic lymph nodes. Clin Radiol 1996;51(3):186–190

Ahuja A, Ying M, King W, Metreweli C. A practical approach to ultrasound of cervical lymph nodes. J Laryngol Otol 1997;111(3):245–256

Ahuja A, Leung SF, Ying M, Metreweli C. Echography of metastatic nodes treated by radiotherapy. J Laryngol Otol 1999;113(11):993–998

Ahuja AT, King AD, Metreweli C. Second branchial cleft cysts: variability of sonographic appearances in adult cases. AJNR Am J Neuroradiol 2000;21(2):315–319

Ahuja AT, King AD, Metreweli C. Sonographic evaluation of thyroglossal duct cysts in children. Clin Radiol 2000;55(10):770–774

Ahuja AT, Marshall JN, Roebuck DJ, King AD, Metreweli C. Sonographic appearances of preauricular sinus. Clin Radiol 2000;55(7):528–532

Ahuja AT, Ying M, Yuen HY, Metreweli C. "Pseudocystic" appearance of non-Hodgkin's lymphomatous nodes: an infrequent finding with high-resolution transducers. Clin Radiol 2001;56(2):111–115

Ahuja AT, Ying M, Ho SS, Metreweli C. Distribution of intranodal vessels in differentiating benign from metastatic neck nodes. Clin Radiol 2001;56(3):197–201

Ahuja AT, Ying M, Ho SY, et al. Ultrasound of malignant cervical lymph nodes. Cancer Imaging 2008;8:48–56 Review

Alberico RA, Husain SH, Sirotkin I. Imaging in head and neck oncology. Surg Oncol Clin N Am 2004;13(1):13–35

Arens C, Weigt J, Schumacher J, Kraft M. Ultrasound of the larynx, hypopharynx and upper esophagus. HNO 2011;59(2):145–154

Ariji Y, Kimura Y, Hayashi N, et al. Power Doppler sonography of cervical lymph nodes in patients with head and neck cancer. AJNR Am J Neuroradiol 1998;19(2):303–307

Arning Ch. Ultrasonographic imaging of carotidynia: syndrome or entity?. [Article in German]. Nervenarzt 2004;75(12):1200–1203

Attie JN, Setzin M, Klein I. Thyroid carcinoma presenting as an enlarged cervical lymph node. Am J Surg 1993;166(4):428–430

Baatenburg de Jong RJ, Rongen RJ, Laméris JS, Harthoorn M, Verwoerd CD, Knegt P. Metastatic neck disease. Palpation vs ultrasound examination. Arch Otolaryngol Head Neck Surg 1989;115(6):689–690

Benzel W, Zenk J, Iro H. [Color Doppler ultrasound studies of parotid tumors]. HNO 1995;43(1):25–30

de Bondt RBJ, Nelemans PJ, Hofman PAM, et al. Detection of lymph node metastases in head and neck cancer: a meta-analysis comparing US, USgFNAC, CT and MR imaging. Eur J Radiol 2007;64(2):266–272

Bozzato A, Zenk J, Gottwald F, Koch M, Iro H. [Influence of thyroid cartilage ossification in laryngeal ultrasound]. Laryngorhinootologie 2007;86(4):276–281

Bozzato A, Zenk J, Greess H, et al. Potential of ultrasound diagnosis for parotid tumors: analysis of qualitative and quantitative parameters. Otolaryngol Head Neck Surg 2007;137(4):642–646

Bozzato A, Hertel V, Bumm K, Iro H, Zenk J. Salivary simulation with ascorbic acid enhances sonographic diagnosis of obstructive sialadenitis. J Clin Ultrasound 2009;37(6):329–332

Bozzato A, Loika A, Hornung J, et al. Comparison of conventional B-scan, tissue harmonic imaging, compound imaging and tissue harmonic compound imaging in neck lesion characterisation. Eur Arch Otorhinolaryngol 2010;267(10):1593–1598

van den Brekel MW, Stel HV, Castelijns JA, et al. Cervical lymph node metastasis: assessment of radiologic criteria. Radiology 1990;177(2):379–384

Bruneton JN, Normand F. Cervical lymph nodes. In: Bruneton JN, ed. Ultrasonography of the Neck. Berlin: Springer; 1987:81

Bruneton JN, Roux P, Caramella E, Demard F, Vallicioni J, Chauvel P. Ear, nose, and throat cancer: ultrasound diagnosis of metastasis to cervical lymph nodes. Radiology 1984;152(3):771–773

Bruneton JN, Caramella E, Héry M, Aubanel D, Manzino JJ, Picard JL. Axillary lymph node metastases in breast cancer: preoperative detection with US. Radiology 1986;158(2):325–326

Bruneton JN, Normand F, Balu-Maestro C, et al. Lymphomatous superficial lymph nodes: US detection. Radiology 1987;165(1):233–235

Bruneton JN, Balu-Maestro C, Marcy PY, Melia P, Mourou MY. Very high frequency (13 MHz) ultrasonographic examination of the normal neck: detection of normal lymph nodes and thyroid nodules. J Ultrasound Med 1994;13(2):87–90

Callen PW, Marks WM. Lymphomatous masses simulating cysts by ultrasonography. J Can Assoc Radiol 1979;30(4):244–246

Capaccio P, Cuccarini V, Ottaviani F, et al. Comparative ultrasonographic, magnetic resonance sialographic, and videoendoscopic assessment of salivary duct disorders. Ann Otol Rhinol Laryngol 2008;117(4):245–252

Carrig CB, Pyle RL. Anatomic models and phantoms for diagnostic ultrasound instruction. Vet Radiol Ultrasound 2001;42(4):320–328

Cervin JR, Silverman JF, Loggie BW, Geisinger KR. Virchow's node revisited. Analysis with clinicopathologic correlation of 152 fine-needle aspiration biopsies of supraclavicular lymph nodes. Arch Pathol Lab Med 1995;119(8):727–730

Chang DB, Yuan A, Yu CJ, Luh KT, Kuo SH, Yang PC. Differentiation of benign and malignant cervical lymph nodes with color Doppler sonography. AJR Am J Roentgenol 1994;162(4):965–968

Chikui T, Yonetsu K, Nakamura T. Multivariate feature analysis of sonographic findings of metastatic cervical lymph nodes: contribution of blood flow features revealed by power Doppler sonography for predicting metastasis. AJNR Am J Neuroradiol 2000;21(3):561–567

De Jong SA, Demeter JG, Jarosz H, Lawrence AM, Paloyan E. Primary papillary thyroid carcinoma presenting as cervical lymphadenopathy: the operative approach to the "lateral aberrant thyroid". Am Surg 1993;59(3):172–176, discussion 176–177

Delorme S. Sonography of enlarged cervical lymph nodes. [Article in German]. Bildgebung 1993;60(4):267–272

DePeña CA, Van Tassel P, Lee YY. Lymphoma of the head and neck. Radiol Clin North Am 1990;28(4):723–743

Dragoni F, Cartoni C, Pescarmona E, et al. The role of high resolution pulsed and color Doppler ultrasound in the differential diagnosis of benign and malignant lymphadenopathy: results of multivariate analysis. Cancer 1999;85(11):2485–2490

Esen G. Ultrasound of superficial lymph nodes. Eur J Radiol 2006;58(3):345–359

Evans RM, Ahuja A, Metreweli C. The linear echogenic hilus in cervical lymphadenopathy—a sign of benignity or malignancy? Clin Radiol 1993;47(4):262–264

Fischer T, Paschen CF, Slowinski T, et al. Differentiation of parotid gland tumors with contrast-enhanced ultrasound. Rofo 2010;182(2):155–162

Forsberg F. Ultrasonic biomedical technology; marketing versus clinical reality. Ultrasonics 2004;42(1–9):17–27

Gallipoli A, Manganella G, De Lutiodi di Castelguidone E, et al. Ultrasound contrast media in the study of salivary gland tumors. Anticancer Res 2005;25(3c):2477–2482

Gritzmann N. Sonography of the neck: current potentials and limitations. Ultraschall Med 2005;26(3):185–196

Gritzmann N, Czembirek H, Hajek P, Karnel F, Frühwald F. [Sonographic anatomy of the neck and its importance in lymph node staging of head and neck cancer]. Rofo 1987;146(1):1–7

Gritzmann N, Czembirek H, Hajek P, Karnel F, Türk R, Frühwald F. Sonography in cervical lymph node metastases. [Article in German]. Radiologe 1987;27(3):118–122

Gritzmann N, Hollerweger A, Macheiner P, Rettenbacher T. Sonography of soft tissue masses of the neck. J Clin Ultrasound 2002;30(6):356–373

Groppo ER, Glastonbury CM, Orloff LA, Kraus PE, Eisele DW. Vascular malformation masquerading as sialolithiasis and parotid obstruction: a case report and review of the literature. Laryngoscope 2010;120(Suppl 4):S130

Hajek PC, Salomonowitz E, Turk R, Tscholakoff D, Kumpan W, Czembirek H. Lymph nodes of the neck: evaluation with US. Radiology 1986;158(3):739–742

Ho SS, Ahuja AT, Yeo W, Chan TC, Kew J, Metreweli C. Longitudinal colour Doppler study of superficial lymph nodes in non-Hodgkin's lymphoma patients on chemotherapy. Clin Radiol 2000;55(2):110–113

Hollerweger A, Macheiner P, Neureiter D, Dietze O. Uncommon cystic appearance of lymph nodes in malignant lymphoma. [Article in German]. Ultraschall Med 2008;29(3):308–310

Holtel MR. Emerging technology in head and neck ultrasonography. Otolaryngol Clin North Am 2010;43(6):1267–1274, vii

Ishii J, Fujii E, Suzuki H, Shinozuka K, Kawase N, Amagasa T. Ultrasonic diagnosis of oral and neck malignant lymphoma. Bull Tokyo Med Dent Univ 1992;39(4):63–69

Ishii JI, Amagasa T, Tachibana T, Shinozuka K, Shioda P. US and CT evaluation of cervical lymph node metastasis from oral cancer. J Craniomaxillofac Surg 1991;19:123

Jakobsen JA. Ultrasound contrast agents: clinical applications. Eur Radiol 2001;11(8):1329–1337

Jeong HS, Baek CH, Son YI, et al. Use of integrated ^{18}F-FDG PET/CT to improve the accuracy of initial cervical nodal evaluation in patients with head and neck squamous cell carcinoma. Head Neck 2007;29(3):203–210

Johnson JT. A surgeon looks at cervical lymph nodes. Radiology 1990;175(3):607–610

Kalyvas D, Tsiklakis K, Rentis A. [Ultrasonography. Interpretation of physiologic structures of the neck and face]. Odontostomatol Proodos 1990;44(1):37–43

King AD, Tse GMK, Ahuja AT, et al. Necrosis in metastatic neck nodes: diagnostic accuracy of CT, MR imaging, and US. Radiology 2004;230(3):720–726

Kiricuta IC, Willner J, Kölbl O, Bohndorf W. The prognostic significance of the supraclavicular lymph node metastases in breast cancer patients. Int J Radiat Oncol Biol Phys 1994;28(2):387–393

Klem C. Head and neck anatomy and ultrasound correlation. Otolaryngol Clin North Am 2010;43(6):1161–1169, v

Koischwitz D, Gritzmann N. Ultrasound of the neck. Radiol Clin North Am 2000;38(5):1029–1045

Komisar A. Treatment of the node negative neck. In: Vogl SE, ed. Head and Neck Cancer. New York: Churchill Livingstone; 1988:19

Kotecha S, Bhatia P, Rout PG. Diagnostic ultrasound in the head and neck region. Dent Update 2008;35(8):529–530, 533–534

Lamont JP, McCarty TM, Fisher TL, Kuhn JA. Prospective evaluation of office-based parotid ultrasound. Ann Surg Oncol 2001;8(9):720–722

Lee YLP, Antonio GE, Ho SSY, et al. Serial dynamic sonographic contrast enhancement changes in cervical lymph nodes: before and after treatment for lymphoma. International & 9th National Head and Neck Cancer Conference, 7–11 September 2007, Urumqi, China; 2007

Lee YY, Van Tassel P, Nauert C, North LB, Jing BS. Lymphomas of the head and neck: CT findings at initial presentation. AJR Am J Roentgenol 1987;149(3):575–581

Lefor AT, Ord RA. Multiple synchronous bilateral Warthin's tumors of the parotid glands with pleomorphic adenoma. Case report and review of the literature. Oral Surg Oral Med Oral Pathol 1993;76(3):319–324

Leicher-Dueber A, Bleier R, Dueber C, Thelen M. [Cervical lymph node metastases: a histologically controlled comparison of palpation, sonography and computed tomography.] Rofo 1990;153:575–579

Lewin PA. Quo vadis medical ultrasound? Ultrasonics 2004;42(1–9):1–7

Liao LJ, Wang CT, Young YH, Cheng PW. Real-time and computerized sonographic scoring system for predicting malignant cervical lymphadenopathy. Head Neck 2010;32(5):594–598

Lindberg R. Distribution of cervical lymph node metastases from squamous cell carcinoma of the upper respiratory and digestive tracts. Cancer 1972;29(6):1446–1449

McCurdy JA Jr, Nadalo LA, Yim DW. Evaluation of extrathyroid masses of the head and neck with gray scale ultrasound. Arch Otolaryngol 1980;106(2):83–87

Mäurer J, Willam C, Schroeder R, et al. Evaluation of metastases and reactive lymph nodes in Doppler sonography using an ultrasound contrast enhancer. Invest Radiol 1997;32(8):441–446

Moritz JD, Ludwig A, Oestmann JW. Contrast-enhanced color Doppler sonography for evaluation of enlarged cervical lymph nodes in head and neck tumors. AJR Am J Roentgenol 2000;174(5):1279–1284

Na DG, Lim HK, Byun HS, Kim HD, Ko YH, Baek JH. Differential diagnosis of cervical lymphadenopathy: usefulness of color Doppler sonography. AJR Am J Roentgenol 1997;168(5):1311–1316

Nakamura T, Sumi M. Nodal imaging in the neck: recent advances in US, CT and MR imaging of metastatic nodes. Eur Radiol 2007;17(5):1235–1241

Oeppen RS, Gibson D, Brennan PA. An update on the use of ultrasound imaging in oral and maxillofacial surgery. Br J Oral Maxillofac Surg 2010;48(6):412–418

van Overhagen H, Laméris JS, Berger MY, et al. Supraclavicular lymph node metastases in carcinoma of the esophagus and gastroesophageal junction: assessment with CT, US, and US-guided fine-needle aspiration biopsy. Radiology 1991;179(1):155–158

van Overhagen H, Laméris JS, Zonderland HM, Tilanus HW, van Pel R, Schütte HE. Ultrasound and ultrasound-guided fine needle aspiration biopsy of supraclavicular lymph nodes in patients with esophageal carcinoma. Cancer 1991;67(3):585–587

van Overhagen H, Laméris JS, Berger MY, et al. Improved assessment of supraclavicular and abdominal metastases in oesophageal and gastro-oesophageal junction carcinoma with the combination of ultrasound and computed tomography. Br J Radiol 1993;66(783):203–208

Probst R, Grevers G, Iro H. Hals-Nasen-Ohren-Heilkunde. 3rd ed. Stuttgart: Thieme; 2008

Restrepo R, Oneto J, Lopez K, Kukreja K. Head and neck lymph nodes in children: the spectrum from normal to abnormal. Pediatr Radiol 2009;39(8):836–846

Rettenbacher T. Sonography of peripheral lymph nodes part 1: normal findings and B-image criteria. Ultraschall Med 2010/ 31/(4):344–362

Rettenbacher T, Tzankov A, Hollerweger A. [Sonographic appearances of subcutaneous and cutaneous oedema—correlation with histopathology]. Ultraschall Med 2006;27(3):240–244

Richards PS, Peacock TE. The role of ultrasound in the detection of cervical lymph node metastases in clinically N0 squamous cell carcinoma of the head and neck. Cancer Imaging 2007;7:167–178

Rottey S, Petrovic M, Bauters W, et al. Evaluation of metastatic lymph nodes in head and neck cancer: a comparative study between palpation, ultrasonography, ultrasound-guided fine needle aspiration cytology and computed tomography. Acta Clin Belg 2006;61(5):236–241

Rubaltelli L, Proto E, Salmaso R, Bortoletto P, Candiani F, Cagol P. Sonography of abnormal lymph nodes in vitro: correlation of sonographic and histologic findings. AJR Am J Roentgenol 1990;155(6):1241–1244

Rubaltelli L, Khadivi Y, Tregnaghi A, et al. Evaluation of lymph node perfusion using continuous mode harmonic ultrasonography with a second-generation contrast agent. J Ultrasound Med 2004;23(6):829–836

Sakaguchi T, Yamashita Y, Katahira K, et al. Differential diagnosis of small round cervical lymph nodes: comparison of power Doppler US with contrast-enhanced CT and pathologic results. Radiat Med 2001;19(3):119–125

Sakai F, Kiyono K, Sone S, et al. Ultrasonic evaluation of cervical metastatic lymphadenopathy. J Ultrasound Med 1988;7(6):305–310

Schade G. Use of Ensemble tissue harmonic imaging to improve the resolution in ultrasound investigations of the head and neck area. [Article in German]. Laryngorhinootologie 2002;81(6):413–417

Scheible W. Recent advances in ultrasound: high-resolution imaging of superficial structures. Head Neck Surg 1981;4(1):58–63

Scheipers U, Siebers S, Gottwald F, et al. Sonohistology for the computerized differentiation of parotid gland tumors. Ultrasound Med Biol 2005;31(10):1287–1296

Schulte-Altedorneburg G, Demharter J, Linné R, Droste DW, Bohndorf K, Bücklein W. Does ultrasound contrast agent improve the diagnostic value of colour and power Doppler sonography in superficial lymph node enlargement? Eur J Radiol 2003;48(3):252–257

Shimizu M, Ussmüller J, Hartwein J, Donath K, Kinukawa N. Statistical study for sonographic differential diagnosis of tumorous lesions in the parotid gland. Oral Surg Oral Med Oral Pathol Oral Radiol Endod 1999;88(2):226–233

Shozushima M, Suzuki M, Nakasima T, Yanagisawa Y, Sakamaki K, Takeda Y. Ultrasound diagnosis of lymph node metastasis in head and neck cancer. Dentomaxillofac Radiol 1990;19(4):165–170

Silverman PM. Lymph node imaging: multidetector CT (MDCT). Cancer Imaging 2005;23(5) Spec No A:S57–S67

Sniezek JC. Head and neck ultrasound: why now? Otolaryngol Clin North Am 2010;43(6):1143–1147, v

Soeding P, Eizenberg N. Review article: anatomical considerations for ultrasound guidance for regional anesthesia of the neck and upper limb. Can J Anaesth 2009;56(7):518–533

Sofferman RA. Interpretation of ultrasound. Otolaryngol Clin North Am 2010;43(6):1171–1202, v–vi

Solbiati L, Rizzatto G, Bellotti E, Montali G, Cioffi V, Croce F. High-resolution sonography of cervical lymph nodes in head and neck cancer. Radiology 1988;169(P):113

Solbiati L, Rizzatto G, Bellotti E, et al. High resolution sonography of cervical lymph nodes in head and neck cancer: criteria for differentiation of reactive versus malignant nodes. Proceedings of the 74th Meeting of the Radiologic Society of North America, Chicago; 1988:113

Solbiati L, Cioffi V, Ballarati E. Ultrasonography of the neck. Radiol Clin North Am 1992;30(5):941–954

Som PM. Lymph nodes of the neck. Radiology 1987;165(3):593–600

Som PM. Detection of metastasis in cervical lymph nodes: CT and MR criteria and differential diagnosis. AJR Am J Roentgenol 1992;158(5):961–969

Som PM, Brandwein M, Lidov M, Lawson W, Biller HF. The varied presentations of papillary thyroid carcinoma cervical nodal disease: CT and MR findings. AJNR Am J Neuroradiol 1994;15(6):1123–1128

Som PM, Curtin HD, Mancuso AA. Imaging-based nodal classification for evaluation of neck metastatic adenopathy. AJR Am J Roentgenol 2000;174(3):837–844

Steinhart H, Zenk J, Sprang K, Bozzato A, Iro H. Contrast-enhanced color Doppler sonography of parotid gland tumors. Eur Arch Otorhinolaryngol 2003;260(6):344–348

Steinkamp HJ, Mäurer J, Cornehl M, Knöbber D, Hettwer H, Felix R. Recurrent cervical lymphadenopathy: differential diagnosis with color-duplex sonography. Eur Arch Otorhinolaryngol 1994;251(7):404–409

Steinkamp HJ, Teske C, Knöbber E, Schedel H, Felix R. Sonography in tumor after-care of head-neck tumor patients. Value of sonomorphologic criteria and sonographic M/Q quotients. [Article in German]. Ultraschall Med 1994;15(2):81–88

Steinkamp HJ, Mueffelmann M, Böck JC, Thiel T, Kenzel P, Felix R. Differential diagnosis of lymph node lesions: a semiquantitative approach with colour Doppler ultrasound. Br J Radiol 1998;71(848):828–833

Steinkamp HJ, Wissgott C, Rademaker J, Felix R. Current status of power Doppler and color Doppler sonography in the differential diagnosis of lymph node lesions. Eur Radiol 2002;12(7):1785–1793

Steinkamp HJ, Beck A, Werk M, Rademaker J, Felix R. Extracapsular spread of cervical lymph node metastases: diagnostic relevance of ultrasound examinations. [Article in German]. Ultraschall Med 2003;24(5):323–330

Sugama Y, Kitamura S. Ultrasonographic evaluation of neck and supraclavicular lymph nodes metastasized from lung cancer. Intern Med 1992;31(2):160–164

Sumi M, Ohki M, Nakamura T. Comparison of sonography and CT for differentiating benign from malignant cervical lymph nodes in patients with squamous cell carcinoma of the head and neck. AJR Am J Roentgenol 2001;176(4):1019–1024

Sumi M, Van Cauteren M, Nakamura T. MR microimaging of benign and malignant nodes in the neck. AJR Am J Roentgenol 2006;186(3):749–757

Swartz JD, Yussen PS, Popky GL. Imaging of the neck: nodal disease. Crit Rev Diagn Imaging 1991;31(3-4):413–469

Teymoortash A, Schrader C, Shimoda H, Kato S, Werner JA. Evidence of lymphangiogenesis in Warthin's tumor of the parotid gland. Oral Oncol 2007;43(6):614–618

Tiedjen KU, Hildmann H. [Sonography of the neck—indications and value]. HNO 1988;36(7):267–276

To EW, Tsang WM, Cheng J, et al. Is neck ultrasound necessary for early stage oral tongue carcinoma with clinically N0 neck? Dentomaxillofac Radiol 2003;32(3):156–159

Tohnosu N, Onoda S, Isono K. Ultrasonographic evaluation of cervical lymph node metastases in esophageal cancer with special reference to the relationship between the short to long axis ratio (S/L) and the cancer content. J Clin Ultrasound 1989;17(2):101–106

Tregnaghi A, De Candia A, Calderone M, et al. Ultrasonographic evaluation of superficial lymph node metastases in melanoma. Eur J Radiol 1997;24(3):216–221

Tschammler A, Wirkner H, Ott G, Hahn D. Vascular patterns in reactive and malignant lymphadenopathy. Eur Radiol 1996;6(4):473–480

Vassallo P, Wernecke K, Roos N, Peters PE. Differentiation of benign from malignant superficial lymphadenopathy: the role of high-resolution US. Radiology 1992;183(1):215–220

Vassallo P, Edel G, Roos N, Naguib A, Peters PE. In-vitro high-resolution ultrasonography of benign and malignant lymph nodes. A sonographic—pathologic correlation. Invest Radiol 1993;28(8):698–705

Wu CH, Chang YL, Hsu WC, Ko JY, Sheen TS, Hsieh FJ. Usefulness of Doppler spectral analysis and power Doppler sonography in the differentiation of cervical lymphadenopathies. AJR Am J Roentgenol 1998;171(2):503–509

Yang WT, Ahuja A, Tang A, Suen M, King W, Metreweli C. Ultrasonographic demonstration of normal axillary lymph nodes: a learning curve. J Ultrasound Med 1995;14(11):823–827

Yao ZH, Wu AR. Supraclavicular lymph node metastasis from carcinoma of the uterine cervix after radiotherapy—analysis of 219 patients. [Article in Chinese]. Zhonghua Zhong Liu Za Zhi 1988;10(3):230–232

Ying MTC. Ultrasound evaluation of cervical lymph nodes in a Chinese population. [MPhil thesis]. Hong Kong: Department of Optometry and Radiography, The Hong Kong Polytechnic University; 1996. 235 p.

Ying MTC. Power Doppler sonography of normal and abnormal cervical lymph nodes. [PhD thesis]. Hong Kong: Department of Optometry and Radiography, The Hong Kong Polytechnic University; 2002. 236 p.

Ying M, Ahuja A, Brook F, Brown B, Metreweli C. Sonographic appearance and distribution of normal cervical lymph nodes in a Chinese population. J Ultrasound Med 1996;15(6):431–436

Ying M, Ahuja AT, Evans R, King W, Metreweli C. Cervical lymphadenopathy: sonographic differentiation between tuberculous nodes and nodal metastases from non-head and neck carcinomas. J Clin Ultrasound 1998;26(8):383–389

Ying M, Ahuja A, Metreweli C. Diagnostic accuracy of sonographic criteria for evaluation of cervical lymphadenopathy. J Ultrasound Med 1998;17(7):437–445

Ying M, Ahuja A, Brook F, Brown B, Metreweli C. Nodal shape (S/L) and its combination with size for assessment of cervical lymphadenopathy: which cut-off should be used? Ultrasound Med Biol 1999;25(8):1169–1175

Ying M, Ahuja A, Brook F, Metreweli C. Power Doppler sonography of normal cervical lymph nodes. J Ultrasound Med 2000;19(8):511–517

Ying M, Ahuja A, Brook F, Metreweli C. Vascularity and grey-scale sonographic features of normal cervical lymph nodes: variations with nodal size. Clin Radiol 2001;56(5):416–419

Ying M, Ahuja A, Brook F. Repeatability of power Doppler sonography of cervical lymph nodes. Ultrasound Med Biol 2002;28(6):737–744

Ying M, Ahuja A, Brook F. Sonographic appearances of cervical lymph nodes: variations by age and sex. J Clin Ultrasound 2002;30(1):1–11

Yonetsu K, Ohki M, Kumazawa S, Eida S, Sumi M, Nakamura T. Parotid tumors: differentiation of benign and malignant tumors with quantitative sonographic analyses. Ultrasound Med Biol 2004;30(5):567–574

Yuan WH, Hsu HC, Chou YH, Hsueh HC, Tseng TK, Tiu CM. Gray-scale and color Doppler ultrasonographic features of pleomorphic adenoma and Warthin's tumor in major salivary glands. Clin Imaging 2009;33(5):348–353

Zajkowski P, Białek EJ. [Ultrasound imaging in laryngology]. Otolaryngol Pol 2007;61(4):544–549

Zajkowski P, Jakubowski W, Białek EJ, Wysocki M, Osmólski A, Serafin-Król M. Pleomorphic adenoma and adenolymphoma in ultrasonography. Eur J Ultrasound 2000;12(1):23–29

Zenk J, Bozzato A, Steinhart H, Greess H, Iro H. Metastatic and inflammatory cervical lymph nodes as analyzed by contrast-enhanced color-coded Doppler ultrasonography: quantitative dynamic perfusion patterns and histopathologic correlation. Ann Otol Rhinol Laryngol 2005;114(1 Pt 1):43–47

Zenk J, Bozzato A, Hornung J, et al. Neck lymph nodes: prediction by computer-assisted contrast medium analysis? Ultrasound Med Biol 2007;33(2):246–253

Zenk J, Iro H, Klintworth N, Lell M. Diagnostic imaging in sialadenitis. Oral Maxillofac Surg Clin North Am 2009;21(3):275–292

Subject Index

Notes: Page numbers in *italics* refer to material in figures, whilst numbers in **bold** refer to material in tables.
vs. indicates a comparison or differential diagnosis.